Pancreas and Biliary Disease

Kulwinder Dua • Reza Shaker

Editors

Pancreas and Biliary Disease

A Point of Care Clinical Guide

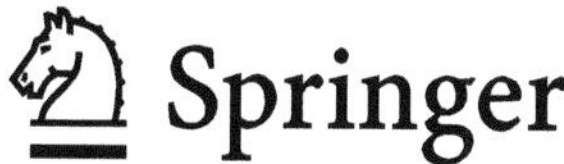 Springer

Editors
Kulwinder Dua
Division of Gastroenterology &
  Hepatology
Medical College of Wisconsin
Milwaukee, WI, USA

Reza Shaker
Division of Gastroenterology &
  Hepatology
Medical College of Wisconsin
Milwaukee, WI, USA

ISBN 978-3-319-28087-5   ISBN 978-3-319-28089-9   (eBook)
DOI 10.1007/978-3-319-28089-9

Library of Congress Control Number: 2016944235

Printed on acid-free paper

This Springer imprint is published by Springer Nature
The registered company is Springer International Publishing AG Switzerland

Preface

Pancreas and bile duct disorders can be benign, premalignant, and malignant. Patients present with a variety of symptoms that not only create anxiety and fear in the patient but also can be confusing to the treating primary care provider or the internist. The spectrum of clinical presentation can range from nonspecific symptoms to a severely sick patient admitted to the ICU. Several patients are also referred with incidental findings on imaging studies or blood tests done for other reasons. The gastroenterology provider is often faced with patient questions like "What is going on?" "Why did this happen to me?" "Is this serious?" "Do I have cancer?" "Will I develop cancer?" "Can this be treated without surgery?" "Will this happen again?" "How long will I live?" and so on. These questions, while seemingly straightforward, require current, and frequently contradictory knowledge of the recommended guidelines (if any) to formulate a reasonable answer that the patient can understand. This book is a point-of-care reference for a busy clinician who needs the best evidence-based answers to patient questions. The general format of the chapters is focused around patient questions followed by a summary of pertinent literature. For example "What happened and why did this happen?" "What tests am I going to have?" "Are there any complications from the test?" will cover the *Diagnosis and differential diagnosis*; "Why did this happen to me?" will address *Epidemiology, genetics, environment, and pathogenesis*; "Do I need surgery?" "I don't want surgery" "Can you treat me only with medicines?" "How experienced is the doctor you are referring me to?" will describe the *Treatment and management*; and last but not the least, "Will it happen again?" "Will I develop cancer?" "How long am I going to live?" "What if I don't take any treatment?" will describe the *Prognosis*. National and international experts in the field have contributed to this book providing answers to these questions followed by an evidence-based summary of the particular disorder. This book will provide clinicians with state-of-the-art information at their fingertips when caring for patients with diseases of the pancreas and the bile ducts.

Milwaukee, WI, USA   Kulwinder Dua
Milwaukee, WI, USA   Reza Shaker

Contents

Contributors

Douglas G. Adler, M.D., F.A.C.G., A.G.A.F. Gastroenterology and Hepatology, Huntsman Cancer Center, University of Utah School of Medicine, Salt Lake City, UT, USA

Chad Barnes, M.D. Department of Surgery, Medical College of Wisconsin, Milwaukee, WI, USA

Omer Basar, M.D. Pancreas Biliary Center, Gastrointestinal Unit, Massachusetts General Hospital, Boston, MA, USA

Department of Gastroenterology, University of Hacettepe, Ankara, Turkey

Nicholas G. Berger, M.D. Department of Surgery, The Medical College of Wisconsin, Milwaukee, WI, USA

Yan Bi Division of Gastroenterology and Hepatology, Mayo Clinic, Rochester, MN, USA

William R. Brugge, M.D. Pancreas Biliary Center, Gastrointestinal Unit, Massachusetts General Hospital, Boston, MA, USA

Jennifer A. Cahill, M.D. Department of Medicine, Medical College of Wisconsin, Milwaukee, WI, USA

Suresh Chari Division of Gastroenterology and Hepatology, Mayo Clinic, Rochester, MN, USA

Kathleen K. Christians, M.D. Division of Surgical Oncology, Department of Surgery, Medical College of Wisconsin, Milwaukee, WI, USA

Douglas B. Evans, M.D. Division of Surgical Oncology, Department of Surgery, Medical College of Wisconsin, Milwaukee, WI, USA

José Franco Division of Gastroenterology and Hepatology, Medical College of Wisconsin, Milwaukee, WI, USA

Srinivas Gaddam, M.D., M.P.H. Digestive Diseases Center, Cedars-Sinai Medical Center, Los Angeles, CA, USA

T. Clark Gamblin, M.D., M.S., M.B.A. Department of Surgery, The Medical College of Wisconsin, Milwaukee, WI, USA

Nalini M. Guda, M.D., F.A.S.G.E., A.G.A.F. Aurora St. Luke's Medical Center, Milwaukee, WI, USA

University of Wisconsin School of Medicine and Public Health, Madison, WI, USA

Abdulrahman Y. Hammad, M.D. Division of Surgical Oncology, Department of Surgery, The Medical College of Wisconsin, Milwaukee, WI, USA

Walter J. Hogan, M.D. Department of Gastroenterology, Froedtert and the Medical College of Wisconsin, Froedtert Specialty Clinics, Milwaukee, WI, USA

Abdul H. Khan, M.D. Division of Gastroenterology and Hepatology—Froedtert, Medical College of Wisconsin, Milwaukee, WI, USA

Simon Lo, M.D., F.A.C.P. Digestive Diseases Center, Cedars-Sinai Medical Center, Los Angeles, CA, USA

Venkata N. Muddana, M.D. Aurora St. Luke's Medical Center, Milwaukee, WI, USA

Saurabh Mukewar Division of Gastroenterology and Hepatology, Mayo Clinic, Rochester, MN, USA

Sheeva K. Parbhu, M.D. Gastroenterology and Hepatology, University of Utah School of Medicine, Salt Lake City, UT, USA

Nicolo' de Pretis Division of Gastroenterology and Hepatology, Mayo Clinic, Rochester, MN, USA

Brian Rajca, M.D. Aurora St. Luke's Medical Center, Milwaukee, WI, USA

D. Nageshwar Reddy Asian Institute of Gastroenterology, Hyderabad, Telangana, India

Raghuwansh P. Sah Division of Gastroenterology and Hepatology, Department of Medicine, Mayo Clinic, Rochester, MN, USA

Natesh Shivakumar Division of Surgical Oncology, Medical College of Wisconsin, Milwaukee, WI, USA

Rupjyoti Talukdar Asian Institute of Gastroenterology, Hyderabad, Telangana, India

Asian Healthcare Foundation, Hyderabad, Telangana, India

Susan Tsai, M.D., M.H.S. Division of Surgical Oncology, Department of Surgery, Medical College of Wisconsin, Milwaukee, WI, USA

Santhi Swaroop Vege, M.D. Division of Gastroenterology and Hepatology, Department of Medicine, Mayo Clinic, Rochester, MN, USA

Travis P. Webb Department of Surgery, Medical College of Wisconsin, Milwaukee, WI, USA

George Younan Department of Surgery, Division of Surgical Oncology, Medical College of Wisconsin, Milwaukee, WI, USA

Chapter 1
Elevated Amylase and Lipase: Physiology Including Non-pancreatitis related Elevations

Brian Rajca and Nalini M. Guda

Introduction

Acute pancreatitis is a disease of considerable morbidity and mortality with an annual incidence that appears to be increasing [1]. There is a wide variability in the clinical presentation, and although serological testing of amylase and lipase is readily done, at times interpretation of these results is challenging due to other clinical situations that can mimic pancreatitis. This chapter briefly reviews pancreas physiology, with a particular emphasis on serum amylase and lipase, and then addresses a few common clinical scenarios where one needs to exercise caution in interpreting these results.

B. Rajca, M.D.
Aurora St. Luke's Medical Center,
Milwaukee, FL, USA

N.M. Guda, M.D., F.A.S.G.E., A.G.A.F. (✉)
Aurora St. Luke's Medical Center, Milwaukee, WI, USA

University of Wisconsin School of Medicine and Public Health,
Madison, WI, USA
e-mail: nguda@wisc.edu

© Springer International Publishing Switzerland 2016
K. Dua, R. Shaker (eds.), *Pancreas and Biliary Disease*,
DOI 10.1007/978-3-319-28089-9_1

Pancreas Physiology

The pancreas is a soft, elongated gland with both exocrine and endocrine functions. The main functional unit of the pancreas is the acinus with the associated ductule. The acinar cells are specialized to synthesize, store, and secrete digestive enzymes. Hormones and neurotransmitters bind to receptors on the basolateral membrane, stimulating the pancreas to secrete enzymes [2]. These receptors are cyclic adenosine monophosphate (cAMP) linked and result in increases in intracellular free Ca^{2+} [3]. As hormones bind to the receptors this intracellular cascade activates the nearby endoplasmic reticulum to increase protein synthesis. Enzymes then transit to the apical cell membrane where they are released through zymogen granules [4]. As the enzymes are released the secretions transit through the acinar ductule, into the interlobular ducts and ultimately into the main pancreatic duct [5]. The exocrine products of the pancreas can be classified into organic and inorganic constituents. The principal inorganic components are water, sodium, potassium, chloride, and bicarbonate [5]. These secretions are clear, alkaline, and isotonic and serve to deliver the digestive enzymes to the duodenal lumen. The flow of pancreatic secretions can increase from 0.2 ml/min at rest to 4 ml/min when stimulated, with a total daily secretion volume of 2.5 L [5].

The organic constituents consist of the digestive enzymes, including the amylase and lipase. Human amylase is primarily secreted by the salivary gland and pancreas and is the main enzyme to digest starch and glycogen. When food is ingested, salivary amylase initiates the cleavage of glycogen linkages and continues as food transits to the stomach where the enzyme activity is buffered by gastric contents and the mucous layer. Pancreatic lipase consists of three main types: triglyceride lipase, phospholipase A_2, and carboxylesterase [5]. Although salivary and gastric lipases exist, they are typically minor contributors of fat digestion. Lipase binds to the triglyceride droplet but requires bile acids as well as colipase to achieve full enzymatic activity. Bile acids serve to emulsify the triglycerides, leading to an increase in the surface area while colipase assists with lipolysis by forming a complex between the bile salts and lipase [6]. Several proteases exist that are secreted by the pancreas to assist in protein degradation but are not discussed in this chapter.

Pancreatic exocrine secretion occurs during the fasting and the fed states. The fasting, or interdigestive, pattern is cyclic and follows the pattern of the migrating motor complex (MMC) [7]. This pattern cycles every 1–2 h and assists in clearance of residual intestinal contents. The fed, or digestive, state mimics gastric secretion in that it displays a cephalic, gastric, and intestinal phase [5]. The cephalic phase is mediated by the vagal nerve with maximal stimulation once the gastric contents reach the duodenum. The gastric phase results mainly from gastric distention once food reaches the stomach while the intestinal phase begins once food reaches the duodenum. Duodenal stimulation results in the release of secretin by the duodenal mucosa which results in a large increase in pancreatic bicarbonate secretion aimed at neutralizing the intestinal pH. This normalization is necessary to achieve optimal enzyme activity. Cholecystokinin (CCK) is the main mediator of pancreatic enzyme secretion and similarly is released from the duodenal mucosa during the intestinal phase. These enzymes remain active until the CCK cascade is deactivated by trypsin. During meals trypsin cannot complex with CCK due to the presence of food but once food is cleared trypsin rapidly inactivates CCK resulting in cessation of pancreatic enzyme secretion. The concept of duodenal mediated stimulation of pancreatic secretion is the basis behind jejunal tube feeds. The intent is to administer enteral nutrition in the jejunum in an attempt to bypass duodenal mediated pancreatic stimulation. Although theoretically this concept seems correct, studies have shown that gastric feeding in acute pancreatitis can be equally safe [8].

Patients with pancreatic insufficiency have slightly altered physiology due to the decreased ability to produce and secrete digestive enzymes. These patients have lower levels of pancreatic lipase secretion. As a compensatory mechanism gastric lipase secretion from the chief cells of the stomach is increased and becomes the main source of active lipase. These patients also have a reduced ability to secrete pancreatic amylase. Although salivary amylase activity is preserved in chronic pancreatitis, a compensatory mechanism to increase activity does not exist as it does for gastric lipase [4]. Medium chain triglycerides have been found to have comparable nutritional value to long chain triglycerides but do not lead to the increase in CCK and pancreatic secretion that occurs with long chain triglycerides. They are therefore useful as an energy source for patients that cannot tolerate pancreatic stimulation.

Common Clinical Questions

Can Serum Amylase and Lipase Be Normal in Acute Pancreatitis?

Yes, and perhaps more problematic is that both serum amylase and lipase can be normal even in episodes of severe acute pancreatitis complicated by pancreatic necrosis. When using a cut off of three times the upper limits of normal both tests show a high specificity but the sensitivity remains poor. Unfortunately combining both tests have not shown to improve the diagnostic accuracy. When directly compared, the serum lipase outperforms serum amylase. This likely results from the short half-life of serum amylase and the much longer half-life of serum lipase. During an acute episode both the amylase and lipase will elevate within a few hours. The amylase will typically normalize within 24 h whereas the lipase will remain elevated for several days. As a result if there is any delay in the patient presentation the serum amylase may normalize and the diagnosis missed if only serum amylase was assessed.

Two other main scenarios exist where the serum amylase and lipase may be normal in acute pancreatitis. These are acute alcoholic pancreatitis and hypertriglyceridemia as a result of technical issues with the assay. If there is a high clinical suspicion for acute pancreatitis in the setting of a normal serum amylase or lipase, particularly in the above scenarios, abdominal cross-sectional imaging should be considered. Hence the revised Atlanta criteria for acute pancreatitis suggest two of the following three features should be present to diagnose acute pancreatitis [9]. These include abdominal pain, greater than threefold elevation of amylase and/or lipase, or abdominal imaging consistent with acute pancreatitis.

> Typically one would see a threefold elevation of amylase and/or lipase in a setting of acute pancreatitis. Patients with acute on chronic pancreatitis, alcoholic pancreatitis, and pancreatitis due to hypertriglyceridemia may have mild or severe pancreatitis without significant enzyme elevations.

What Are the Most Common Non-pancreatic Causes of Elevated Amylase and Lipase?

Despite the high specificity several non-pancreatic causes of enzyme elevation still exist. The most frequently encountered is in the setting of renal insufficiency due to decreased renal clearance of the enzymes. Critically ill patients often display elevations of lipase and amylase but independently this does not change the clinical course and appears to be secondary to end-organ dysfunction. This has similarly been shown in patients who undergo cardiac surgery with cardiopulmonary bypass [10]. It has been shown that pancreatic enzymes are frequently elevated postoperatively with an increased risk if the levels are elevated preoperatively. This seems most likely due to a result of alterations in perfusion intra-operatively but has not been shown to have clinical significance.

Other causes, in no particular order, are biliary tract disease (choledocholithiasis, cholecystitis or cholangitis), bowel obstruction, medications, viral infections (cytomegalovirus and human immunodeficiency virus), over-tube assisted deep enteroscopy, liver failure, celiac disease, malignancy, macroamylasemia, parotitis, inflammatory bowel disease and gastroenteritis.

Patients who undergo endoscopic retrograde cholangio-pancreatography (ERCP) are likely to have elevations in the serum amylase and lipase post procedure but if not accompanied by nausea, vomiting, or abdominal pain are likely secondary to instrumentation and not reflective of post-ERCP pancreatitis ("biochemical pancreatitis"). Patients with chronic asymptomatic elevation of the amylase and lipase have been described. The clinical relevance of this is unclear though these patients are more likely to show pancreatic abnormalities that may warrant further evaluation. Despite these abnormalities this usually does not influence the acute management of the patient. Clinicians should consider an alternative diagnosis in patients with an elevated serum amylase and lipase that lack clinical or radiographic evidence of pancreatitis.

> Elevation in the pancreatic enzymes can be seen in several other non-pancreatic disease states. One should be careful in the interpretation of serum amylase and lipase in a setting of liver failure, renal insufficiency, pregnancy, hypertriglyceridemia, biliary disease and bowel obstruction. In the appropriate clinical setting these enzyme elevations help make a diagnosis of pancreatitis but pursuing an isolated hyper-enzymemia is often misleading.

Can Amylase and Lipase Be Used to Follow the Clinical Course of Pancreatitis or Predict the Severity of the Disease?

Although it would be useful if this were true, there unfortunately is no role for serial amylase and lipase levels as they do not correlate with the clinical course. Asymptomatic patients with elevated enzymes may experience marked fluctuations in the daily enzyme levels despite no change in symptoms. Similarly, patients may display clinical improvement despite worsening of the enzymes or clinical deterioration despite normalization of the enzymes. Often clinicians are concerned when the amylase or lipase rises after initiation of enteral feeds; however, this does not correlate with a worsening of the pancreatitis. Provided the patient does not experience a worsening in nausea, vomiting, or abdominal pain the enteral feedings can be continued regardless of a rise in the enzymes.

A single serum amylase and lipase is useful for the diagnosis but there is no role for repeated measurements once a diagnosis of acute pancreatitis has been established. Serum enzymes can be normal in severe acute pancreatitis and even in the presence of pancreatic necrosis. The degree of amylase or lipase elevation does not predict a more mild or severe disease process and cannot be used for prognostication. There is evidence to suggest that the lipase to amylase ratio may help to differentiate a pancreatic versus a biliary etiology, but this is not adequately reliable and should not be relied on in clinical practice. Other information, such as the clinical history and imaging studies, should be used to help identify the likely etiology. Disease severity can only be determined with an accepted scoring system such as the Ranson's criteria or the Acute Physiology and Chronic Health Evaluation (APACHE) II score. These scoring systems are problematic due to the multiple components and prolonged time over which data are collected but remain the only reliable way to assess the severity of the disease.

> The degree of enzyme elevation does not correspond to the severity or help prognosticate the clinical course of pancreatitis. Pancreatic enzymes are helpful to establish the diagnosis but have no role in the ongoing management of the patient.

Brief Review of the Literature

The diagnosis of acute pancreatitis is suspected in the setting of acute onset abdominal pain associated with nausea and vomiting. The classical presentation is pain located in the epigastrium radiating into the back and can be seen in 40–70 % of patients [11]. The diagnosis is supported by elevations in the amylase and lipase and the finding of acute pancreatic inflammation on cross-sectional imaging. Generally the serum lipase should be elevated to greater than three times the upper limit of normal to differentiate pancreatitis from non-pancreatic abdominal pain [12]. Diagnostic difficulties occur in patients with normal or minimally elevated pancreatic enzymes or in patients without abdominal pain but with significant elevations in the pancreatic enzymes.

In acute pancreatitis the serum amylase rises as a result of both increased release and reduced catabolism of the enzyme [13]. Although the serum amylase and lipase are routinely used in the diagnosis of acute pancreatitis, they are not perfect and can be misleading. Historically the preferred laboratory test was amylase but has been gradually replaced with serum lipase due to the increased sensitivity, particularly in acute alcoholic pancreatitis. There are over 200 different techniques to measure serum amylase which creates confusion in identifying the ideal technique and determining what a normal level should be [13]. The reported performance of the serum amylase and lipase varies considerably based on the study. The sensitivity for amylase and lipase has ranged from 45 to 72 % and 55–100 %, and specificity from 97 to 99 % and 96–99 %, respectively [11, 12]. The performance characteristics of each test was thoroughly assessed in a prospective study where amylase and lipase levels were measured on presentation and on days 1, 2, and 3 following admission [14]. Receiver operating characteristics for each test were assessed individually and combined at each time point. There was no evidence to suggest that combining the serum amylase or lipase increased the diagnostic accuracy for acute pancreatitis. The study concluded that the serum lipase alone, both early and late in the presentation, was the single recommend test for diagnosis.

There are three major reasons the serum amylase may be normal during an episode of acute pancreatitis. Those are the time interval since the onset of the attack, in the setting of acute alcoholic pancreatitis, and in patients with hypertriglyceridemia [13]. There also exist several less frequently encountered causes of reduced amylase and lipase. Reduced levels of enzymes can occur during first trimester of pregnancy suggesting that pregnant patients may have normal or mildly elevated enzymes during an episode of acute pancreatitis [15]. In addition, conditions which increase pancreatic inflammation will result in a reduction in the levels of amylase and lipase. This is most commonly seen in chronic pancreatitis where patients can present with an exacerbation despite having normal levels of the pancreatic enzymes [14]. Similarly, lower levels of amylase and lipase can be seen in patients with recurrent acute pancreatitis without chronic pancreatitis as the more frequent episodes result in subclinical residual pancreatic inflammation [16].

The duration of time the serum amylase and lipase remain elevated in acute pancreatitis varies and results in the different sensitivity for each assay. The serum amylase typically rises within the first few hours of the attack and normalizes within 24 h. The serum lipase similarly rises rapidly within the first 4–8 h after the onset of symptoms but can potentially remain elevated for several days to a week after the episode [13]. After the onset of symptoms if there is any delay in the patient seeking medical attention or in evaluation of the serum amylase by the provider the amylase may have normalized and the diagnosis missed. The serum lipase, however, would remain elevated and thus is the more reliable laboratory test in diagnosing acute pancreatitis.

Patients with acute alcoholic pancreatitis, including severe pancreatitis, can present with only mild elevations in the serum amylase and lipase. In one study of 68 patients admitted with acute alcoholic pancreatitis confirmed by imaging the serum amylase was normal in 32 % of patients [17]. This was also shown in a retrospective review of 284 consecutive patients where patients with acute alcoholic pancreatitis were more likely to present with minimal (less than three times the upper limit of normal) elevations in the pancreatic enzymes [18]. Although acute alcoholic pancreatitis may present with a normal amylase, the serum lipase has been shown to be more reliably elevated in this setting, making it the preferred test in patients with alcohol induced pancreatitis [13]. This feature, combined with the longer half-life, contributes to the improved sensitivity of the serum lipase.

Hypertriglyceridemia has been shown to result in lower serum amylase levels; however, this is more the result of a limitation of the assay [19]. A circulatory inhibitor of serum amylase exists in the setting of hypertriglyceridemia which interferes with the assay though it can be corrected if recognized by the laboratory and serial dilution techniques are performed [13]. Although hypertriglyceridemia is a known cause of acute pancreatitis the diagnosis can be difficult to detect as the triglyceride levels can rapidly normalize once the patient has ceased eating and intravenous resuscitation has begun. If hypertriglyceridemia is not considered then diluting the serum to correct the amylase assay would likely not be performed. As a result of these issues the diagnosis of acute pancreatitis can be missed when hypertriglyceridemia is present if not recognized by the astute clinician.

Patients frequently present to the healthcare system with complaints of acute abdominal pain. There has been an interest in the triage of these patients with routine serum amylase and lipase but this approach has not been shown to be cost effective [20]. In this study amylase and lipase assays were performed in patients presenting with acute abdominal pain regardless of whether the presentation was consistent with acute pancreatitis or not. Of the 1598 patients included only 1 % of patients were identified with acute pancreatitis resulting in a number needed to treat that was not cost effective. The study concluded that the serum amylase and lipase levels should only be assessed in patients with a clinical presentation consistent with acute pancreatitis and not used as a screening tool for all patients with abdominal pain.

Serum Amylase and lipase should not be used as routine tests in evaluation of abdominal pain.

More common than a normal amylase or lipase in acute pancreatitis is finding elevated enzymes in a patient without clinical evidence of acute pancreatitis. This entity and the various causes are well documented in several studies and case reports. The most commonly encountered and documented cause of an elevated serum amylase and lipase is renal insufficiency as a result of reduced urinary excretion [11,21,22]. There appears to be a direct correlation between the degree of renal insufficiency and the likelihood of elevation of the amylase and lipase. A study of 128 patients with varying degrees of renal insufficiency noted that the serum amylase and lipase remained normal provided the creatinine clearance remained above 50 ml/min but at lower levels the enzymes were more likely to be elevated [21]. A second study of 24 controls and 47 patients with renal insufficiency studied six pancreatic enzymes including amylase and lipase [22]. They found that the lipase was less frequently elevated than the amylase at a creatinine clearance between 13 and 39 ml/min suggesting there may be a diagnostic advantage to the serum lipase in patients with moderate renal insufficiency. The upper limit of normal for the serum amylase and lipase in patients with renal insufficiency has not been determined and clinical judgment is needed to determine the likelihood of a pancreatic process. If there is any concern about the diagnosis cross-sectional imaging should be obtained.

Several other non-pancreatic etiologies for elevated amylase and lipase have been reported. Due to the presence of amylase and lipase in the gastrointestinal tract elevated enzymes can be seen in the setting of bowel obstruction, colitis, celiac disease, inflammatory bowel disease, and gastroenteritis [23–27]. In addition, several viral etiologies such as cytomegalovirus and human immunodeficiency virus infection may lead to an enzyme elevation [28, 29]. Endoscopic instrumentation of the gastrointestinal tract, particularly with deep balloon assisted enteroscopy, have also been implicated presumably from stimulation of the gastrointestinal wall though rarely are these enzyme elevations accompanied by acute pancreatitis [30, 31]. Hyperamylasemia has also been reported in patients with acute liver failure as shown in a study by the Acute Liver Failure Study Group registry [32]. Elevated amylase was associated with increased mortality; however, when assessed by itself it was not found to be an independent predictor. The hyperamylasemia of acute liver failure is likely secondary to its association with renal impairment and multiorgan dysfunction and by itself does not have clinical significance. This same conclusion was reached by a prospective study of 160 critically ill patients with elevated lipase where the clinical relevance and imaging findings were assessed [33]. Hyperlipasemia was frequently encountered but the majority of these patients displayed no pancreatic abnormalities on imaging and those that did showed only mild morphologic changes. There did not appear to be any change to the hospital course regardless of the findings again concluding that the enzyme elevation itself was not of clinical significance.

> One should be careful in the interpretation of serum amylase and lipase in a setting of liver failure, renal insufficiency, pregnancy, hypertriglyceridemia, biliary disease, and bowel obstruction.

Endoscopic retrograde cholangiopancreatography is now readily available and the potential for post-ERCP pancreatitis is a well-known complication. Although identifying patients with post-ERCP pancreatitis early is critical, the serum amylase and lipase levels post-ERCP are not reliable in predicting which patients will develop pancreatitis. Post-procedural hyperamylasemia can occur in nearly 50 % of patients post-ERCP with pancreatitis occurring in only 5 % [34, 35]. The majority of patients with elevated amylase and lipase post-ERCP are secondary to instrumentation. There is evidence that an elevated serum amylase greater than five times the upper limit of normal 4 h post procedure may be predictive of patients who will develop post-ERCP pancreatitis but this has not been universally adopted [35]. Overall, there is no role for routinely following the amylase or lipase after an ERCP unless there is a strong clinical suspicion for post-ERCP pancreatitis though it must be remembered that even patients with post-procedural abdominal pain and elevated lipase and amylase may not progress to acute pancreatitis.

It is well accepted that the serum amylase and lipase may be normal during an exacerbation of chronic pancreatitis. There are patients, however, with chronic pancreatitis with elevated serum amylase or lipase despite remaining asymptomatic. In a prospective study in patients with chronic pancreatitis and elevated enzymes 11 % were shown to have macroamylasemia of no clinical consequence again suggesting that asymptomatic patients with elevated amylase and lipase may not have an underlying pancreatic process [36].

Chronic asymptomatic pancreatic hyperenzymemia (CAPH) is an entity that has been reported and results in an abnormal increase in the serum amylase and lipase without pancreatic symptoms or radiologic evidence of pancreatic disease. These patients typically undergo an extensive evaluation of laboratory, radiologic, and even invasive procedures as part of the evaluation. To better assess this, a prospective study of 163 patients was performed where all patients underwent a thorough evaluation including abdominal magnetic resonance imaging [37]. Interestingly the study found that 50 % of the patients had pathologic findings on secretin-enhanced magnetic resonance imaging. The most common findings were dilation of the main pancreatic duct (19.4 %) or diffuse pancreatic side branch dilation (25.6 %). In 23 of the patients (14.4 %) the diagnosis resulted in a change in clinical management requiring either a surgical intervention or close surveillance imaging. Although asymptomatic elevation of the amylase and lipase may not be reflective of acute pancreatitis, it may be suggestive of other underlying pathology which may require further evaluation; however, discretion should be used to determine when an adequate evaluation has been completed.

> For those with persistent elevation of enzymes without clinical features of acute pancreatitis one should consider noninvasive testing especially secretin enhanced MRCP.

Once a patient is admitted with acute pancreatitis they are followed clinically for improvement. There is no utility in following the serum amylase and lipase as the enzyme levels do not correlate with the clinical course [38]. A patient may develop resolution of symptoms despite worsening of the amylase or lipase or may clinically deteriorate despite improvements or even normalization of the enzymes. The serum amylase and lipase are useful for diagnosis on admission but should not be serially followed throughout the hospitalization. Clinicians are often concerned when the serum amylase or lipase rises after initiation of enteral feeding but this elevation does not correlate with worsening of the pancreatitis. When enteral feeds are restarted the patient should be clinically followed and provided there is not an exacerbation of nausea, vomiting, or abdominal pain enteral feeding may be continued.

Previous studies have attempted to assess if the amylase and lipase levels have a role in determining the etiology of the pancreatitis. Patients with acute alcoholic pancreatitis have been shown to have a significantly lower amylase than patients with a biliary etiology [39]. Despite this a low serum amylase does not reliably predict a pancreatic process as low serum amylase can be seen in all etiologies of pancreatitis. The lipase to amylase ratio has also been studied as a potential indicator of the etiology and severity of the pancreatitis and has been shown that patients with acute alcoholic pancreatitis have lower levels of amylase and lipase [40]. However, when the combined pancreatic and biliary group was compared to the non-pancreatic, non-biliary pancreatitis group there was no difference. It appears that although a lower amylase and lipase level may be seen in acute alcoholic pancreatitis, it does not reliably predict whether the pancreatitis is of a pancreaticobiliary etiology. That determination can only be made after a thorough review of the clinical history, laboratory data, and available imaging studies.

Acute pancreatitis can have a complicated course which is best identified early in the hospitalization. Unfortunately the serum amylase and lipase are also unable to accurately predict the severity of the pancreatitis. Patients with severe acute pancreatitis with multiorgan failure requiring an admission to the intensive care unit may present with only a minimal elevation in the amylase and lipase [18]. On the contrary, patients with significant elevations in the amylase and lipase may have mild pancreatitis that can resolve within 24 h. Not only is the degree of lipase and amylase elevation unreliable in predicting the severity of the pancreatitis but it is also unreliable in predicting day to day changes in the clinical course. To help with prognosis and to better determine the severity of the pancreatitis several scoring systems have been developed and are widely available. They are generally laborious and require multiple laboratory values and calculations. They are beyond the scope of this chapter and are discussed elsewhere in this book.

> An elevation of pancreatic enzymes helps confirm the diagnosis of acute pancreatitis but does not predict the severity of the disease. The daily trend of the pancreatic enzymes does not correlate with clinical improvement or deterioration and once the diagnosis is confirmed measurements of amylase and lipase should not be repeated.

Future Directions

Our understanding of acute pancreatitis and pancreatic physiology has improved drastically over the past two decades. Despite this our ability to identify and treat patients with pancreatic disease remains suboptimal. This is partly due to the high variability in patient presentations and also due to the quality of literature. There is a lack of well designed, randomized controlled trials evaluating acute pancreatitis. As a result the majority of the management is based on expert opinion. In addition, the fact that a large percentage of patients with severe pancreatitis can present with normal or minimal elevations in amylase and lipase also complicates the field as these patients are often excluded from research studies as a result of the normal levels [18]. Future studies need to include not only patients with elevated pancreatic enzymes but also patients with radiologic evidence of acute pancreatitis.

Serum amylase and lipase have improved our abilities to diagnose patients with acute pancreatitis; however, better markers are still needed. Other markers have been evaluated, including pancreatic isoamylase, immunoreactive trypsinogen, and elastase 1; however, the results have not proven superior than the serum amylase and lipase [13]. We lack a cost-effective and safe test to track the clinical course of a patient through the hospitalization. At the present time the patient's symptoms and radiographic studies are the only means to assess improvement. If a reliable serum test were available to track the clinical course, we would be better able to predict clinical changes and potentially improve patient outcomes. Additional bench and translational research is needed to identify new diagnostic markers that yield improved sensitivity and hence improved accuracy compared to the currently available amylase and lipase assays.

Conclusion

Serum amylase and lipase are helpful markers in the diagnosis of acute pancreatitis. In the proper clinical setting with appropriate symptoms or radiologic evidence of acute pancreatic inflammation, elevated pancreatic enzymes are consistent with a diagnosis of acute pancreatitis. Elevated pancreatic enzymes by themselves are not diagnostic of the disease. Patients with a clinical or radiologic presentation consistent with acute pancreatitis with normal pancreatic enzymes should not be discounted and a diagnosis of acute pancreatitis should be considered. The three major explanations for this scenario are in patients with a delayed presentation, in acute alcoholic pancreatitis, and in hypertriglyceridemia. To help avoid the diagnostic dilemmas created by these the recommended diagnostic test for acute pancreatitis is the serum lipase due to the longer half-life and higher levels seen in patients with acute alcoholic pancreatitis.

An elevated amylase or lipase in a patient without abdominal pain and with normal imaging is unlikely to reflect a diagnosis of acute pancreatitis. These patients may have another underlying diagnosis that would explain the enzyme elevation though this may not be discovered until a thorough evaluation is performed. For patients with a persistent elevation of the amylase and lipase but without a clear explanation the diagnosis of chronic asymptomatic pancreatic hyperenzymemia should be considered. In this subset of patients pancreatic imaging with secretin enhanced magnetic resonance imaging is reasonable due to the frequent finding of pancreatic abnormalities. If normal, then continued evaluation is not indicated and the hyperenzymemia is most likely a benign finding. Once a diagnosis of acute pancreatitis is established further measurements of the amylase and lipase are not helpful as they do not correlate with clinical improvement and are not predictive of the severity of the disease.

Although the management of acute pancreatitis has improved considerably, there is still a need for well-designed translational and clinical trials to improve our diagnostic abilities and therapeutic understanding. Until then clinicians will have to rely on their clinical judgment augmented by laboratory and radiologic studies to properly care for the patient with acute pancreatitis.

References

1. Lowenfels AB, Sullivan T, Fiorianti J, Maisonneuve P. The epidemiology and impact of pancreatic diseases in the United States. Curr Gastroenterol Rep. 2005;7(2):90–5.
2. Williams JA. Intracellular signaling mechanisms activated by cholecystokinin-regulating synthesis and secretion of digestive enzymes in pancreatic acinar cells. Annu Rev Physiol. 2001;63: 77–97.
3. Williams JA. Regulation of acinar cell function in the pancreas. Curr Opin Gastroenterol. 2010;26:478–83.
4. Whitcomb DC, Lowe ME. Human pancreatic digestive enzymes. Dig Dis Sci. 2007;52(1):1–17.
5. Sleisenger and Fordtran's Gastrointestinal and Liver Disease. 9th ed. Saunders Elsevier; 2010.
6. Frank B, Gottlieb K. Amylase normal, lipase elevated: is it pancreatitis? A case series and review of the literature. Am J Gastroenterol. 1999;94(2):463–9.
7. DiMagno EP, Hendricks JC, Go VL, Dozois RR. Relationships among canine fasting pancreatic and biliary secretions, pancreatic duct pressure, and duodenal phase III motor activity— Boldyreff revisited. Dig. 1979;24(9):689–93.
8. Eatock FC, Chong PS, Menezes N, Imrie CW, McKay CJ, Carter R. Nasogastric feeding in severe acute pancreatitis is safe and avoids the risks associated with the nasojejunal route: a randomised controlled trial. Gastroenterology. 2001;120(5):A469.

9. Banks PA, Bollen TL, Deryenis C, Gooszen HG, Johnson CD, Sarr MG, et al. Classification of acute pancreatitis—2012: revision of the Atlanta classification and definitions by international consensus. Gut. 2013;62(1):102–11.

10. Nys M, Venneman I, Deby-Dupont G, Preiser JC, Vanbelle S, Albert A, et al. Pancreatic cellular injury after cardiac surgery with cardiopulmonary bypass: frequency, time course and risk factors. Shock. 2007;27(5):474–81.

11. Forsmark CE, Baillie J. AGA institute technical review on acute pancreatitis. Gastroenterology. 2007;132(5):2022–44.

12. Gumaste VV, Roditis N, Mehta D, Dave PB. Serum lipase levels in nonpancreatic abdominal pain versus acute pancreatitis. Am J Gastroenterol. 1993;88(12):2051–5.

13. Yadav D, Agarwal N, Pitchumoni CS. A critical evaluation of laboratory tests in acute pancreatitis. Am J Gastroenterol. 2002;97(6):1309–18.

14. Treacy J, Williams A, Bais R, Willson K, Worthley C, Reece J, et al. Evaluation of amylase and lipase in the diagnosis of acute pancreatitis. J Surg. 2001;71(10):577–82.

15. Karsenti D, Bacq Y, Brechot J, Mariotte N, Vol S, Tichet J. Serum amylase and lipase activities in normal pregnancy: a prospective case-control study. Am J Gastroenterol. 2001;96(3):697–9.

16. Clavien P, Robert J, Meyer P, Borst F, Hauser H, Herrmann F, et al. Acute pancreatitis and normoamylasemia not an uncommon combination. Ann Surg. 1989;210(5):614–20.

17. Spechler SJ, Dalton JW, Robbins AH, Gerzof SG, Stern JS, Johnson WC, et al. Prevalence of normal serum amylase levels in patients with acute alcoholic pancreatitis. Dig Dis Sci. 1983;28(10):865–9.

18. Lankisch PG, Burchard-Reckert S, Lehnick D. Underestimation of acute pancreatitis: patients with only a small increase in amylase/lipase levels can also have or develop severe acute pancreatitis. Gut. 1999;44:542–4.

19. Fallat RW, Vester JW, Glueck CJ. Suppression of amylase activity by hypertriglyceridemia. JAMA. 1973;225(11):1331–4.

20. Sutton PA, Humes DJ, Purcell G, Smith JK, Whiting F, Wright T, et al. The role of routine assays of serum amylase and lipase for the diagnosis of acute abdominal pain. Ann R Coll Surg Engl. 2009;91:381–4.

21. Collen MJ, Ansher AF, Chapman AB, Mackow RC, Lewis JH. Serum amylase in patients with renal insufficiency and renal failure. Am J Gastroenterol. 1990;85(10):1377–80.

22. Seno T, Harada H, Ochi K, Tanaka J, Matsumoto S, Choudhury R, et al. Serum levels of six pancreatic enzymes as related to the degree of renal dysfunction. Am J Gastroenterol. 1995;90(11):2002–5.
23. Choung BS, Kim SH, Seo SY, Kim IH, Kim SW, Lee S-O, et al. Pancreatic hyperenzymemia is associated with bacterial culture positive, more severe and right-sided colitis. Dig Dis Sci. 2014;59(9):2272–9.
24. Ben-Horin S, Farfel Z, Mouallem M. Gastroenteritis-associated hyperamylasemia. Arch Intern Med. 2002;162(6):689–92.
25. Venkataraman D, Howarth L, Beattie RM, Afzal NA. A very high amylase can be benign in paediatric Crohn's disease. BMJ Case Reports 2012
26. Liu Z, Wang J, Qian J, Tang F. Hyperamylasemia, reactive plasmacytosis, and immune abnormalities in a patient with celiac disease. Dig Dis Sci. 2007;52(6):1444–7.
27. Pieper-Bigelow C, Strocchi A, Levitt MD. Where does serum amylase come from and where does it go? Gastroenterol Clin North Am. 1990;19(4):793–810.
28. Argiris A, Mathur-Wagh U, Wilets I, Mildvan D. Abnormalities of serum amylase and lipase in HIV-positive patients. Am J Gastroenterol. 1999;94(5):1248–52.
29. Tomonari A, Takahashi S, Takasugi K, Ooi J, Tsukada N, Konuma T, et al. Pancreatic hyperamylasemia and hyperlipasemia in association with cytomegalovirus infection following unrelated cord blood transplantation for acute myelogenous leukemia. Int J Hematol. 2006;84(5):438–40.
30. Teshima CW, Aktas H, Kuipers EJ, Mensink PB. Hyperamylasemia and pancreatitis following spiral enteroscopy. Can J Gastroenterol. 2012;26(9):603–6.
31. Zepeda-Gomez S, Barreto-Zuniga R, Ponce-de-Leon S, Meixueiro-Daza A, Herrera-Lopez JA, Camacho J, et al. Risk of hyperamylasemia and acute pancreatitis after double-balloon enteroscopy: a prospective study. Endoscopy. 2011;43(9):766–70.
32. Cote GA, Gottstein JH, Daud A, Lee WM, Blei AT. The acute liver failure study group. The role of etiology in the hyperamylasemia of acute liver failure. Am J Gastroenterol. 2009;104(3):592–7.
33. Denz C, Siegel L, Lehman K, Dagorn J, Fiedler F. Is hyperlipasemia in critically ill patients of clinical importance? An observational CT study. Intensive Care Med. 2007;33(9):1633–6.

34. Gottlieb K, Sherman S, Pezzi J, Esber E, Lehman GA. Early recognition of post-ERCP pancreatitis by clinical assessment and serum pancreatic enzymes. Am J Gastroenterol. 1996;91(8):1553–7.
35. Testoni PA, Bagnolo F, Caporuscio S, Lella F. Serum amylase measured four hours after endoscopic sphincterotomy is a reliable predictor of postprocedure pancreatitis. Am J Gastroenterol. 1999;94(5):1235–41.
36. Gubergrits N, Golubova O, Lukashevich G, Fomenko P. Elevated serum amylase in patients with chronic pancreatitis: acute attack or macroamylasemia? Pancreatology. 2014;14(2):114–6.
37. Amodio A, Manfredi R, Katsotourchi AM, Gabbrielli A, Benini L, Mucelli RP, et al. Prospective evaluation of subjects with chronic asymptomatic pancreatic hyperenzymemia. Am J Gastroenterol. 2012;107(7):1089–95.
38. Gullo L. Day-to-day variations of serum pancreatic enzymes in benign pancreatic hyperenzymemia. Clin Gastroenterol Hepatol. 2007;5(1):70–4.
39. Hiatt JR, Calabria RP, Passaro Jr E, Wilson SE. The amylase profile: a discriminant in biliary and pancreatic disease. Am J Surg. 1987;154(5):490–2.
40. Pezzilli R, Billi P, Miglioli M, Gullo L. Serum amylase and lipase concentrations and lipase/amylase ratio in assessment of etiology and severity of acute pancreatitis. Dig Dis Sci. 1993;38(7): 1265–9.

Part 1
Clinical Scenario:
Abdominal Pain With or Without Elevated Amylase and Lipase

Chapter 2
Acute Pancreatitis

Raghuwansh P. Sah and Santhi Swaroop Vege

What Causes Acute Pancreatitis?

Suggested response to patient: About 4 in 10 cases are caused by gall stones. In these cases, small (<5 mm) stones escape from the gall bladder and pass into the ducts that drain pancreatic juices causing blockade. This results in damage to the pancreas resulting in inflammation and pancreatitis. Another 3 in 10 cases are caused by heavy alcohol drinking. Exactly how alcohol causes pancreatitis in not well known. There are many other known causes that account for the rest although in many patients no cause can be found by current methods. It is thought that damage to the pancreas results from auto-digestion by action of powerful pancreatic enzymes that get activated within the pancreas. Inflammatory cells from the blood are recruited to the area of damage. These cells along with the cells of the pancreas lead to systemic inflammatory response. This can lead to fluid leakage into various spaces in the body including into the lungs causing problems in breathing, low blood pressure,

R.P. Sah • S.S. Vege, M.D. (✉)
Division of Gastroenterology and Hepatology,
Department of Medicine, Mayo Clinic, 200 First Street SW,
Rochester, MN 55905, USA
e-mail: Vege.santhi@mayo.edu

© Springer International Publishing Switzerland 2016
K. Dua, R. Shaker (eds.), *Pancreas and Biliary Disease*,
DOI 10.1007/978-3-319-28089-9_2

and damage to multiple organs. With current aggressive treatment, this inflammatory response can be managed in as many as 70–80 % of the patients resulting in quick recovery. However, 15–30 % of patients will go on to develop moderately severe or severe disease.

Brief Review of the Literature

Introduction

Acute pancreatitis (AP) is an inflammatory disorder of the pancreas which often affects many organ systems. Historically, AP was associated with a high mortality. While the overall mortality rate has dropped to 2–4 %, patients with severe disease continue to have a high mortality with estimates ranging from 20 % to 40 % for specific subgroups [1]. In the US, it affects about 40 individuals per 100,000 each year and its incidence is estimated to be increasing [2]. Based on US data from 2009 [3], AP was the most common gastroenterology discharge diagnosis with more than 275,000 hospitalizations, an estimated 2.6 billon US dollars in direct and indirect costs and 2600 deaths, making it the fifth leading cause of in-hospital deaths.

Diagnosis

AP is diagnosed clinically when any two of the following are present: (1) abdominal pain consistent with the disease, (2) serum amylase and/or lipase greater than three times the upper limit of normal, (3) consistent radiologic imaging (CT or MRI) findings [4].

The pain is typically described in the epigastric region or left upper quadrant and usually severe in intensity. Patients may describe pain radiating to the back, flank or chest although this is nonspecific. Serum lipase has better specificity than amylase and remains elevated longer making it preferable over amylase measurements. It is to be emphasized that neither the severity of the pain or the degree of enzyme elevations correlates with severity of the disease [4]. Imaging is not required for establishing diagnosis and should be reserved for patients in whom diagnosis is not clear or who fail to show improvement within 48–72 h or to evaluate for development of complications in the later stages of the disease [4]. Diffuse or localized swelling of the pancreas is consistent for AP on imaging with or without varying degree of peripancreatic fat stranding.

Etiology

Gall stones account for ~40 % and heavy alcohol abuse accounts for another ~30 % of cases of AP in the US [2, 5]. *An abdominal ultrasound should be performed in all patients with AP* to identify gall stones and biliary dilatation due to possible choledocholithiasis [4]. Heavy alcohol use for greater than 5 years is typically considered necessary for development of pancreatitis. Further, only 5 % of patients with gall stones or heavy alcohol use develop pancreatitis in their lifetime. Pancreatic tumors should be considered as a possible etiology in patients older than 40 or 50 years of age, without gall stone disease or history of alcohol abuse. Intra-ductal papillary mucinous neoplasms (IPMN), usually main duct type but sometimes even side-branch type may cause AP. The other infrequent causes include drugs, following procedures like ERCP (rarely after EUS and fine needle aspiration), hypercalcemia, hypertriglyceridemia (>1000 mg/dl), trauma, ischemia, autoimmune pancreatitis, and certain infections. These are quite uncommon, and caution should be exercised in ascribing one of these uncommon causes as the etiology. Often, these causes, especially drugs, are falsely implicated as the causative agent of AP. Post-ERCP AP is usually obvious and can occur in 5 % of diagnostic ERCPs, 7 % of therapeutic ERCPs and up to 25 % in patients with sphincter of Oddi dysfunction [6].

Idiopathic AP is defined as cases of AP where the etiology is not evident after imaging (trans-abdominal ultrasound and CT/MRI in the appropriate setting) and standard laboratory investigations including calcium and triglyceride levels [4]. Idiopathic AP may account for up to 30 % of all cases. Hereditary pancreatitis accounts for a small proportion of idiopathic AP. There is no clear data on risks and benefits of further endoscopic examination for evaluation of etiology of idiopathic AP. Further, no causative etiology may ever be identified in many of these patients. Current guidelines recommend referral of idiopathic AP to centers of expertise for further work-up of etiology [4].

Natural Course and Complications

Regardless of the etiology, AP involves an early phase usually lasting a week or two which can progress in some patients into a late phase lasting weeks to months [4]. The early phase correlates to the time-course and effects of intense systemic inflammatory response elicited due to pancreatic injury. The late phase correlates to development of local complications from pancreatic injury. Persistent dysfunction of one or more organ systems can occur in both phases. Among the patients who succumb to AP, approximately half of them die during the first week or two (early phase) and another half in the late phase [7–10]. Deaths in the early phase occur due to organ failure and complications related to the severe inflammatory response. In the late phase, deaths occur due to local complications including infection of pancreatic necrosis or interventions for these complications [11].

Development of local complications and persistent organ failure are both associated with increased mortality, prolonged course of illness and increased rate of complications [1, 12]. This understanding has been the basis of the evolution of strategies for classifying patients with AP. The concepts of local complications and of organ failure are explained in detail below. The long-standing 1992 Atlanta Classification has been recently revised in 2013, resulting in a widely accepted classification system that has three groups—mild, moderately severe, and severe AP [12]. Another parallel classification system with an additional group of critical AP was developed around the same time, known as Determinant Based Classification (DBC) of AP [13]. Initial validation studies have shown both strategies to be effective in classifying patients appropriately with the aim of identifying patients at the highest risk of mortality and morbidity [14, 15]. In this chapter we discuss this Revised Atlanta Classification of AP in detail.

Organ failure conceptually refers to failure of cardiovascular, pulmonary, or renal systems commonly associated with conditions resulting in profound systemic inflammatory response. For objective assessment of organ failure, a modified Marshall scoring system (the following Web based resource may be used: http://www.pmidcalc.org/?sid=23100216&newtest=Y) is recommended in the Revised Atlanta Classification [12]. A score of 0–4 is assigned for each organ system depending on the severity of dysfunction assessed by worst observations over a 24 h period for PaO2/FiO2 for pulmonary, creatinine rise for renal, and hypotension for cardiovascular system. A score of 2 or more in any system (corresponds to PaO2/FiO2≤300, creatinine >1.9 mg/dl, and systolic blood pressure < 90 not fluid responsive) defines *organ failure*. While organ failure may be transient, its persistence for greater than 48 h is defined as *persistent organ failure*.

Local complications refer to *acute necrotic collections* and *acute peripancreatic fluid collections* and their morphologic counterparts: *walled-off necrosis (WON)* and *pseudocyst*, respectively, which evolve over 4–6 weeks [12]. These are defined in Table 2.1. In the early phase of AP, acute necrotic or peripancreatic fluid collections can be diagnosed by CT scan or MRI. However, it is unreliable to determine the extent of necrosis within the first few days, and the extent of morphological changes does not necessarily correlate with the severity of organ failure. Further, an acute fluid collection may occur in 30–50 % of the patients but are not predictive of organ failure as most of them resolve spontaneously. Because of the above reasons, assessment of local complications by multi-detector contrast enhanced CT is most reliable when performed at least after 5–7 days after admission [4]. In patients with renal failure, MRI without contrast can be used

TABLE 2.1 Definitions for local complications in acute pancreatitis (AP)

Type of AP →	Acute interstitial pancreatitis		Acute necrotizing pancreatitis	
Time course ↓	Complication	Imaging[a] (CECT features)	Complication	Imaging (CECT features)
Early (<4 weeks)				
	Acute peripancreatic fluid collection	• Homogenous collection with fluid density • Confined by normal peripancreatic fascial planes • No definable encapsulating wall • No intrapancreatic extension • No pancreatic necrosis	*Pancreatic necrosis*	Lack of pancreatic parenchymal enhancement by IV contrast affecting > 30 % or 3 cm of pancreas;
			Acute necrotic collection	• Collection containing variable amounts of fluid and necrosis • Variable heterogeneous and non-liquid density as the necrotic collection evolves • No encapsulating wall • Intra- or extra-pancreatic
Late (>4 weeks)				
	Pancreatic pseudocyst	• Well-circumscribed oval or round collection • Usually outside the pancreas • Little or no necrosis (no non-liquid component) • Homogenous density • Definable encapsulating wall	*Walled-off necrosis (WON)*	• Well-defined encapsulating wall with heterogenous liquid and non-liquid density • Intra or extra pancreatic.

[a]CECT: Contrast enhanced CT scan

to evaluate pancreatic necrosis on T2 weighted imaging. Local complications should be suspected when there is lack of expected clinical improvement.

The presence of pancreatic and/or peripancreatic necrosis defines **acute necrotizing pancreatitis** [12]. Its absence defines **acute interstitial pancreatitis** [12]. Brief hospital stay and early recovery are typical in acute interstitial pancreatitis although some patients may have acute peripancreatic fluid collections and a small proportion may develop pseudocysts late in the disease. Although useful in understanding the natural course of AP, this morphologic classification is not evident in the early stage of AP and therefore not effective in predicting outcomes.

(Peri-)pancreatic necrosis can be sterile or infected. Infection of (peri-)pancreatic necrosis typically occurs 7–10 days after admission in the late phase of AP. Infected necrosis should be suspected in patients with persistent organ failure or signs of sepsis exceeding beyond 7 days [4]. Both sterile and infected necrosis can result in persistent organ failure. Infected necrosis is usually associated with higher mortality rates [1]. However, many patients with infected necrosis may lack persistent organ failure and infected necrosis without persistent organ failure has significantly lesser mortality than those with persistent organ failure.

Other local complications of AP include gastric outlet obstruction which can delay enteral nutrition, biliary obstruction, splenic and portal vein thrombosis, celiac and splenic artery pseudo-aneurysms that can lead to brisk bleeding, disruption of main pancreatic duct leading to refractory fluid collections, and rarely colon necrosis. Recurrent AP can be seen in about 15–20 % of patients with AP related to heavy alcohol abuse and also in a few patients with idiopathic AP [16].

Prognosis, Risk Stratification, and the Revised Atlanta Classification

Historically, AP has been associated with a high mortality and adverse outcomes. Advances in management including aggressive supportive care for patients with AP has led to significant improvement in the outcomes of AP overall. With institution of current management recommendations, about 70–80 % patients with AP have a mild course requiring only a brief hospitalization and showing good recovery without progressing to the late phase of the disease. However, a subset of patients (estimates ranging from 15 to 30 %) will go on to develop moderately severe or severe disease with high morbidity (prolonged hospital stay and/or need for interventions), and mortality rates of 25–40 % [1, 12, 17, 18]. Predicting which patient will show mild disease with good outcomes and who will develop moderately severe or severe disease has historically been a challenge and continues to be very challenging today despite decades of efforts aimed at developing prediction tools and strategies. There have been no studies about predicting the moderately severe disease and those that addressed severe disease lacked high positive predictive value.

Many prediction tools including Ranson's criteria, BISAP score, APACHE-II score, Harmless AP score, and other lab values in various combinations including BUN, hematocrit, CRP have been tested extensively for their utility of predicting severity [4, 6]. Most of these require 48 h for predicting severe disease by which time the clinical condition of the patient makes the severity obvious. None of the presenting symptoms or signs on physical exam or initial CT/MRI is helpful in predicting severity of AP.

Local complications and persistent organ failure are the most important determinants of mortality and outcomes in AP and therefore form the backbone of strategy to classify AP patients into high risk and low risk groups [12]. It is to be emphasized that none of these features can be defined at admission, full characterization of local complications may not be possible in the early stages of AP and persistent organ failure can only be defined at 48 h or later. In the Revised Atlanta Classification [12] (Table 2.2), persistent organ failure (or death) defines **severe AP** while lack of any local complications or organ failure defines **mild AP**. Transient organ failure and/or local complications define **moderately severe AP**.

TABLE 2.2 Revised Atlanta classification of acute pancreatitis (AP)

Group	Defining features
Mild	No local complication or organ failure
Moderately severe	Local complications and/or transient organ failure (<48 h)
Severe	Persistent organ failure (>48 h)

Local complications refer to pancreatic necrosis or necrotic collection and peripancreatic fluid collection in the early stages (<4 weeks from onset of illness) and their respective counterparts: Walled-off necrosis or pseudocyst, respectively. Organ failure defined by modified Marshall score (≥ 2 score in any one of respiratory, renal, or cardiovascular systems assessed by worst observation over 24 h, corresponding to PaO2/FiO2$\leq$300, creatinine >1.9 mg/dl, and systolic blood pressure <90 not fluid responsive, respectively)

The mortality for mild AP is <1 % while that for severe AP is estimated to be between 20 and 40 % [4, 12, 17]. The mortality rate of moderately severe AP is similar to mild AP but is associated with much higher morbidity with local complications needing interventions and prolonged hospital stays [18].

Management

(a) Initial assessment

As discussed above, none of the clinical or imaging or scoring systems are predictive of severity of AP. *For all practical purposes, for the initial 48 h, all patients with AP should be considered as severe AP.* Frequently patients without local complications evident on initial imaging are mislabeled as mild AP leading to adverse outcomes. For initial assessment, a careful attention should be paid to general high risk features in the patient characteristics (age >55, obesity), presence of SIRS, signs of hypovolemia, features of focal infections, altered mental status, and presence of other comorbid conditions. While most patients can be aggressively managed in medical wards, patients with hemodynamic instability or respiratory decompensation or altered mental status needing intubation should be admitted to ICU. In general, providers should maintain a low threshold for ICU transfer, and patients with persistent SIRS or organ failure in the first 24 h in particular should be considered for ICU care when possible or for intermediary care setting at the minimum [4].

(b) Hydration

Aggressive hydration is most beneficial within the first 12–24 h [4]. The importance of early aggressive hydration cannot be overemphasized. A rate of 250–500 ml/h or 5–10 ml/h/kg of isotonic crystalloid (lactated Ringer's solution preferred) should be provided unless cardiac, renal, or other comorbidities are prohibitive in which case the rate should be tailored to the patient's comorbid conditions [4]. In patients with severe volume depletion, rapid boluses may be needed initially. An objective measure of early fluid resuscitation should be to decrease hematocrit, BUN and maintain good hourly urine output [4]. Fluid requirement should be reassessed frequently within initial 6 h and for the next 24–48 h.

(c) Need for ERCP

In patients presenting with AP who concurrently have acute cholangitis (fever, jaundice, elevated alkaline phosphatase), ERCP should be performed within 24 h [4]. In most AP patients with gall stones without evidence of ongoing biliary obstruction, ERCP is not beneficial. When choledocholithiasis is suspected but there is no cholangitis or jaundice, MRCP or EUS can be performed for evaluation rather than a diagnostic ERCP. In patients who require ERCP, rectal indomethacin or prophylactic pancreatic duct stents should be used to reduce the risk of post-ERCP pancreatitis [4].

(d) Supportive care

Oxygen by nasal cannula (or additional respiratory support as needed) is recommended in all patients with AP. In patients with organ failure, supportive care targeted to each affected organ system should be administered. Antibiotics should only be given when an extra-pancreatic infection is suspected or established. Prophylactic use of antibiotics in severe AP or in patients with sterile necrosis is not recommended [4].

(e) Nutrition

Traditionally, the concept of resting the pancreas in AP by avoiding enteral route has been floated. On the other hand, increased intestinal and colonic permeability due to disruption of gut mucosal barrier because of absence of food in the gut is thought to increase infectious complications in AP. In most patients with mild AP, oral feeding with soft low fat diet can be started as soon as nausea, vomiting, and pain have lessened and advanced as tolerated [4]. A recent trial showed that oral feeding initiated at 72 h with provision for nasoenteric feeding if oral route not tolerated was as effective as early nasoenteric feeding enteral feeding initiated within 24 h in preventing infectious complications in AP with high risk of complications [19]. Parenteral feeding should be avoided unless enteral route is not feasible or effective. Nasogastric and nasojejunal feeding appear to be comparable in tolerability and efficacy.

(f) Steps for prevention of recurrent episodes

In AP patients with gall stones, cholecystectomy is recommended within the index admission for mild AP and should be performed after active inflammation subsides and fluid collections resolve or stabilize in moderate or severe AP [4]. In patients with AP related to alcohol abuse, counseling and support for alcohol cessation should be offered.

(g) Management of local complications

Local complications can lead to lack of expected clinical improvement or even relapse of symptoms, especially pain, nausea, and failure of oral intake. No intervention is necessary for asymptomatic local complications including fluid collections, pseudocysts, or pancreatic necrosis regardless of size, location, or extension [4]. These patients can be safely followed.

Infected necrosis should be suspected after 7–10 days in patients with persistent organ failure or obvious sepsis or in patients who deteriorate after initial improvement.

A contrast enhanced CT should be obtained if not already performed to evaluate for presence of gas in the necrotic collection which can establish the diagnosis of infected necrosis. In the absence of CT features, either empiric approach with necrosis penetrating antibiotics (Ciprofloxacin, metronidazole, imipenem or piperacillin/tazobactam) or occasionally CT guided FNA sampling for gram stain and culture are appropriate [4]. Role of FNA is diminishing in recent years and either empiric antibiotics for suspected infection or intervention if there is no improvement seems to be more commonly used. Traditionally, infected necrosis was managed with surgical necrosectomy. However, recent studies demonstrated higher mortality in stable patients with infected necrosis treated surgically (~50 %) compared to minimally invasive methods of intervention (15–20 %) [11, 20, 21]. Prompt surgical debridement should only be performed in unstable patients with infected necrosis. In otherwise stable patients with infected necrosis, conservative approach is to administer antibiotics as noted above and closely monitor clinical status with a plan to perform minimally invasive necrosectomy (endoscopic, percutaneous, or surgical) after 4 weeks once the collection is walled off (WON) and the necrotic contents have liquefied (which otherwise is cement like and not amenable to minimally invasive debridement) [4, 20]. A subgroup of patients may be managed by antibiotics alone without needed minimally invasive debridement if on close follow-up, the patients continue to be asymptomatic. However, it is to be emphasized that patients with infected necrosis have a high mortality and therefore should be clinically monitored very closely [4, 11, 21].

If further improvements in morbidity and mortality were to be seen, a drug that can be used safely at presentation to prevent organ failure and necrosis is highly necessary. Pentoxifylline has been recently reported to have some effect in a small pilot study [22] and a large NIH funded study is currently in progress.

Conclusion

Acute Pancreatitis is an inflammatory disorder of the pancreas which can cause a severe disease with high mortality and morbidity. With advances in management, the outcomes of acute pancreatitis have improved considerably. Local complications and organ failure are important determinants of mortality. Patients can be classified into mild acute pancreatitis in the absence of local complications or organ failure and severe acute pancreatitis in the presence of persistent organ failure. The remainder with local complications and/or transient organ failure is classified into moderately severe acute pancreatitis. Aggressive management including hydration, feeding, and treatment of complications are crucial in acute pancreatitis.

References

1. Petrov MS, Shanbhag S, Chakraborty M, Phillips AR, Windsor JA. Organ failure and infection of pancreatic necrosis as determinants of mortality in patients with acute pancreatitis. Gastroenterology. 2010;139(3):813–20.
2. Yadav D, Lowenfels AB. The epidemiology of pancreatitis and pancreatic cancer. Gastroenterology. 2013;144(6):1252–61.
3. Peery AF, Dellon ES, Lund J, Crockett SD, McGowan CE, Bulsiewicz WJ, et al. Burden of gastrointestinal disease in the United States: 2012 update. Gastroenterology. 2012;143(5):1179–87 e1–3.
4. Tenner S, Baillie J, DeWitt J, Vege SS. American College of Gastroenterology guideline: management of acute pancreatitis. Am J Gastroenterol. 2013;108(9):1400–15. 16.
5. Lowenfels AB, Maisonneuve P, Sullivan T. The changing character of acute pancreatitis: epidemiology, etiology, and prognosis. Curr Gastroenterol Rep. 2009;11(2):97–103.
6. Lankisch PG, Apte M, Banks PA. Acute pancreatitis. Lancet. 2015;386(9988):85–96.
7. Mutinga M, Rosenbluth A, Tenner SM, Odze RR, Sica GT, Banks PA. Does mortality occur early or late in acute pancreatitis? Int J Pancreatol. 2000;28(2):91–5.

8. Renner IG, Savage 3rd WT, Pantoja JL, Renner VJ. Death due to acute pancreatitis. A retrospective analysis of 405 autopsy cases. Dig Dis Sci. 1985;30(10):1005–18.

9. McKay CJ, Buter A. Natural history of organ failure in acute pancreatitis. Pancreatology. 2003;3(2):111–4.

10. Gloor B, Muller CA, Worni M, Martignoni ME, Uhl W, Buchler MW. Late mortality in patients with severe acute pancreatitis. Br J Surg. 2001;88(7):975–9.

11. Mouli VP, Sreenivas V, Garg PK. Efficacy of conservative treatment, without necrosectomy, for infected pancreatic necrosis: a systematic review and meta-analysis. Gastroenterology. 2013;144(2):333–40. e2.

12. Banks PA, Bollen TL, Dervenis C, Gooszen HG, Johnson CD, Sarr MG, et al. Classification of acute pancreatitis--2012: revision of the Atlanta classification and definitions by international consensus. Gut. 2013;62(1):102–11.

13. Dellinger EP, Forsmark CE, Layer P, Levy P, Maravi-Poma E, Petrov MS, et al. Determinant-based classification of acute pancreatitis severity: an international multidisciplinary consultation. Ann Surg. 2012;256(6):875–80.

14. Choi JH, Kim MH, Oh D, Paik WH, Park do H, Lee SS, et al. Clinical relevance of the revised Atlanta classification focusing on severity stratification system. Pancreatology. 2014; 14(5):324–9.

15. Nawaz H, Mounzer R, Yadav D, Yabes JG, Slivka A, Whitcomb DC, et al. Revised Atlanta and determinant-based classification: application in a prospective cohort of acute pancreatitis patients. Am J Gastroenterol. 2013;108(12):1911–7.

16. Yadav D, O'Connell M, Papachristou GI. Natural history following the first attack of acute pancreatitis. Am J Gastroenterol. 2012;107(7):1096–103.

17. Spanier BW, Dijkgraaf MG, Bruno MJ. Epidemiology, aetiology and outcome of acute and chronic pancreatitis: an update. Best Pract Res Clin Gastroenterol. 2008;22(1):45–63.

18. Vege SS, Gardner TB, Chari ST, Munukuti P, Pearson RK, Clain JE, et al. Low mortality and high morbidity in severe acute pancreatitis without organ failure: a case for revising the Atlanta classification to include "moderately severe acute pancreatitis". Am J Gastroenterol. 2009;104(3):710–5.

19. Bakker OJ, van Brunschot S, van Santvoort HC, Besselink MG, Bollen TL, Boermeester MA, et al. Early versus on-demand nasoenteric tube feeding in acute pancreatitis. N Engl J Med. 2014;371(21):1983–93.

20. Freeman ML, Werner J, van Santvoort HC, Baron TH, Besselink MG, Windsor JA, et al. Interventions for necrotizing pancreatitis: summary of a multidisciplinary consensus conference. Pancreas. 2012;41(8):1176–94.
21. van Santvoort HC, Besselink MG, Bakker OJ, Hofker HS, Boermeester MA, Dejong CH, et al. A step-up approach or open necrosectomy for necrotizing pancreatitis. N Engl J Med. 2010;362(16):1491–502.
22. Vege SS, Atwal T, Bi Y, Chari ST, Clemens MA, Enders FT. Pentoxifylline treatment in severe acute pancreatitis: a pilot, double-blind, placebo-controlled, randomized trial. Gastroenterology. 2015;149(2):318–20. e3.

Chapter 3
Chronic Pancreatitis

Rupjyoti Talukdar and D. Nageshwar Reddy

Patient Questions

1. Will I get complete relief from pain?

   Chronic pancreatitis is a disease characterized by progressive inflammation that results in fibrosis of the pancreatic tissue culminating in exocrine and endocrine dysfunction. Pain results from pancreatic ductal obstruction by stones or stricture, and pancreatic neuropathy. Oxidative stress could also drive the intrapancreatic inflammation and thereby contribute to pain.

   Pain can be ameliorated by relieving the pancreatic duct of obstruction by endoscopic therapy. However, since the inflammation in CP is progressive, pain might recur.

R. Talukdar
Asian Institute of Gastroenterology, 6-3-661, Somajiguda, Hyderabad 500082, Telangana, India

Asian Healthcare Foundation, Hyderabad 500082, Telangana, India

D.N. Reddy (⊠)
Asian Institute of Gastroenterology, 6-3-661, Somajiguda, Hyderabad 500082, Telangana, India
e-mail: aigindia@yahoo.co.in

© Springer International Publishing Switzerland 2016
K. Dua, R. Shaker (eds.), *Pancreas and Biliary Disease*,
DOI 10.1007/978-3-319-28089-9_3

2. How can I prevent painful episodes?

Abstinence from alcohol and smoking can prevent recurrence of episodes of pain. Intake of antioxidant rich food and avoidance of fatty diet might help.

3. How long do I have to take medications?

There is no specific duration for therapy; and the treatment regimen needs to be individualized. Single modality therapy is unlikely to provide long term treatment. Antioxidants needs to be initiated early and should be taken at least for 6 months following which it may be titrated or stopped according to the clinical response. If pain relapses after endotherapy or surgery, the pain could be neuropathic predominant and should be treated with pregabalin (β-isobutyl-γ-aminobutyric acid).

Introduction

Chronic pancreatitis (CP) is characterized by recurrent abdominal pain, exocrine insufficiency, and endocrine dysfunction that results from progressive inflammation and fibrosis of the pancreas. CP does not have a definitive treatment and currently available treatments are directed toward management of complications.

Epidemiology and Etiology

The epidemiology and etiology of CP differ across the globe [1]. Its estimated incidence and prevalence in the USA are 4.05/100,000 and 41.76/100,000 population, respectively. Finland has the highest incidence among the European countries (13.4/100,000). While Japan has reported the prevalence of CP of 45/100,000 population, the prevalence of CP has increased from 3.08/100,000 to 13.52/100,000 between 1996 and 2003. CP is endemic in South India with a prevalence of 126/100,000 population as shown in population based studies in Kerala [2]. The distinctive characteristics of CP in these patients were collectively described as an entity called tropical chronic pancreatitis (TCP). CP is also prevalent in other parts of India and the phenotype currently seen all over the country (including South India) does not always match the one described as TCP, with only 3.8–5.8 % patients satisfying the criteria.

In the west CP is associated primarily with alcohol, though its role as a distinct etiological factor is currently questioned. Even though smoking was earlier considered as a cofactor with alcohol in the pathogenesis of CP, recent population based studies have demonstrated smoking as an independent risk factor [3]. Among the Asia-Pacific countries, alcohol is the etiology in 95 % of CP in Australia, 70 % in the Republic of Korea and 54 % in Japan. In India and China, on the other hand, over 70 % of patients with CP have idiopathic chronic pancreatitis [4]. Oxidative stress and genetic mutations are the predominant factors that have emerged as the risk factors in patients with idiopathic CP in India.

Median survival for alcohol related CP was 20–24 years in an earlier European study but more recently it was found to be 15.5 years from all cause CP. A study form India reported an 83 % probability of surviving for 35 years after the onset of CP [5].

Natural History and Clinical Manifestations

CP is believed to develop after a series acute pancreatic injury at the acinar (trypsinogen activation) or ductal (improper bicarbonate secretion) level. This is the Sentinel Acute Pancreatitis Event (SAPE) hypothesis; and the first or subsequent acute episode may not necessarily be clinically detectable. The clinical course of CP is very variable and can be arbitrarily divided into early (first 5 years), intermediate (5–10 years), and late stages (beyond 10 years), though there can be significant overlap between the three. Recurrent acute pain (with acute pancreatitis) marks the early phase while development of morphological changes such as pancreatic calculi, ductal strictures, and pseudocysts are predominantly seen in the intermediate phase. Pancreatic exocrine insufficiency (PEI) and diabetes manifest by the late stage, although these begins to develop earlier [6].

Abdominal pain is the dominant clinical manifestation. A small proportion of patients with CP may run a painless course. Even though it appears that with gross parenchymal destruction the pain would decrease or even disappear, this appears unlikely and pain could progress even after pancreatic atrophy. Analgesic requirement in up to 40 % of patients even after total pancreatectomy is a testimony to this [7]. Patients who have early onset CP (onset <35 years of age) appear to have a longer duration of pain. With recent understanding of the mechanisms of pain in CP, it would be important to identify neuropathic pain since this could have therapeutic implications. Even though there are currently no specific clinical tools to confirm neuropathy, the pain DETECT questionnaire (available in the internet) is a semiquantitative tool that could suggest the development of neuropathic pain.

Clinical manifestations of PEI appear after the post-prandial output of pancreatic exocrine secretion into the duodenum falls to below 10 % of normal. This can occur either after development of gross pancreatic atrophy or obstructing ductal calculi in the head region. However, since CP is a progressive condition, subclinical PEI sets in much earlier. Steatorrhea is the most conspicuous manifestation of PEI. Other manifestations could be progressive weight loss and deficiency of fat soluble vitamins and micronutrients.

Diabetes secondary to CP is now termed as Type 3c diabetes. Western data show that diabetes in CP usually occurs 10 years after the onset of disease. However, clinical observations and experimental studies suggest that beta-cell dysfunction and diabetes develop much earlier in India, occasionally with diabetes preceding the diagnosis of CP [8].

Diarrhea in patients with CP could result from fat malabsorption, diabetic autonomic neuropathy, small intestinal bacterial overgrowth, and CP associated intestinal dysmotility.

Pathogenesis

Genetics of Chronic Pancreatitis

Foremost among the genetic mutations and polymorphisms recognized in CP are the cationic trypsinogen gene (PRSS1), pancreatic secretory trypsin inhibitor gene (SPINK1) and cystic fibrosis transmembrane conductance regulator gene (CFTR). Studies have demonstrated chymotrypsinogen C (CTRC), cathepsin B (CTSB), calcium-sensing receptor (CaSR), and carboxypeptidase 1 (CPA1) also to be associated with the disease [9]. Recently, genome wide association studies (GWAS) have demonstrated a strong association of the polymorphisms in the claudin 2 and PRSS1-PRSS2 genes with alcoholic recurrent acute and chronic pancreatitis [9–11]. The mechanisms by which genetic polymorphisms could result in CP are varied and involve intraacinar and intraductal mechanisms based on the genetic polymorphism that is operating.

Fibrosis

Progressive fibrosis, which is the pathological hallmark of CP is primarily mediated by the pancreatic stellate cell (PSC) [12]. PSCs are cells that reside in the pancreas surrounding the basolateral surfaces of the pancreatic acini and constitute about 10 % of all resident cells in the pancreas. In the healthy state, PSCs remain in a quiescent state, maintain the pancreatic extracellular matrix, and contribute to physiological exocrine secretion from the pancreas via a cholecystokinin mediated mechanism. After exposure to oxidative stresses (cigarette smoking and alcohol metabolites), and after recurrent acinar injuries, the PSCs transform into an activated phenotype that secrete a wide array of cytokines which are capable of triggering an inflammatory cascade. The cytokine that primarily drives fibrosis is TGF-beta. As a result of the paracrine and autocrine activation, activated PSCs lay down excess amounts of collagen I in the extracellular matrix thereby resulting in the imbalance between the matrix deposition and degradation towards a pro-fibrogenic state.

Pain

Pain is the most debilitating clinical manifestation of CP. An important pain mechanism that has emerged from recent clinical and experimental studies is oxidative stress and inflammation induced pancreatic nociception and neuro-immune alterations [13]. Experimental evidence supports that PSCs can generate oxidative stress in response to pressure. This observation makes it plausible that pancreatic ductal/interstitial hypertension from obstructing stones and/or strictures could activate PSCs and result in a pro-inflammatory milieu within the pancreas.

Studies have shown that nociceptors (pain receptors) such as the proteinase-activated receptor 2 (PAR-2), the transient receptor potential vanilloid 1 (TRPV-1) receptors and the ligand-gated cation channel transient receptor potential ankyrin 1 (TRPA-1) are expressed in the pancreas specific sensory nerves and dorsal root ganglia. Trypsin and mast cell tryptase (that is known to be secreted in the pancreas in CP) can bind to and activate these receptors. Other receptors that are also shown to be expressed on different neural components include trkA, P75, and GFRα3. These receptors are activated by their ligands, namely nerve growth factor (NGF), brain derived neurotropic factor (BDNF), and artimin, respectively. In addition, several neuroimmune alterations have been described in CP. Predominant among these includes: infiltration of inflammatory cells (especially mast cells and eosinophils); neural edema and perineural disruption; Schwann cell (glial cell in peripheral nerves) proliferation; neural hypertrophy and sprouting and expression of nestin and growth-associated protein (GAP43), which are indicators of neuroplasticity. Several factors namely, glutamine, calcitonin gene related polypeptide (CGRP), substance P, and fractalkine (a neural cytokine) have been implicated in the causation of the neural infiltration. The persistent inflammation and neuroplastic changes in the pancreatic nerves leading to continuous depolarization of these nerves result in a state of spinal hypersensitivity, a phenomenon known as global sensitization. These result in mechanical allodynia, i.e., generation of pain after a physiological or non-noxious stimulus, and inflammatory hyperalgesia, meaning amplified pain response to normal or minimal pain stimuli. Eventually, these events bring about a change in the entire cortical pain modulating neural network in the brain [14]. These events could explain why patients with long standing CP could develop pain even after total pancreatectomy.

Diabetes

Even though diabetes secondary to CP (Type 3C DM) has long been ascribed to pancreatic parenchymal fibrosis and islet destruction, recent experimental studies have demonstrated that beta cell dysfunction is noticed in patients with CP even in the absence of significant beta cell death (apoptosis). The beta cells do not secrete insulin in response to glucose challenge. This lack of response appears to be mediated by the inflammatory milieu contributed by PSCs and T-helper subsets that infiltrate into the islets [15]. Observations from these studies have important implications in that if the inflammatory milieu can be altered, the functional capacity of the islets could possibly be revived.

Diagnosis

Diagnosis of CP includes evaluation of the morphologic and functional (exocrine and endocrine) alterations. Transabdominal ultrasonography (USG) can show pancreatic atrophy and a dilated pancreatic duct. Contrast enhanced computed tomography (CECT) scan of the abdomen provides reliable evidence of the pancreatic parenchymal volume, localization of pancreatic stones and calcifications, complications such as pseudocyst, and presence of a cancer. MRI/MRCP is helpful in identifying altered ductal anatomy such as dilatation, strictures, leaks, and communication between the pancreatic duct and pseudocysts. In addition, it has the advantage of avoidance of radiation exposure. The above tests are however, not sensitive enough to detect very early changes of CP, in which case endoscopic ultrasonography (EUS) plays an important role. EUS is an operator dependent procedure which requires expertise and experience. With increasing experience it is becoming apparent though that EUS has the tendency to over diagnose early CP. Endoscopic retrograde cholangiopancreatography (ERCP) is seldom used as a diagnostic tool.

Pancreatic function tests (direct and indirect) can be used to assess secretory function of the pancreas. The direct function tests are used to access pancreatic bicarbonate or exocrine enzyme secretion in response to secretin and cholecystokinin stimulation respectively. Pancreatic secretions are collected through specialized tubes (e.g., Dreiling tube), through a conventional upper GI endoscope or directly from the pancreatic duct after cannulation. Even though the sensitivity and specificity of these tests reach over 80 %, they are invasive, technically challenging, time consuming, expensive, and not available widely. Furthermore, the capability of these tests to diagnose early CP is not clear. The secretin-MRCP test is another direct function test that has the advantage of evaluating the function and structure of the pancreas simultaneously. Indirect pancreatic function tests include 72 h fecal fat estimation, fecal elastase test and the ^{13}C mixed triglyceride test. Of these, the ^{13}C mixed triglyceride test has the best diagnostic capability, but requires a mass spectroscopy technique that may not be universally available. Elastase is a pancreatic exocrine enzyme that is biologically stable throughout the intestinal transit and its level in stool accurately reflects the amount secreted by the pancreas. The sensitivity of this test to detect mild and severe disease ranges from 0 to 47 % and 73 to 100 %, respectively [16]. The advantage of this test is that the currently available exogenous pancreatic enzyme supplementation does not affect the results since human monoclonal antibody is used for detection, while the supplemented enzymes are from procine source. Presence of diarrhea might however, result in a falsely low fecal elastase concentration.

Evaluation of Type 3c diabetes should begin with testing for fasting blood glucose and HbA1c. Presence of glutamic acid decarboxylase (GAD) antibodies and hyperinsulinemia can distinguish Type 3c diabetes from Type 1 and Type 2 diabetes respectively. In the presence of ambiguity, an absent polypeptide secretory response after insulin induced hypoglycemia or secretin infusion provides a diagnosis of Type 3c diabetes [17]. Plasma C-peptide levels during an oral glucose tolerance or mixed-nutrient meal testing can ascertain functional beta cell reserve.

Treatment

Goals of treatment for CP include pain relief, pancreatic enzyme replacement, nutritional support, and glycemic control. Abstinence from alcohol and smoking is essential and these patients require constant counselling.

Treatment of Pain

Causes of pain in CP includes: the disease process itself; and complications such as pancreatic pseudocyst, duodenal/biliary obstruction, and pancreatic cancer. It is therefore important to assess the disease morphology prior to initiation of treatment. Several options including medical, endoscopic, and surgical are currently available for pain management.

Medical management: In the setting of acute pain, the WHO pain ladder may be followed beginning with a nonsteroidal anti-inflammatory drug (NSAID). Low potency selective μ-opiate receptor agonist such as tramadol hydrochloride has been shown to be as effective as higher potency narcotics but with a significantly better safety profile. High potency narcotics such as morphine and analogues should be avoided [13].

Currently, there is ample evidence to show a significant reduction of antioxidant defense mechanisms in patients with CP. Therefore, supplementation of antioxidants can be tried for pain management [18]. The primary aim of antioxidant therapy in CP is to supply methyl and thiol moieties for the intra-acinar transulfuration pathway which is essential for protection against oxidative stress. Even though the efficacy of antioxidants in CP has been debatable, two recently published meta-analyses have shown that an antioxidant combination containing organic selenium, ascorbic acid, β-carotene, α-tocopherol, and methionine is effective in improving pain. All the components are required at a higher dose and the most important among them appears to be methionine at a dose of 2–4 g daily [19, 20].

Since there is a neuropathic component to the pain in longstanding CP, neural modulators could have an important role in pain management. Of the several neuromodulators that have been used in clinical practice, only pregabalin has been tested in a randomized controlled setting. An increasing dose from 150 mg to 600 mg per day of pregabalin demonstrated significant reduction in pain in patients with CP when treated for 3 weeks [21]. However, a significantly higher proportion of patients receiving pregabalin experienced adverse events compared with placebo.

A recently completed double blinded placebo controlled RCT demonstrated that a combination of methionine containing antioxidants and pregabalin resulted in a significant reduction of pain in patients with CP who had recurrence of pain after ductal clearance with endotherapy or drainage surgery [22]. Pain recurrence after clearance of ductal obstruction is difficult to treat, and this combination appears to be a viable treatment option for this group of patients.

Pancreatic enzyme supplementation is often used for pain in CP in clinical practice. This is based on the premise that proteins in the food chyme bind to duodenal CCK receptors that results in pancreatic enzyme secretion, which could eventually result in ductal hypertension and pain; and that the protease in the supplemented enzyme cause a negative feedback loop by binding to the CCK receptors. However, a recent systematic review of RCTs showed that pancreatic enzymes did not confer any analgesic benefit. Interestingly, significant pain relief was observed in the individual studies that used non-enteric coated enzyme preparation, thus implying that the binding of non-enteric preparations with CCK receptors is better [23]. However, all the currently available pancreatic enzyme preparations, except Viokase, are enteric coated and are unlikely to be beneficial for pain.

Endoscopic management: Endoscopic management in CP is indicated for obstructing ductal stones, pancreatic and biliary strictures, pseudocyst drainage, and celiac block [24]. Extracorporeal shock wave lithotripsy (ESWL) with or without endoscopic retrograde cholangiopancreatograpgy (ERCP) and stenting is currently the recommended standard of care for the treatment of large obstructive pancreatic ductal stones, especially those located in the head and body region. The primary goal of ESWL is to reduce the stones to fragments below 3 mm size. Best results with ESWL are obtained with the third generation lithotriptors with dual focusing system (fluoroscopy with ultrasonography). Fragmented stones can be removed at ERCP by flushing or using accessories such as baskets and balloons. In a study by Tandan et al. [25] on a cohort of 636 patients, complete pain relief was observed in 68.7 % of patients on intermediate follow-up (2–5 years) and in 60.3 % on long-term follow-up (>5 years) after ESWL. Patients were followed for as long as 96 months. Stone clearance was complete in 77.5 % and 76 % in the intermediate and long-term follow-up groups respectively. Interestingly, 50 % of patients who had recurrence of pain did not have recurrence of stones, implying that a majority of pain recurrences is related to mechanism such as pancreatic neuropathy. In another retrospective study of 120 patients by Seven et al. [26] complete pain relief was observed in 50 % patients, along with a significant improvement in quality of life scores (VAS) [7.3 (2.7) vs. 3.7 (2.4); $p < 0.001$). The longest follow-up duration in this study was 7 years, and 85 % patients had pain relief pain after the mean follow-up of 4.3 years. In another study, injection of IV secretin (16 mcg) before the procedure resulted in a better stone clearance (63 % vs. 46 %; $p = 0.021$), possibly by release of pancreatic ductal secretion that results in a fluid-stone interface [27]. On multiple logistic regression analysis, secretin use and pre-ESWL pancreatic stenting emerged as independent predictors of complete or near complete stone clearance.

Symptomatic pancreatic ductal strictures, especially the ones located in the head of the pancreas are best treated with a single 10Fr polyethylene stent with planned stent exchanges within 1 year even in the absence of symptoms [28]. Many of the dominant strictures require prior dilatation with bougies, balloons, or a Soehendra stent retriever. Pancreatic stenting was technically successful in 85–98 % cases [29–32] and was associated with immediate pain relief in 65–95 % patients that was sustained in 32–68 % of patients on follow-up of up to 14–58 months [29–34]. Even though there is no consensus on the definition of long-term clinical success, absence of pain at 1 year after stent retrieval may be considered as clinical success [29]. Cessation of further stenting during ERCP can be assessed by demonstrating adequate pancreatico-duodenal flow of contrast medium within 1–2 min after filling the pancreatic duct upstream to the stricture and/or easy passage of a 6 Fr catheter through the stricture. Since pancreatic stents run the risk of clogging and migration, several modifications in the shapes and types of stents (multiple plastic and covered expandable metallic stents) are being studied; unfortunately none has been established as a standard of care. Pancreatic duct strictures that persist despite 12 months of single plastic stenting can be treated with multiple plastic stents placed side-by-side simultaneously [35]. Even though excellent technical (100 %) and functional (97.4 %) success could be achieved, stent migration may be seen in 10.5 % patients while 15.8 % patient may require reinterventions. Technical success in placing covered self-expanding metal stents (SEMS) can be as high as 100 % with 80 % functional success in relieving pain on short-term follow-up [36]. Stent migration and reintervention may be required in 8.2 % and 9.8 % patients respectively. Currently, use of SEMS is recommended only under clinical trial settings. Multiple strictures and those located upstream towards the tail are difficult to manage endoscopically. These strictures are best treated with surgery in the presence of symptoms. It is important to be vigilant on the possibility of a cancer in the presence of stricture/s in the background of CP. Pancreatic ductal stenting is also indicated in the treatment of pancreatic duct leaks. However, complete ductal disruption might require pancreatic resection.

Symptomatic pancreatic pseudocyst can be treated endoscopically by transpapillary or transmural (cystogastrostomy and cystojejunostomy) drainage. With linear echoendoscope, drainage is now possible even for pseudocysts that do not produce a bulge in the stomach or the duodenum, and also for those located away from the gastrointestinal lumen. Biliary stricture in CP results from pancreatic fibrosis, pancreatic edema and compression by a pseudocyst. It is important to rule out malignancy as a cause. Biliary strictures require treatment if the patients have evidence of cholestatic symptoms and/or cholangitis or if there is elevation of serum alkaline phosphatase by twofold for more for more than a month. These strictures are usually treated with single or multiple plastic biliary stents that are exchanged every 3 months for a total of 1 year. The long-term results of using a single 10 Fr plastic stent are poor (25 % sustained benefit after 46 months follow-up) [37]. Presence of pancreatic calcification is one of the major factors responsible for long-term failure of single plastic stents [38]. In order to circumvent the poor long-term outcome of placement of single plastic stent, multiple plastic stents can be placed side-by-side for 1-year with scheduled exchanges every three months [29]. Scheduled exchanges are important in order to prevent cholangitis from stent clogging [39]. Successful long-term treatment with placement of multiple simultaneous stents has been shown to be 92 % compared to 24 % with single stent for similar follow-up durations [40]. FCSEMS has also been attempted for biliary strictures, but the current data is not robust enough to incorporate this modality into the routine treatment.

Blocking the celiac plexus is considered as one of the treatment modalities of intractable pain in CP. Celiac plexus block can be achieved with a local anesthetic agent (bupivacaine) with or without steroid (triamcinolone). EUS-guided or percutaneous approaches can be used. However, the overall benefits of celiac plexus block in CP are about 55 % after 4–8 weeks that falls to 10 % by 24 weeks.

Surgical management: Surgical options for pain management in CP include drainage procedures (lateral pancreaticojejunostomy and Frey's procedure), classical (Kausch Whipple) or pylorus preserving (Traverso–Longmire) pancreaticoduodenectomy, distal pancreatectomy, and total pancreatectomy [13]. Pancreaticoduodenectomy is particularly useful in pain with an associated inflammatory mass in the head of the pancreas, especially if a pancreas cancer cannot be excluded in the background of CP. A significant proportion of patients who undergo resection procedures develop exocrine and endocrine insufficiencies. Total pancreatectomy with auto islet-cell transplantation (TPIAT) is being practised in select centers for patients with intractable pain [7, 41]. However, even after removing the entire pancreas, 30–40 % of patients may still experience pain [7]. A lateral pancreaticojejunostomy could be beneficial for painful pancreatic ductal stone located throughout the pancreatic duct.

Treatment of Pancreatic Exocrine Insufficiency (PEI)

The mainstay of treatment for PEI in CP is pancreatic enzyme replacement therapy (PERT) which entails supplementation of lipase, protease, and amylase. Of these three, lipase supplementation is the most important component. To avoid proteolytic digestion, lipase should be administered in enteric coated form. It is important that the pancreatic enzyme supplements are delivered into the duodenum along with the chyme from the antrum. This can be achieved if the enzyme preparations are loaded into pellets of 2 mm or less in size (microsphere and mini microsphere). Pancreas secretes around 600,000 units of lipase daily and 10 % of this is required for fat digestion [42]. Therefore, the minimum daily requirement of lipase in CP is at least 60,000 units. The approximate dose requirement can be calculated on the basis of fat content of the meal; and an ideal beginning daily dose of 40,000 units of lipase or higher should be sufficient. Starting with a higher dose is important because of bile acid denaturation and high proteolytic activity of proteases on the supplemented lipase. The enzyme doses can be titrated thereafter based on the response and fat content in the diet. Since it is important for the supplemented enzymes to mix well with the food chyme for optimal action, pancreatic enzymes should be taken along with meal. Furthermore, it is advisable to co-prescribe a proton pump inhibitor (PPI) so that the supplemented enzymes get an additional protection from acid degradation besides the enteric coating [43]. The benefit of PERT in patients without clear evidence of exocrine insufficiency is not known. Even though substantial emphasis is given on pain management and PERT in clinical practice, nutritional advice and counselling are frequently overlooked. It is important to realize that any enzyme requires a substrate to exert optimal action. Hence, it is not essential to restrict the patient to an unpalatable fat free diet. Therefore, patients on PERT should take normal amount of dietary fat. In the absence of expected improvement of the nutritional status after PERT, it is important to evaluate for other factors such as noncompliance, high fat content in diet, high duodenal acidity, and small intestinal bacterial overgrowth.

Nutritional Support

A thorough nutritional assessment is essential. Dietary supplements should include antioxidants containing food, multivitamins and diets with high complex carbohydrates. Deep frying of food depletes the naturally occurring antioxidants, and therefore, these kinds of food should be avoided [44]. Medium chain triglycerides (MCT) containing diets have an unpalatable taste and might be a cause for noncompliance to dietary advice and are not routinely recommended. Furthermore, a recent randomized controlled trial has shown that good dietary counselling on homemade food could be as good as commercially available MCT containing diet in improving nutritional status in documented malnourished patients with CP [45]. Food with high dietary fibers could interfere with the action of pancreatic enzymes and should be avoided in patients on pancreatic enzyme replacement therapy [46].

Conclusion and Future Directions

CP is a complex illness and does not have definitive cure so far. Pain is the most common clinical symptom that mandates aggressive treatment. It is essential to assess the disease morphology adequately and rule out an underlying cancer especially in the elderly patient with long standing disease. Presence of obstructive ductal calculi or a major stricture should be managed with endotherapy as the first line. The right preparation of antioxidant formulation at the optimal dose and neuromodulators (e.g., pregabalin) can offer significant pain relief. PERT should include at least 20,000 units or higher of lipase and should be taken along with each meals and the dose titrated according to response. Nutritional assessment and supplementation is mandatory. Finally, continuous counselling, reassurance, and advice to abstain from smoking and consuming alcohol are of paramount importance.

Further research needs to be conducted on the genotype–phenotype associations of the disease and pain mechanisms at the molecular level so that effective personalized prognostication and pain management tools can be developed.

References

1. Garg PK. Chronic pancreatitis in India and Asia. Curr Gastroenterol Rep. 2012;14:118–24.
2. Tandon RK, Sato N, Garg PK. Chronic pancreatitis: Asia pacific Consensus report. J Gastroenterol Hepatol. 2002;17:508–18.
3. Yadav D, Lowenfels AB. The epidemiology of pancreatitis and pancreatic cancer. Gastroenterology. 2013;144:1252–61.
4. Garg PK, Tandon RK. Survey on chronic pancreatitis in the Asia Pacific region. J Gastroenterol Hepatol. 2004;19:998–1004.
5. Midha S, Khajuria R, Shastri S, Kabra M, Garg PK. Chronic pancreatitis in India: Phenotypic characterization and strong genetic susceptibility due to SPINK1 and CFTR gene mutation. Gut. 2010;59:800–7.
6. Lévy P, Domínguez-Muñoz E, Imrie C, Löhr M, Maisonneuve P. Epidemiology of chronic pancreatitis: burden of the disease and consequences. United European Gastroenterol J. 2014;2:345–54.
7. Sutherland DE, Radosevich DM, Bellin MD, Hering BJ, Beilman GJ, Dunn TB, et al. Total pancreatectomy and islet autotransplantation for chronic pancreatitis. J Am Coll Surg. 2012;214:409–24.
8. Talukdar R, Rao GV, Reddy DN. Risk factors for development of secondary diabetes in chronic pancreatitis and impact of ductal decompression. Pancreatology. 2013;13:S27.
9. Avanthi SU, Ravi Kanth VV, Agarwal J, Lakhtakia S, Gangineni K, Rao GV, et al. Association of Claudin2 and PRSS1-PRSS2 polymorphisms with idiopathic recurrent acute and chronic pancreatitis: a case-control study from India. J Gastroenterol Hepatol. 2015;30(12):1796–801. doi:10.1111/jgh.13029.
10. Whitcomb DC, LaRusch J, Krasinskas AM, Klei L, Smith JP, Brand RE, et al. Common genetic variants in the CLDN2 and PRSS1-PRSS2 loci alter risk for alcohol-related and sporadic pancreatitis. Nat Genet. 2012;44:1349–54.
11. Derikx MH, Kovacs P, Scholz M, Masson E, Chen JM, Ruffert C, et al. Polymorphisms at PRSS1-PRSS2 and CLDN2-MORC4

loci associate with alcoholic and non-alcoholic chronic pancreatitis in a European replication study. Gut. 2015;64(9):1426–33. doi:10.1136/gutjnl-2014-307453.

12. Talukdar R, Tandon RK. Pancreatic stellate cells: a new target in the treatment of chronic pancreatitis. J Gastroenterol Hepatol. 2008;23:34–40.

13. Talukdar R, Reddy DN. Pain management in chronic pancreatitis: beyond the pancreatic duct. World J Gastroenterol. 2013;19:6319–28.

14. Dimcevski G, Sami SA, Funch-Jensen P, Le Pera D, Valeriani M, Arendt-Nielsen L, et al. Pain in chronic pancreatitis: the role of reorganization in the central nervous system. Gastroenterology. 2007;132:1546–56.

15. Talukdar R, Sasikala M, Pavan Kumar P, Rao GV, Rabella P, Reddy DN. T-helper cell mediated islet inflammation contributes to β-cell dysfunction in chronic pancreatitis. Pancreas. 2016;45(3):434–42.

16. Lankisch PG, Schmidt I. Fecal elastase 1 is not the indirect pancreatic function test we have been waiting for. Dig Dis Sci. 2000;45:166–7.

17. Rickels MR, Bellin M, Toledo FG, Robertson RP, Andersen DK, Chari ST, et al. Detection, evaluation and treatment of diabetes mellitus in chronic pancreatitis: recommendations from PancreasFest 2012. Pancreatology. 2013;13:336–42.

18. Tandon RK, Garg PK. Oxidative stress in chronic pancreatitis: pathophysiological relevance and management. Antioxid Redox Signal. 2011;15:2757–66.

19. Cai GH, Huang J, Zhao Y, Chen J, Wu HH, Dong YL, et al. Antioxidant therapy for pain relief in patients with chronic pancreatitis: systematic review and meta-analysis. Pain Physician. 2013;16:521–32.

20. Talukdar R, Murthy HVV, Reddy DN. Role of methionine containing antioxidants in pain management in chronic pancreatitis: a systematic review and meta-analysis. Pancreatology. 2015;15:136–44.

21. Olesen SS, Bouwense SA, Wilder-Smith OH, van Goor H, Drewes AM. Pregabalin reduces pain in patients with chronic pancreatitis in a randomized, controlled trial. Gastroenterology. 2011;141:536–43.

22. Talukdar R, Lakhtakia S, Pradeep R, Rao GV, Reddy DN. Combination of antioxidant cocktail and pregabalin in the management of pain in chronic pancreatitis after ductal clearance:

A randomized, double-blinded, placebo-controlled trial. Clin Gastroenterol Hepatol. 2015;13:1386.

23. Shafiq N, Rana S, Bhasin D, Pandhi P, Srivastava P, Sehmby SS, et al. Pancreatic enzymes for chronic pancreatitis. Cochrane Database Syst Rev. 2009;4, CD006302.

24. Talukdar R, Nageshwar RD. Endoscopic therapy for chronic pancreatitis. Curr Opin Gastroenterol. 2014;30:484–9.

25. Tandan M, Reddy DN, Talukdar R, Vinod K, Santosh D, Lakhtakia S, et al. Long-term clinical outcomes of extracorporeal shockwave lithotripsy in painful chronic calcific pancreatitis. Gastrointest Endosc. 2013;78:726–33.

26. Seven G, Schreiner MA, Ross AS, Lin OS, Gluck M, Gan SI, et al. Long-term outcomes associated with pancreatic extracorporeal shock wave lithotripsy for chronic calcific pancreatitis. Gastrointest Endosc. 2012;75:997–1004.

27. Choi EK, McHenry L, Watkins JL, Sherman S, Fogel EL, Coté GA, et al. Use of intravenous secretin during extracorporeal shock wave lithotripsy to facilitate endoscopic clearance of pancreatic duct stones. Pancreatology. 2012;12:272–5.

28. Tandan M, Nageshwar RD. Endotherapy in chronic pancreatitis. World J Gastroenterol. 2013;19:6156–64.

29. Dumonceau JM, Delhaye M, Tringali A, Dominguez-Munoz JE, Poley JW, Arvanitaki M, et al. Endoscopic treatment of chronic pancreatitis: European Society of Gastrointestinal Endoscopy (ESGE) Clinical Guideline. Endoscopy. 2012;44:784–800.

30. Cremer M, Deviere J, Delahaye M, Baize M, Vandermeeren A. Stenting in severe chronic pancreatitis: results in medium-term follow up in seventy six patients. Endoscopy. 1991;23:171–6.

31. Ponchon T, Bory RM, Hedelius F, Roubein LD, Paliard P, Napoleon B, et al. Endoscopic stenting for pain relief in chronic pancreatitis: results of a standardized protocol. Gastrointest Endosc. 1995;42:452–6.

32. Weber A, Schneider J, Neu B, Meining A, Born P, Schmid RM, et al. Endoscopic stents for patients with chronic pancreatitis: results from a prospective follow-up study. Pancreas. 2007;34:287–94.

33. Farnbacher MJ, Muhldorfer S, Wehler M, Fischer B, Hahn EG, Schneider HT. Interventional endoscopic therapy in chronic pancreatitis in chronic pancreatitis including temporary stenting: a definitive treatment? Scand J Gastroenterol. 2006;41:111–7.

34. Binmoeller KF, Jue P, Seifert H, Nam WC, Izbicki J, Soehendra N. Endoscopic stent drainage in chronic pancreatitis and a dominant stricture: long-term results. Endoscopy. 1995;27:638–44.

35. Moon SH, Kim MH, Park do H, Song TJ, Eum J, Lee SS, et al. Modified fully-covered self-expandable metal stents with anti migration features for benign pancreatic duct strictures in advanced chronic pancreatitis, with a focus on safety profile and reducing migration. Gastrointest Endosc. 2010;72:86–91.
36. Shen Y, Liu M, Chen M, Li Y, Lu Y, Zou X. Covered metal stent or multiple plastic stents for refractory pancreatic ductal strictures in chronic pancreatitis: A systematic review. Pancreatology. 2014;14:87–90.
37. Barthet M, Bernard JP, Duval JL, Affriat C, Sahel J. Biliary stenting in benign biliary stenosis complicating chronic calcifying pancreatitis. Endoscopy. 1994;26:569–72.
38. Kahl S, Zimmermann S, Genz I, Glasbrenner B, Pross M, Schulz HU, et al. Risk factors for failure of endoscopic stenting of biliary strictures in chronic pancreatitis: a prospective follow-up study. Am J Gastroenterol. 2003;98:2448–53.
39. Pozsar J, Sahin P, Laszlo F, Forró G, Topa L. Medium-term results of endoscopic treatment of common bile duct strictures in chronic calcifying pancreatitis with increasing number of stents. J Clin Gastroenterol. 2004;38:118–23.
40. Catalano MF, Linder JD, George S, Alcocer E, Geenen JE. Treatment of symptomatic distal common bile duct stenosis secondary to chronic pancreatitis: comparison of single vs. multiple simultaneous stents. Gastrointest Endosc. 2004;60:945–52.
41. Robertson RP. Total pancreatectomy and islet autotransplantation for chronic pancreatitis: breaking down barriers. J Clin Endocrinol Metab. 2015;100(5):1762–3. doi:10.1210/jc.2015-1876.
42. Layer P, Keller J. Lipase supplementation therapy: standards, alternatives, and perspectives. Pancreas. 2003;26:1–7.
43. Sarner M. Treatment of pancreatic exocrine deficiency. World J Surg. 2003;27:1192–5.
44. Braganza JM. A framework for the aetiogenesis of chronic pancreatitis. Digestion. 1998;59 Suppl 4:1–12.
45. Singh S, Midha S, Singh N, Joshi YK, Garg PK. Dietary counseling versus dietary supplements for malnutrition in chronic pancreatitis: a randomized controlled trial. Clin Gastroenterol Hepatol. 2008;6:353–9.
46. Dunaif G, Schneeman BO. The effect of dietary fiber on human pancreatic enzyme activity in vitro. Am J Clin Nutr. 1981;34:1034–5.

Chapter 4
Recurrent Acute Pancreatitis

Venkata N. Muddana and Nalini M. Guda

Patient Questions

What should I do? Should I go for surgery or Endoscopic treatments or should I wait and watch? Are there any specific treatments?

The diagnosis of recurrent acute pancreatitis should be made carefully. One should have significant abdominal pain and should have either pancreatic enzymes that are at least three times above the normal limit or should have at least a CT scan showing changes of pancreatitis. Most (80 %) of the times a diagnosis can be established and is usually related to either gall stones (large) or very minute sand like stones, alcohol use, elevated triglycerides, certain congenital abnormalities and/or medications. All offending agents should be eliminated. For obvious stone disease, gall bladder surgery is warranted. Surgery for presumed small stones is not unreasonable and may prevent future attacks. Though genetic abnormalities and

V.N. Muddana, M.D.
Aurora St. Luke's Medical Center, Milwaukee, WI, USA

N.M. Guda, M.D., F.A.S.G.E., A.G.A.F. (⊠)
Aurora St. Luke's Medical Center, Milwaukee, WI, USA
University of Wisconsin School of Medicine and Public Health, Madison, WI, USA
e-mail: nguda@wisc.edu

© Springer International Publishing Switzerland 2016
K. Dua, R. Shaker (eds.), *Pancreas and Biliary Disease,*
DOI 10.1007/978-3-319-28089-9_4

environmental influences play a significant role there are no specific interventions available and testing is limited. Endoscopic therapies have a role in certain conditions and should be done only after careful evaluation at an expert facility. Certain congenital abnormalities such as pancreas divisum could cause recurrent attacks of pancreatitis. Endoscopic treatment may or may not prevent future attacks and again this should be done at an "expert" center. One must avoid smoking as this can lead to progressive gland injury and scarring leading to chronic pancreatitis. Every acute episode should be evaluated and supportive care provided.

Introduction

Acute pancreatitis (AP) can be associated with significant morbidity and mortality. The annual incidence is on the rise [1]. AP is an acute inflammatory process of pancreas that frequently involves peripancreatic tissue and remote organ systems. AP has many causes of which alcohol abuse and Gallstones account for 70 %. The exact mechanisms by which these factors initiate AP are unclear. Genetic and environmental factors seem to play a role in the onset, severity, and outcome of the pancreatic disease [2]. If not corrected, any factor responsible for pancreatitis is capable of producing recurrent attacks of AP, and hence it is important to carefully evaluate the patient and address the underlying issue [3]. Because of the significant interplay between the known risk factors, patient's genetic factors, and the environmental factors, elimination or modification of one of these risk factors does not necessarily result in elimination of future risk. Due to the complex interplay between these factors, establishment of the etiology of AP often requires expensive and sometimes invasive evaluation, some of which entails risk for significant complications, including further pancreatitis [4].

Exact incidence of recurrent acute pancreatitis (RAP) is difficult to estimate due to variation in geographic location, etiologies, and evaluation approach used. Prevalence in various retrospective studies varies from 10 to 30 % [5–7]. In one study evaluating the natural history after the first attack of acute pancreatitis, recurrent attacks were seen in up to 16.5 % of the patients at a mean follow up of 7.8 years [8].

Recent evidence suggests that a continuum exists between RAP and chronic pancreatitis (CP) [9–11]. Ten percent of patients with first episode of AP and 36 % with RAP develop CP [12]. When thoroughly investigating with newer sensitive techniques—such as endoscopic ultrasound (EUS), secretin-enhanced magnetic resonance (S-MRCP), and pancreatic function tests (PFTs)—many patients presenting with isolated RAP and a minority of those presenting with their sentinel attack are found to have morphological evidence of CP, ranging from subtle "minimal change" disease to obvious disease with calcifications. It is not clear if a sentinel event starts an inflammatory process that cannot be turned off (Sentinel acute pancreatitis event SAPE hypothesis) [11], or if the pathology simply represents accumulated damage from prior attacks that has not fully healed [13]. Few of the patients with RAP and normal morphological gland may suffer with intractable chronic pain.

Definition

RAP is defined as two or more well-documented separate attacks of AP with complete resolution for more than three months between the attacks [14–16]. It usually occurs in the setting of normal appearing and functional pancreas. Evidence of underlying CP can be identified either at the time of the first attack or during follow up attacks. At the current time the exact cause of recurrent acute pancreatitis is unclear in up to 30 % and this group of patients is termed as idiopathic recurrent acute pancreatitis (IRAP).

Etiology

Major causes for RAP are gallstones and alcohol abuse. Other causes include hypercalcemia, hypertriglyceridemia, pancreas divisum, post-endoscopic retrograde cholangiopancreatography (ERCP), sphincter of Oddi dysfunction (SOD), viral infections, congenital abnormalities, microlithiaisis, tumors, genetic disorders, and autoimmune pancreatitis. Any condition causing a single episode of AP has the potential to cause a recurrent episode, unless the inciting factor has been corrected. Recurrence in patients with AP due to etiologies mentioned above depends on how effectively the etiology has been treated. Either by eliminating or treating the underlying cause recurrent attacks can be reduced. Patients with idiopathic cause and those with genetic abnormality are at risk for developing subsequent attacks of pancreatitis [17]. Thus, it is reasonable to consider relapsing pancreatitis as a complex syndrome associated with numerous etiologies, clinical variables, and complications.

Gallstones: Gallstone disease is the most common cause for AP around the world accounting for 35–40 % [18]. In addition to obtaining liver function tests, all patients presenting with sentinel attack of AP should undergo right upper quadrant ultrasound to search for biliary cause of AP. If gallstone etiology is suspected, patients should undergo cholecystectomy or ERCP with biliary sphincterotomy to prevent recurrent attacks [19].

> When stones in the bile duct or gall bladder are detected, one should undergo cholecystectomy and/or ERCP, sphincterotomy alone is not adequate unless one is deemed a poor surgical risk

Biliary Sludge or Microlithiasis: Sludge is a viscous suspension of crystals, mucin, glycoproteins, and proteinaceous material in gallbladder that may contain small stones, or microlithiasis (<3 mm in diameter) [20]. On ultrasound it is seen as mobile, low amplitude echoes that do not produce a shadow and layers in most dependent part of the gallbladder. It occurs in functional or mechanical bile stasis. Common associations are a prolonged fast, TPN, and distal bile duct obstruction.

Microlithiasis: A cut off of 3 mm has been taken because abdominal ultrasound can diagnose stones > 3 mm in size. They are predominantly composed of cholesterol. Microlithiasis and sludge are often used interchangeably. Sludge may regress spontaneously but microlithiasis does not. These are best detected on EUS with sensitivity of 96 % which is found to be superior to bile crystal analysis [21]. Studies have shown that in patients with suspected microlithiasis, there were detectable gallstones on follow-up ultrasound [22, 23]. The prevalence of these as the cause for RAP has varied across the studies. Some studies showed high prevalence 60–73 % using bile microscopy in gall bladder in situ patients and RAP has been eliminated by removal of gallbladder [22–25]. A study from India has reported low prevalence (13 %) of microlithiasis. In this particular study EUS was used for diagnosis instead of bile microscopy [26]. Ideal situation to label microlithiasis as cause of RAP would be detection of these by EUS in patients with suspected biliary etiology. Recurrence rates of AP are approximately 33–60 % if biliary etiology is not treated properly [26, 27]. There is definite risk of AP during waiting period for cholecystectomy [28]. Early cholecystectomy (<72 h) from the time of hospitalization is preferred in the setting of mild AP and not to wait for normalization of enzymes [29, 30].

> When biliary etiology is suspected early cholecystectomy is preferred and not all patients need an ERCP. ERCP should be done only in those with concern for presence of stones in the bile ducts as shown by liver function tests or imaging studies. In the setting of acute biliary pancreatitis ERCP is indicated only for ongoing biliary obstruction and or ascending cholangitis.

Alcohol and Smoking: Excess alcohol consumption is responsible for 30 % of all cases of AP in the USA [31]. Recurrent episodes of acute pancreatitis typically occur in those patients who continue to drink and in those with underlying chronic calcific pancreatitis [32]. Prevalence estimates for RAP in alcoholics are about 16.9 % in men and 5.5 % in women [33]. Recent data has shown that smoking is an independent and dose dependent risk factor for AP, RAP, and CP [34–36]. The effects of smoking are enhanced in the presence of alcohol consumption. Risk for progression to CP in patients with AP and RAP are higher among smokers and alcoholics [12]. Therefore, it is important to elicit a proper social history and provide necessary counseling.

Drug induced Pancreatitis: Several drugs have been implicated as a cause of AP, but ascertaining a true case and effect relationship can be difficult. In addition, some may cause pancreatitis through an intermediary, like hypertriglyceridemia. Evidence of pancreatitis on rechallenge is not seen in all the implicated drugs, and the weight of evidence is variable for different drugs. Latency periods for development of pancreatitis can be unpredictable. A review of medications and cessation of drugs that have a temporal relationship with the attack, or have more evidence of being casual, with or without a trial of that medicine, is beneficial in some patients [37].

Genetic Factors: Genetic factors have long been suspected to play a role in the cause, clinical course and outcomes of RAP and development of CP overtime. In a Danish study, the cationic trypsinogen gene (*PRSS1*), serine protease inhibitor Kazal type 1 (*SPINK1*), and the cystic fibrosis transmembrane conductance regulator gene (*CFTR*) were present in up to 50 % of patients with idiopathic CP [38].

CFTR-gene mutations: *CFTR*-gene induces a defect in chloride ion transport at the level of the apical membrane-chloride channels of epithelial cells, resulting in an abnormally viscous exocrine secretion that leads to persistently high intraductal pancreatic pressure. There are many clinical features associated with *CFTR*-gene mutation phenotype: exocrine pancreatic insufficiency with no inflammatory changes, RAP, asymptomatic patient with elevated pancreatic enzymes, and normal morpho-functional gland. Even when etiology is obvious (e.g., in pancreas divisum), an interplay with genetic factors apparently occurs (increased incidence of *CFTR*), thus accounting for RAP only in a subset of patients [39].

SPINK1 gene mutations: *SPINK1* have been associated with RAP, but are not common findings in those with initial/sentinel attacks of pancreatitis in the North American population [40]. *SPINK1* may be responsible for much of "tropical pancreatitis," and both *CFTR* and *SPINK1* appear to increase the risk of alcohol-related pancreatitis.

PRSS1-gene mutations: Hereditary pancreatitis is an autosomal dominant disorder with penetrance rates up to 80 %. Mutations of the *PRSS1* are most often responsible, with impaired activation of trypsin and continuous activation of the digestive enzymes predisposes individuals to recurrent bouts of pancreatitis in childhood and frequent progression to CP. Lifetime risk of pancreatic cancer in this population is about 40 %. Management of threes patients are similar to that for AP or CP of other etiologies, although interest is increasing in total pancreatectomy with auto islet cell transplantation, partly because of cancer risk [41]. Genetic counseling may be important for family members and patients.

> Current evidence does not suggest routine genetic testing. Facilities are not available at all centers and may be done in an appropriate research/clinical settings

Metabolic causes: Up to 4 % of episodes of AP are thought to be related to hypertriglyceridemia. In general, to cause AP, it is felt that fasting serum triglycerides must be present in excess of 1000 mg/dl. It is less clear how acute transient rises in serum triglycerides after meals can affect the pancreas, because patients with moderately elevated fasting levels may still have toxic levels after meals. Recurrent rates of AP in patients with hypertriglyceridemia can be prevented if triglyceride levels are controlled within normal limits with diet and medications [42]. Mutations in LPL proteins and higher frequency *of CFTR* gene polymorphisms have been identified in hypertriglyceridemia related pancreatitis [43, 44]. Control of diabetes mellitus, weight loss and lipid lowering drugs will reduce the triglyceride levels, but noncompliance is frequent and many of these patients progress towards CP.

Hyperparathyroidism can cause AP, RAP, and CP. Felderbauer et al. have shown that genetic mutations involving *SPINK1, CFTR*, and *CTRC* genes are seen in patients with hyperparathyroidism associated pancreatitis [45].

Celiac disease: Celiac disease is thought to be a possible cause of RAP by causing papillary inflammation and obstruction.

However, data are scant. Treatment is usually endoscopic sphincterotomy for relief of obstruction, along with necessary dietary counseling for celiac disease [46].

Autoimmune Pancreatitis: Autoimmune pancreatitis (AIP) is a systemic fibroinflammatory disease that can affect the pancreas. AIP is divided into type 1 (lymphoplasmacytic sclerosing pancreatitis), which is related to IgG4, and type 2 (idiopathic duct centric pancreatitis), which is associated with granulocyte epithelial lesions [47]. AIP may present in a variety of ways, including biliary and pancreatic obstructive disease with or without a pancreatic mass, sometimes mimicking pancreatic cancer; it may also present as RAP, especially in young women with inflammatory bowel disease. The clinical profile and relapse differ for type 1 versus type 2 AIP. The proportion of patients who present with IRAP and have AIP is relatively very low [48]. Data are limited, but suggest that clinical or biochemical autoimmune stigmata can be present in up to 40 % of patients labeled as having idiopathic CP. In the presence of abnormal imaging suggestive of AIP it is reasonable to assess further for presence of AIP. Sensitivity of serum IgG4 levels in US patients is very low, generally under 20 %, and is probably lower for those with RAP. Because the diagnosis can be elusive, several criteria have been proposed to diagnose AIP. The most widely used in the USA is the HISORt criteria (histology, imaging, serology, other organ involvement, and response to therapy) [49] . Histologic confirmation is desirable, but can be difficult and potentially risky to obtain. Histologic confirmation can be obtained by EUS-guided Tru-Cut biopsy of the pancreas; however this method is generally reserved for IgG4-negative patients with a strong clinical suspicion. Ampullary biopsy with IgG4 staining may be a safer option, and specificity approaches 100 %, although sensitivity is about 50 % [50]. Treatment is usually with corticosteroids, although spontaneous resolution without therapy has been reported; relapses are relatively common with type 1. Long-term consequences of steroids and other immunosuppressive agents are of concern [51].

Congenital Abnormalities of Pancreatic and Biliary Anatomy

Pancreas divisum: Common congenital anomaly of pancreas present in 2.7–22 % of the western populations; it is less common in Asians [52, 53]. Pancreas divisum is certainly associated with RAP and CP but why a few patients are affected while the majority are spared is unknown [54, 55]. Studies have shown that minor papillotomy decreases the risk of recurrence of AP if CP is not already established [56, 57]. Once CP is present, minor papillotomy may benefit only 40–50 %. Although one retrospective series found no correlation between pancreas divisum and RAP [58]. It is well recognized now that pancreas divisum with RAP is associated with increased prevalence of genetic abnormalities. Several studies have suggested that a heterozygous defect in the *CFTR* gene may predispose patients with pancreas divisum to RAP [39, 59, 60]. At this time, pancreas divisum should be considered as a possible causative factor for RAP. ERCP solely for the purpose of ductography should be avoided, and alternate imaging techniques should be used instead to establish the anatomy. Although the sensitivities of MRCP and EUS are modest, the specificities are generally very high. The addition of secretin to MRCP very likely improves accuracy such that it approaches that of ERCP. As with all pancreatic sphincterotomies, restenosis occurs in 20–30 % of patients and repeat interventions may be needed to correct it [61].

> ERCP with minor papillotomy might be of benefit for those with definite recurrent acute pancreatitis. Endoscopic therapy should be done after careful assessment and discussion of the limited efficacy of therapies. Preferably this should be done at an institution with significant expertise and in a research setting.

Choledochocele: Cystic dilation of the biliary system can involve either the extrahepatic or intrahepatic biliary system. There are five types of choledochal cysts; type 3 is by definition choledochocele. In type 3, there is dilation of the intramural segment of the pancreatobiliary junction. Association of choledochocele with RAP is likely from sludge or stones obstructing the pancreatic duct outflow. Diagnosis is often made by MRCP, EUS, or ERCP. Therapy involves endoscopic unroofing of the papilla, with biliary plus or minus additional pancreatic sphincterotomy [62].

Anomalous pancreatobiliary junction involves an unusually long (>1.5 cm) common channel between the bile and pancreatic ducts, caused by failure of descent in embryologic development. This anomaly facilitates fee reflux of bile and pancreatic juice into the alternative ducts, possibly resulting in pancreatitis. The risks of cholangiocarcinoma and gallbladder carcinoma possibly are increased, especially if a choledochal cyst is also present. Diagnosis can be made by EUS or MRCP. The role of ERCP and sphincterotomy in reducing risk is uncertain, as are biliary resection or diversion procedures, and there are very limited data to support this approach [62].

Annular pancreas is defined as a pancreatic tissue partially or completely encircling the duodenum usually at the level of or just proximal to the major papilla [63]. It is often associated with duodenal or biliary obstructive symptoms and/or pancreatitis that may affect the annulus or the remaining pancreas. Treatment consists of gastrojejunostomy in case of duodenal occlusion.

Sphincter of Oddi Dysfunction (SOD): The current "gold standard" to measure biliary and pancreatic sphincter pressure is to perform ERCP using a manometry catheter [64]. Manometrically, SOD is defined as basal biliary or pancreatic sphincter pressures > 40 mmHg which is greater than 3 standard deviations above normal [65]. In patients with well-documented RAP, where a thorough history, routine laboratory testing, and conventional imaging have not found a cause, abnormal manometry is found in 15–72 %. SOD has been classified under three sub types on the basis of clinical and morphological parameters, and manometric findings [66]. This may involve biliary and/or pancreatic segment of the sphincter [67]. Type 1 dysfunction patients have AP (pancreatitis-like pain with high serum pancreatic enzymes) together with a dilated common bile and/or main pancreatic duct and prolonged drainage, suggesting a structural abnormality.

Type II dysfunction patients have pancreatic-like pain, associated with one or two type 1 items, in this group, with either pancreatitis or only pancreatic-like pain patients with functional or structural sphincter disorder are probably evenly distributed. Manometry shows elevated basal pressures but no stenosis in majority of patients. Type III SOD patients have pancreatic-like pain with no rise in serum pancreatic enzymes and bilio-pancreatic morphological abnormalities. However, based upon recent EPISOD study [68] SOD type III does not exist as true pancreatobiliary disease and these patients should be categorized as functional abdominal pain [69], rather than true pancreatobiliary disease. Unfortunately, abnormal findings on Sphincter of Oddi manometry of biliary and/pancreatic sphincters does not necessarily predict consistent relief of symptoms from biliary and/or pancreatic sphincterotomy. As a result, SOD is controversial as an etiology for IRAP, especially in patients who still have intact normal gallbladder. The relative importance of the biliary and pancreatic sphincters to the syndrome, and the added benefit of dual versus single sphincterotomy are also unclear.

> Whether sphincter of Oddi dysfunction causes recurrent acute pancreatitis is very controversial.

Tumors: Pancreatic and Ampullary tumors are an unusual but important cause of RAP. Conventional imaging can easily miss benign and malignant tumors. Pancreatic neuroendocrine, mucinous cystic neoplasms and ductal adenocarcinoma may all present as unexplained pancreatitis, albeit in a small (~2 %) proportion of patients. EUS with high sensitivity is generally indicated for idiopathic pancreatitis, especially in older patients to evaluate for small tumors. Ampullary lesion can be identified on standard endoscopy, EUS or by ERCP. One should pay attention to the minor papilla as well preferably with secretin stimulated MRCP to rule out santorinicele, tumors of the minor papilla. The rate of AP in patients with mucinous cystic neoplasms in the largest published surgical series has varied from 12 % to 67 % [70]. The risk of AP seems to be similar with both main duct and side branch intra ductal papillary mucinous neoplasms (IPMN), although data are controversial. AP seems to happen more often in patients with IPMN then induced with ductal adenocarcinoma possible because of obstruction of main pancreatic duct by thick mucin.

Diagnostic Approach

It is extremely important to establish the cause of AP because by removing the cause we eliminate the risk of further recurrences unless there is chronic underlying disease involved. A proper history (including alcohol smoking history, and medication review) and physical examination are central to the evaluation of unexplained RAP, including IRAP. Standard diagnostic tests such as blood chemistry, trans-abdominal ultrasound, and pancreatic protocol CT scan generally detect the causes of recurrent episodes in about 70–80 % of cases. Transabdominal ultrasound is done to assess presence of gallstones and may need to be repeated after the attack if the ultrasound during the attack was technically limited by pain or ileus. Pancreatic protocol CT of the abdomen is useful selectively to assess the pancreas for abnormalities, including extent and severity of pancreatitis, duct dilation, evidence of chronic or autoimmune pancreatitis and presence of tumor, especially in older patients. With the coronal imaging, routine pancreatic and biliary ductal dilation and anatomy are often apparent.

When no cause is found at the initial diagnostic workup, these patients should have more advanced diagnostic workup that includes specific pancreatic tests, genetic testing, MRCP-Secretin, sphincter of Oddi manometry, EUS, and in selected cases ERCP. In younger patients (<40 years of age) with RAP, it is reasonable to check for genetic markers in the absence of other etiology. The enthusiasm for genetic testing is hampered by the cost, availability and lack of effective genetically tailored treatments. However, it is important to recognize hereditary pancreatitis because it has important clinical implications, including that these individuals would also need screening for pancreatic cancer because of their increased risk. An algorithm of appropriate workup based on current evidence and practice is proposed [71].

> Genetic testing is not routinely done due to lack of availability, costs and lack of specific therapies

Endoscopic Ultrasound

EUS is accurate, low risk diagnostic tool for evaluation of unexplained pancreatitis and should be considered the first-line examination in such patients [72]. EUS has shown to identify microlithiasis or gallstones when standard imaging has failed [73]. EUS has been documented to have a sensitivity of 96 % for diagnosing microlithiasis and has a negative predictive value of 95.4 % for diagnosing CBD stones [74]. Yield of EUS in finding the etiology of pancreatitis is similar for patients with a first attack and those with repeated attacks [75]. Apart from EUS being most sensitive test for gallbladder stones, it is highly accurate for the identification of CP, pancreas divisum, pancreatic IPMNs, and small pancreatic and ampullary masses by experienced operators. The frequency of the diagnosis of CP in patients with RAP on the basis of EUS criteria ranges from 10 to 30 % [75, 76].

> It is reasonable to perform EUS after an unexplained episode of sentinel attack/recurrent acute pancreatitis.

Bile Crystal Analysis

When EUS is unrevealing, duodenal bile aspiration should be considered after administration of intravenous cholecystokinin at the same time session in patients with intact gallbladder [77]. Microscopic analysis reveals crystals in up to 48 % of patients with IRAP and cholesterol crystals or bilirubinate granules in bile are not totally excluded by EUS.

> Very few centers perform bile crystal analysis and EUS is more commonly used to detect microlithiasis

MRCP

MRCP is a noninvasive test that permits evaluation of the parenchyma with T1- and T2-weighted images, and allows three-dimensional reconstruction of the modality to evaluate the biliary and pancreatic ductal anatomy. With EUS, MRCP is usually a second-step procedure in the evaluation of RAP [78]. MRCP with secretin test permits indirect evaluation of sphincter of Oddi motility, as an alternative to more invasive tests such as sphincter of Oddi manometry. However, the secretin test is less sensitive than manometry for intermittent sphincter motility disorders like Type II SOD. In cases of pancreas divisum with non-dilated dorsal duct, the MRCP with secretin test may help detect some minor papilla malfunction.

> MRCP can give similar data as ERCP in most instances except for pressure measurements. It is a noninvasive test and has minimal risks as compared to ERCP

ERCP

With the advances in pancreaticobiliary imaging and availability of EUS and MRCP, ERCP is rarely used for diagnostic purpose only except for Sphincter of Oddi manometry and intraductal EUS. ERCP has the advantage to perform therapeutic measures when mechanical cause of RAP is suspected. Endoscopic ampullectomy may be appropriate for patients with benign localized ampullary neoplasia. Endoscopic biliary and/or pancreatic sphincterotomy may have a role in other obstructive conditions, including congenital anatomic variants (e.g., choledochocele, pancreas divisum, and SOD). Obstructive processes (e.g., parasitic infections, as in ascariasis and clonorchiasis) seem to respond to endoscopic therapy [79]. Relieving obstruction in chronic pancreatitis (strictures/stones) can reduce acute-on-chronic pancreatitis. Well-designed prospective studies are needed to evaluate the efficacy of endoscopic therapies for RAP.

ERCP does have a definite therapeutic role in some situations and all alternatives should be considered prior to performing ERCP

Management

Acute episodes of pancreatitis, irrespective of the etiology, are treated with supportive care, including aggressive hydration and analgesics. If specific cause pertinent to RAP is ascertained than therapy is directed to that etiology. Attempts should be made to correct underlying metabolic disturbances. Contrast enhanced CT scan if permit is generally performed within the first 3 days for patients with more severe attacks. EUS and MRCP are reasonable choices of testing prior to performing ERCP; EUS may be preferred in old patients and in those with gallbladder in place. Appropriate definitive treatment would depend on the results of evaluation and discussion of the risks and benefits with the patient. Abstinence of alcohol significantly reduces the recurrence of alcohol-related pancreatitis, and cholecystectomy is effective at preventing recurrent biliary pancreatitis, thereby addressing the two most common causes of RAP.

If the gallbladder appears normal on EUS and liver chemistries are within normal limits empiric cholecystectomy can be avoided. Those patients who have undergone cholecystectomy and have signs suggesting biliary etiology or SOD, endoscopic sphincterotomy could be considered. A prospective randomized trial comparing biliary to dual sphincterotomy in treatment of SOD in patients with IRAP showed no difference in reducing episodes of RAP [80]. Clinical improvement after endoscopic sphincterotomy has been reported in 55–95 % of patients, depending on the SOD type [76, 81, 82]. In patients with type III SOD based on recent EPISOD trial ERCP should be avoided [83]. Endoscopic and surgical therapies for PD are comparably effective in 70–90 % so endoscopic therapy is preferred in most cases. Endoscopic therapy includes minor papillotomy or stenting, or catheter dilation. Diseases such as SOD and pancreas divisum which are thought to cause an obstruction and hence pancreatitis, have variable outcomes when the obstruction is relieved, bringing etiology into question.

> Sphincterotomy in patients with SOD should be done only in high volume centers preferably in a research setting. A thorough discussion regarding the potential non-relief of symptoms and risk of post procedural complications including higher rate of pancreatitis is required. Sphincterotomy for type III SOD should be avoided. Biliary sphincterotomy alone might be just as beneficial as both biliary and pancreatic sphincterotomies.

Effects of interventions are poorly understood, especially if RAP is thought to have multiple etiologies, such as those with pancreas divisum or microlithiasis, which could have a gene mutation or other environmental influence. For those with frequent RAP without signs of SOD, pancreas divisum, with or without metabolic or genetic abnormality, there are few options. Empiric sphincterotomy is not recommended, nor is long-term stenting. Nonetheless, in patients without other options, with poor quality of life due to these recurrent attacks, total pancreatectomy with auto islet cell transplantation may be a consideration.

Summary

RAP is a common clinical condition. After confirming the attacks truly is pancreatitis, etiology is apparent in at least 70–80 % of cases with standard investigations. In another 10–15 % of cases, a cause can be found with additional advanced investigations. Up to 10 % of cases will remain idiopathic. Empiric cholecystectomy is no longer performed. Genetic predisposition is a common cofactor, but the role of routine testing is still unclear, except in those with a family history of suspected *PRSS1* mutation (which identifies a higher cancer risk). EUS and MRCP are recommended after complete history and physical with the laboratory tests and imaging studies. Endoscopic ultrasound is preferred in unexplained RAP because of its ability to detect small tumors and microlithiasis. ERCP solely for diagnostic purposes (without manometry or divisum-targeted therapy) should be avoided. Strict alcohol abstinence and smoking cessation is encouraged. Establishing subtle evidence of chronic pancreatitis may be worthwhile in patients with intractable pain between attacks. Data on the role of pancreatectomy with auto islet cell transplantation in RAP without CP is are limited but seem to be encouraging.

Future Trends

Well-designed clinical trials looking at the treatment options and outcomes are necessary. Future trials should take into account the complex interplay between genetics and environmental factors and treatments should be individualized. There is a need for comparative effectiveness trials evaluating various treatment options. In the meantime one should exercise cautious enthusiasm and optimism for invasive therapies.

References

1. Lowenfels AB, Maisonneuve P, Sullivan T. The changing character of acute pancreatitis: epidemiology, etiology, and prognosis. Curr Gastroenterol Rep. 2009;11:97–103.
2. Shelton CA, Whitcomb DC. Genetics and treatment options for recurrent acute and chronic pancreatitis. Curr Treat Options Gastroenterol. 2014;12:359–71.
3. Somogyi L, Martin SP, Venkatesan T, Ulrich CD. Recurrent acute pancreatitis: an algorithmic approach to identification and elimination of inciting factors. Gastroenterology. 2001;120: 708–17.
4. Sajith KG, Chacko A, Dutta AK. Recurrent acute pancreatitis: clinical profile and an approach to diagnosis. Dig Dis Sci. 2010;55:3610–6.
5. Gullo L, Migliori M, Pezzilli R, Oláh A, Farkas G, Levy P, et al. An update on recurrent acute pancreatitis: data from five European countries. Am J Gastroenterol. 2002;97:1959–62.
6. Andersson R, Andersson B, Haraldsen P, Drewsen G, Eckerwall G. Incidence, management and recurrence rate of acute pancreatitis. Scand J Gastroenterol. 2004;39:891–4.

7. Zhang W, Shan HC, Gu Y. Recurrent acute pancreatitis and its relative factors. World J Gastroenterol. 2005;11:3002–4.
8. Lankisch PG, Breuer N, Bruns A, Weber-Dany B, Lowenfels AB, Maisonneuve P. Natural history of acute pancreatitis: a long-term population-based study. Am J Gastroenterol. 2009;104:2797–805.
9. Gorry MC, Gabbaizedeh D, Furey W, Gates Jr LK, Preston RA, Aston CE, et al. Mutations in the cationic trypsinogen gene are associated with recurrent acute and chronic pancreatitis. Gastroenterology. 1997;113:1063–8.
10. Whitcomb DC, Gorry MC, Preston RA, Furey W, Sossenheimer MJ, Ulrich CD, et al. Hereditary pancreatitis is caused by a mutation in the cationic trypsinogen gene. Nat Genet. 1996;14:141–5.
11. Whitcomb DC. Value of genetic testing in the management of pancreatitis. Gut. 2004;53:1710–7.
12. Sankaran SJ, Xiao AY, Wu LM, Windsor JA, Forsmark CE, Petrov MS. Frequency of progression from acute to chronic pancreatitis and risk factors: a meta-analysis. Gastroenterology. 2015;149(6):1490–500.
13. Witt H, Apte MV, Keim V, Wilson JS. Chronic pancreatitis: challenges and advances in pathogenesis, genetics, diagnosis, and therapy. Gastroenterology. 2007;132:1557–73.
14. Al-Haddad M, Wallace MB. Diagnostic approach to patients with acute idiopathic and recurrent pancreatitis, what should be done? World J Gastroenterol. 2008;14:1007–10.
15. Romagnuolo J, Guda N, Freeman M, Durkalski V. Preferred designs, outcomes, and analysis strategies for treatment trials in idiopathic recurrent acute pancreatitis. Gastrointest Endosc. 2008;68:966–74.
16. Takuma K, Kamisawa T, Hara S, Tabata T, Kuruma S, Chiba K, et al. Etiology of recurrent acute pancreatitis, with special emphasis on pancreaticobiliary malformation. Adv Med Sci. 2012;57:244–50.
17. Whitcomb DC, Yadav D, Adam S, Hawes RH, Brand RE, Anderson MA, et al. Multicenter approach to recurrent acute and chronic pancreatitis in the United States: the North American Pancreatitis Study 2 (NAPS2). Pancreatology. 2008;8:520–31.
18. Forsmark CE, Baillie J. AGA Institute technical review on acute pancreatitis. Gastroenterology. 2007;132:2022–44.
19. Sharma VK, Howden CW. Metaanalysis of randomized controlled trials of endoscopic retrograde cholangiography and endoscopic sphincterotomy for the treatment of acute biliary pancreatitis. Am J Gastroenterol. 1999;94:3211–4.

20. Ko CW, Sekijima JH, Lee SP. Biliary sludge. Ann Intern Med. 1999;130:301–11.
21. Dahan P, Andant C, Lévy P, Amouyal P, Amouyal G, Dumont M, et al. Prospective evaluation of endoscopic ultrasonography and microscopic examination of duodenal bile in the diagnosis of cholecystolithiasis in 45 patients with normal conventional ultrasonography. Gut. 1996;38:277–81.
22. Ros E, Navarro S, Bru C, Garcia-Puges A, Valderrama R. Occult microlithiasis in 'idiopathic' acute pancreatitis: prevention of relapses by cholecystectomy or ursodeoxycholic acid therapy. Gastroenterology. 1991;101:1701–9.
23. Lee SP, Nicholls JF, Park HZ. Biliary sludge as a cause of acute pancreatitis. N Engl J Med. 1992;326:589–93.
24. Venu RP, Geenen JE, Hogan W, Stone J, Johnson GK, Soergel K. Idiopathic recurrent pancreatitis. An approach to diagnosis and treatment. Dig Dis Sci. 1989;34:56–60.
25. Kaw M, Brodmerkel Jr GJ. ERCP, biliary crystal analysis, and sphincter of Oddi manometry in idiopathic recurrent pancreatitis. Gastrointest Endosc. 2002;55:157–62.
26. Garg PK, Tandon RK, Madan K. Is biliary microlithiasis a significant cause of idiopathic recurrent acute pancreatitis? A long-term follow-up study. Clin Gastroenterol Hepatol. 2007;5:75–9.
27. Frei GJ, Frei VT, Thirlby RC, McClelland RN. Biliary pancreatitis: clinical presentation and surgical management. Am J Surg. 1986;151:170–5.
28. van Baal MC, Besselink MG, Bakker OJ, van Santvoort HC, Schaapherder AF, Nieuwenhuijs VB, et al. Timing of cholecystectomy after mild biliary pancreatitis: a systematic review. Ann Surg. 2012;255:860–6.
29. Bouwense SA, Besselink MG, van Brunschot S, Bakker OJ, van Santvoort HC, Schepers NJ, et al. Pancreatitis of biliary origin, optimal timing of cholecystectomy (PONCHO trial): study protocol for a randomized controlled trial. Trials. 2012;13:225.
30. Nebiker CA, Frey DM, Hamel CT, Oertli D, Kettelhack C. Early versus delayed cholecystectomy in patients with biliary acute pancreatitis. Surgery. 2009;145:260–4.
31. Yang AL, Vadhavkar S, Singh G, Omary MB. Epidemiology of alcohol-related liver and pancreatic disease in the United States. Arch Intern Med. 2008;168:649–56.
32. Migliori M, Manca M, Santini D, Pezzilli R, Gullo L. Does acute alcoholic pancreatitis precede the chronic form or is the opposite true? A histological study. J Clin Gastroenterol. 2004;38:272–5.

33. Coté GA, Yadav D, Slivka A, Hawes RH, Anderson MA, Burton FR, et al. Alcohol and smoking as risk factors in an epidemiology study of patients with chronic pancreatitis. Clin Gastroenterol Hepatol. 2011;9:266–73.
34. Munigala S, Conwell DL, Gelrud A, Agarwal B. Heavy smoking is associated with lower age at first episode of acute pancreatitis and a higher risk of recurrence. Pancreas. 2015;44:876–81.
35. Majumder S, Gierisch JM, Bastian LA. The association of smoking and acute pancreatitis: a systematic review and meta-analysis. Pancreas. 2015;44:540–6.
36. Greer JB, Thrower E, Yadav D. Epidemiologic and mechanistic associations between smoking and pancreatitis. Curr Treat Options Gastroenterol. 2015;13:332–46.
37. Tenner S. Drug induced acute pancreatitis: does it exist? World J Gastroenterol. 2014;20:16529–34.
38. Joergensen M, Brusgaard K, Cruger DG, Gerdes AM, Schaffalitzky de Muckadell OB. Incidence, etiology and prognosis of first-time acute pancreatitis in young patients: a population-based cohort study. Pancreatology. 2010;10:453–61.
39. Gelrud A, Sheth S, Banerjee S, Weed D, Shea J, Chuttani R, et al. Analysis of cystic fibrosis gener product (CFTR) function in patients with pancreas divisum and recurrent acute pancreatitis. Am J Gastroenterol. 2004;99:1557–62.
40. Aoun E, Muddana V, Papachristou GI, Whitcomb DC. SPINK1 N34S is strongly associated with recurrent acute pancreatitis but is not a risk factor for the first or sentinel acute pancreatitis event. Am J Gastroenterol. 2010;105:446–51.
41. Blondet JJ, Carlson AM, Kobayashi T, Jie T, Bellin M, Hering BJ, et al. The role of total pancreatectomy and islet autotransplantation for chronic pancreatitis. Surg Clin North Am. 2007;87:1477–501. x.
42. Athyros VG, Giouleme OI, Nikolaidis NL, Vasiliadis TV, Bouloukos VI, Kontopoulos AG, et al. Long-term follow-up of patients with acute hypertriglyceridemia-induced pancreatitis. J Clin Gastroenterol. 2002;34:472–5.
43. Fortson MR, Freedman SN, Webster III PD. Clinical assessment of hyperlipidemic pancreatitis. Am J Gastroenterol. 1995;90:2134–9.
44. Jap TS, Jenq SF, Wu YC, Chiu CY, Cheng HM. Mutations in the lipoprotein lipase gene as a cause of hypertriglyceridemia and pancreatitis in Taiwan. Pancreas. 2003;27:122–6.
45. Felderbauer P, Karakas E, Fendrich V, Lebert R, Bartsch DK, Bulut K. Multifactorial genesis of pancreatitis in primary

hyperparathyroidism: evidence for "protective" (PRSS2) and "destructive" (CTRC) genetic factors. Exp Clin Endocrinol Diabetes. 2011;119:26–9.
46. Patel RS, Johlin Jr FC, Murray JA. Celiac disease and recurrent pancreatitis. Gastrointest Endosc. 1999;50:823–7.
47. Chari ST, Kloeppel G, Zhang L, Notohara K, Lerch MM, Shimosegawa T. Histopathologic and clinical subtypes of autoimmune pancreatitis: the Honolulu consensus document. Pancreas. 2010;39:549–54.
48. Sah RP, Chari ST, Pannala R, et al. Differences in clinical profile and relapse rate of type 1 versus type 2 autoimmune pancreatitis. Gastroenterology. 2010;139:140–8.
49. Chari ST. Diagnosis of autoimmune pancreatitis using its five cardinal features: introducing the Mayo Clinic's HISORt criteria. J Gastroenterol. 2007;42 Suppl 18:39–41.
50. Moon SH, Kim MH, Park do H, Song TJ, Eum J, Lee SS, et al. IgG4 immunostaining of duodenal papillary biopsy specimens may be useful for supporting a diagnosis of autoimmune pancreatitis. Gastrointest Endosc. 2010;71:960–6.
51. Hart PA, Zen Y, Chari ST. Recent advances in autoimmune pancreatitis. Gastroenterology. 2015;149:39–51.
52. Alempijevic T, Stimec B, Kovacevic N. Anatomical features of the minor duodenal papilla in pancreas divisum. Surg Radiol Anat. 2006;28:620–4.
53. Kin T, Shapiro AM, Lakey JR. Pancreas divisum: a study of the cadaveric donor pancreas for islet isolation. Pancreas. 2005;30:325–7.
54. Bernard JP, Sahel J, Giovannini M, Sarles H. Pancreas divisum is a probable cause of acute pancreatitis: a report of 137 cases. Pancreas. 1990;5:248–54.
55. Cotton PB. Congenital anomaly of pancreas divisum as cause of obstructive pain and pancreatitis. Gut. 1980;21:105–14.
56. Liao Z, Gao R, Wang W, Ye Z, Lai XW, Wang XT, et al. A systematic review on endoscopic detection rate, endotherapy, and surgery for pancreas divisum. Endoscopy. 2009;41:439–44.
57. Kwan V, Loh SM, Walsh PR, Williams SJ, Bourke MJ. Minor papilla sphincterotomy for pancreatitis due to pancreas divisum. ANZ J Surg. 2008;78:257–61.
58. Delhaye M, Engelholm L, Cremer M. Pancreas divisum: congenital anatomic variant or anomaly? Contribution of endoscopic retrograde dorsal pancreatography. Gastroenterology. 1985;89:951–8.

59. Choudari CP, Imperiale TF, Sherman S, Fogel E, Lehman GA. Risk of pancreatitis with mutation of the cystic fibrosis gene. Am J Gastroenterol. 2004;99:1358–63.
60. Bertin C, Pelletier AL, Vullierme MP, Bienvenu T, Rebours V, Hentic O, et al. Pancreas divisum is not a cause of pancreatitis by itself but acts as a partner of genetic mutations. Am J Gastroenterol. 2012;107:311–7.
61. Attwell A, Borak G, Hawes R, Cotton P, Romagnuolo J. Endoscopic pancreatic sphincterotomy for pancreas divisum by using a needle-knife or standard pull-type technique: safety and reintervention rates. Gastrointest Endosc. 2006;64:705–11.
62. Levy MJ, Geenen JE. Idiopathic acute recurrent pancreatitis. Am J Gastroenterol. 2001;96:2540–55.
63. Urayama S, Kozarek R, Ball T, Brandabur J, Traverso L, Ryan J, et al. Presentation and treatment of annular pancreas in an adult population. Am J Gastroenterol. 1995;90:995–9.
64. Fazel A, Geenen JE, MoezArdalan K, Catalano MF. Intrapancreatic ductal pressure in sphincter of Oddi dysfunction. Pancreas. 2005;30:359–62.
65. Pfau PR, Banerjee S, Barth BA, et al. Sphincter of Oddi manometry. Gastrointest Endosc. 2011;74:1175–80.
66. Hogan WJ, Geenen JE, Dodds WJ. Dysmotility disturbances of the biliary tract: classification, diagnosis, and treatment. Semin Liver Dis. 1987;7:302–10.
67. Eversman D, Fogel EL, Rusche M, Sherman S, Lehman GA. Frequency of abnormal pancreatic and biliary sphincter manometry compared with clinical suspicion of sphincter of Oddi dysfunction. Gastrointest Endosc. 1999;50:637–41.
68. Cotton PB, Durkalski V, Romagnuolo J, Pauls Q, Fogel E, Tarnasky P, et al. Effect of endoscopic sphincterotomy for suspected sphincter of Oddi dysfunction on pain-related disability following cholecystectomy: the EPISOD randomized clinical trial. JAMA. 2014;311:2101–9.
69. Behar J, Corazziari E, Guelrud M, Hogan W, Sherman S, Toouli J. Functional gallbladder and sphincter of Oddi disorders. Gastroenterology. 2006;130:1498–509.
70. Sakorafas GH, Smyrniotis V, Reid-Lombardo KM, Sarr MG. Primary pancreatic cystic neoplasms of the pancreas revisited. Part IV: rare cystic neoplasms. Surg Oncol. 2012;21:153–63.
71. Kinney TP, Lai R, Freeman ML. Endoscopic approach to acute pancreatitis. Rev Gastroenterol Disord. 2006;6:119–35.

72. Tandon M, Topazian M. Endoscopic ultrasound in idiopathic acute pancreatitis. Am J Gastroenterol. 2001;96:705–9.
73. Morris-Stiff G, Al-Allak A, Frost B, Lewis WG, Puntis MC, Roberts A. Does endoscopic ultrasound have anything to offer in the diagnosis of idiopathic acute pancreatitis? JOP. 2009;10:143–6.
74. Amouyal P, Palazzo L, Amouyal G, Ponsot P, Mompoint D, Vilgrain V, et al. Endosonography: promising method for diagnosis of extrahepatic cholestasis. Lancet. 1989;2:1195–8.
75. Yusoff IF, Raymond G, Sahai AV. A prospective comparison of the yield of EUS in primary vs. recurrent idiopathic acute pancreatitis. Gastrointest Endosc. 2004;60:673–8.
76. Coyle WJ, Pineau BC, Tarnasky PR, Knapple WL, Aabakken L, Hoffman BJ, et al. Evaluation of unexplained acute and acute recurrent pancreatitis using endoscopic retrograde cholangiopancreatography, sphincter of Oddi manometry and endoscopic ultrasound. Endoscopy. 2002;34:617–23.
77. Delchier JC, Benfredj P, Preaux AM, Metreau JM, Dhumeaux D. The usefulness of microscopic bile examination in patients with suspected microlithiasis: a prospective evaluation. Hepatology. 1986;6:118–22.
78. Mariani A, Arcidiacono PG, Curioni S, Giussani A, Testoni PA. Diagnostic yield of ERCP and secretin-enhanced MRCP and EUS in patients with acute recurrent pancreatitis of unknown aetiology. Dig Liver Dis. 2009;41:753–8.
79. Baillie J. Endoscopic therapy in acute recurrent pancreatitis. World J Gastroenterol. 2008;14:1034–7.
80. Coté GA, Imperiale TF, Schmidt SE, Fogel E, Lehman G, McHenry L, et al. Similar efficacies of biliary, with or without pancreatic, sphincterotomy in treatment of idiopathic recurrent acute pancreatitis. Gastroenterology. 2012;143:1502–9.
81. Toouli J, Di Francesco V, Saccone G, Kollias J, Schloithe A, Shanks N. Division of the sphincter of Oddi for treatment of dysfunction associated with recurrent pancreatitis. Br J Surg. 1996;83:1205–10.
82. Madura JA, Madura JA, Sherman S, Lehman GA. Surgical sphincteroplasty in 446 patients. Arch Surg. 2005;140:504–11.
83. Imler TD, Sherman S, McHenry L, Fogel EL, Watkins JL, Lehman GA. Low yield of significant findings on endoscopic retrograde cholangiopancreatography in patients with pancreatobiliary pain and no objective findings. Dig Dis Sci. 2012;57:3252–7.

Chapter 5
Steroid-Responsive Chronic Pancreatitides: Autoimmune Pancreatitis and Idiopathic Duct-Centric Chronic Pancreatitis

Nicolo' de Pretis, Yan Bi, Saurabh Mukewar, and Suresh Chari

What Is Autoimmune Pancreatitis?

Autoimmune pancreatitis (AIP) is a peculiar form of chronic pancreatitis characterized by dramatic response to steroids. Currently, there are two isoforms that are called type 1 and type 2 AIP. However, these two isoforms have distinct pathological, epidemiological, serological and clinical features, although both show a dramatic response to steroid therapy. While type 1 AIP is commonly seen in elderly patients, and is characterized by other organ involvement and elevated serum IgG4 levels, type 2 AIP is more common in young patients, is pancreas-specific and lacks of serum IgG4 elevation. Over the last few years, AIP type 1 has been considered as the pancreatic manifestation of a multiorgan disease called immunoglobulin G4 (IgG4)-related disease (IgG4-RD) that may virtually involve any organ.

Due to the distinct difference between these two subtypes and the confusion in general practitioners regarding IgG4 and Type 2 AIP, it has recently been suggested that

N. de Pretis • Y. Bi • S. Mukewar • S. Chari (✉)
Division of Gastroenterology and Hepatology, Mayo Clinic, Rochester, MN 55905, USA
e-mail: Chari.Suresh@mayo.edu

© Springer International Publishing Switzerland 2016
K. Dua, R. Shaker (eds.), *Pancreas and Biliary Disease*,
DOI 10.1007/978-3-319-28089-9_5

the term AIP to be used solely for type 1 AIP and the term idiopathic duct-centric chronic pancreatitis (IDCP), the characteristic histopathological changes of Type 2 AIP be used for type 2 AIP. Thus, based on this new terminology, which we follow in this review, steroid-responsive chronic pancreatitis includes two diseases: AIP and IDCP. The main clinical and epidemiological features in AIP and IDCP are summarized in Table 5.1.

How Is AIP Treated?

As mentioned earlier, both AIP and IDCP are characterized by a dramatic response to steroids and the rate of response is close to 100 %. Many different steroid protocols have been proposed. The most frequently reported approach is 40 mg prednisone by mouth daily for 4 weeks, followed by tapering the dose by 5 mg per week. After 4 weeks, and at the end of the treatment, a reassessment of lab work and/or imaging should be performed to confirm response to treatment.

The rate of recurrence of different subtypes of AIP is different. In IDCP, recurrences of the disease after steroid treatment are very uncommon, while the recurrence rate in AIP is between 30 and 50 %.

Multiple strategies to treat recurrent disease have been proposed: (1) Repeat similar protocol of prednisone regimen, followed by a slower taper; (2) Start with the com-

TABLE 5.1 Main clinical and epidemiological features in AIP and IDCP

Type	Mean age (decade)	Gender (male) (%)	Serum IgG4 elevation (%)	OOI (%)	IBD (%)	Steroids response (%)	Relapse (%) after steroids
AIP	Sixth	75	70	20–45	5	100	30–50
IDCP	Fourth	50	15	0	20	100	0–5

OOI other organs involvement, *IBD* inflammatory bowel disease (Crohn's disease and ulcerative colitis)

bination of Prednisone and immunosuppressive drugs (IS) such as azathioprine, mycophenolate mofetil, cyclosporine or methotrexate and then taper down steroid. The IS should be continued after the steroid tapering. (3) The biological agent CD20 inhibitor Rituximab has been reported to be effective in both inducing and maintaining remission, but the experience is currently limited.

Is AIP Associated with Malignancy?

Although AIP patients may suffer from complications of chronic pancreatitis including diabetes and mal-digestion, it has not been associated with shortened life span compared to age-matched controls. Chronic pancreatitis is a well-established risk factor for pancreatic cancer. Although some case reports have been published about the occurrence of cancers, especially pancreatic cancer in AIP, however, due to the rarity of this disease, the true association remains unclear.

Other complications are typically related to AIP in the setting of a diffuse IgG4-related disease that may involve many other organs. The most relevant complications are related to the involvement of the bile ducts and of the urinary tract and are normally well responsive to steroids.

Brief Review of the Literature

AIP

AIP is a rare type of steroid-responsive chronic pancreatitis. It is presumed to be of autoimmune etiology because of its frequent association with elevated gamma globulins and autoantibodies and the dramatic response to steroid therapy. The term of AIP was first coined by Yoshida in 1995 [1] and its association with elevated IgG4 levels was first reported in 2001 by Hamano [2].

Introduction

AIP is the pancreatic manifestation of the multiorgan IgG4-Related Disease (IgG4-RD) which may virtually involve any organ in the body. IgG4-RD is defined as a fibroinflammatory condition characterized by tumefactive lesions in multiple organs, a dense lymphoplasmacytic infiltrate rich in IgG4-positive plasma cells, storiform fibrosis and often, but not always, elevated serum IgG4 concentrations [3].

AIP, despite being the most frequent manifestation of IgG4-RD, is considered a rare disease. The estimated prevalence of AIP in Japan is 2.2/1,00,000 [4, 5]. This disease still remains highly underdiagnosed and the real prevalence may be significantly higher. In Europe [6] and America [7], AIP is 3–4 times more common than IDCP while IDCP is rarely reported in Japan and other eastern countries.

As part of IgG4-RD, AIP is frequently characterized by the involvement of extra-pancreatic organs (Other Organ Involvement (OOI)). The presence of synchronous or metachronous OOI is reported in around two thirds of the cases. The most frequent organs involved are the biliary tree (intra- and extra-hepatic bile ducts), the kidneys, the retroperitoneum, and the salivary glands [3, 6, 7]. Different from AIP, IDCP is not part of IgG4-RD and OOI is rarely reported. However, IBD has been shown in 20–30 % IDCP patients.

Pathogenesis

The pathogens of AIP are incompletely understood. The pathogenesis and pathophysiology of AIP have been studied mainly from immunological approaches and focused for the most part on the role of IgG4.

Elevation of serum IgG4 and a massive infiltration of IgG4-expressing plasma cells in the pancreatic tissue are characteristic of AIP (and of IgG4-RD) [3, 8]. However, it is unclear if IgG4 plays a role in the pathogenesis of AIP or is simply an epiphenomenon of the disease.

Apart from elevated serum IgG4, many antibodies have been reported elevated in AIP suggesting possible autoimmune etiology. About 40 % of patients with AIP have elevated titers of anti-nuclear antibodies (ANA). Other studies have reported elevated serum autoantibodies, such as, those against lactoferrin (75 % of patients), carbonic anhydrase (55 % of patients), ubiquitin ligase, trypsin, and pancreatic secretory trypsin inhibitor [8].

Furthermore, circulating antibodies against antigens of *Helicobacter pylori* have been isolated in AIP patients, suggesting a role for infections in triggering the immunologic response [9].

Currently, none of these antibodies are used in clinical practice and IgG4 still remains the only serological marker clinically useful for diagnosis [10].

Some studies suggest that a genetic predisposition may play a role in the pathogenetic mechanism of AIP. HLA serotypes, such as DRB1*0405, DQB1*0401, are associated with a higher risk of developing AIP, while DQB1*0302 seems associated with a higher risk of relapses after steroid treatment [8]. The rarity of the disease, the limited data, and the costs of genetic analysis limit the validation of these studies and their use in clinical practice.

Clinical Presentation

AIP patients are predominantly male (62–83 %) with a mean age at diagnosis in the sixth and seventh decade of life [8]. AIP has protean clinical presentations. The most frequent symptom reported at the time of diagnosis is painless obstructive jaundice (~60 %), which may be difficult to distinguish from a malignant entity. The majority of AIP patient do not complain of any pain; in those who do the intensity of the pain is usually mild to moderate and not disabling. Other symptoms, less frequently reported, are fatigue, weight loss, hyperglycemia, steatorrhea, acute pancreatitis and symptoms related to the involvement of other organs such as salivary gland, kidneys, retroperitoneum, and lungs. Abnormal imaging findings, such as pancreatic mass or focal/diffuse enlargement of the pancreas, are a more rare first presentation of the disease. Pancreatic atrophy, calcifications, ductal dilation and other features of advanced painless chronic pancreatitis are reported in patients with long-standing AIP.

Marked cachexia, inability to eat, and narcotic-requiring pain are more suggestive of malignant processes and are rarely seen in AIP [8, 11].

Diagnosis

The diagnosis of AIP is frequently challenging and the differential diagnosis with pancreatic cancer or other malignances is crucial. Multiple diagnostic strategies have been proposed with the most commonly used ones are HISORt, Asian Criteria, and the International Consensus Diagnostic Criteria (ICDC) developed in 2011 by the International Association of Pancreatology [10]. These criteria are focused on the diagnosis of AIP and IDCP in an early phase, while the diagnosis in very advanced stages is practically impossible. According to the ICDC, the diagnosis of AIP requires a combination of cardinal features that include:

H Histopathology of the pancreas
I Imaging features of pancreatic parenchyma and pancreatic duct
S Serology
O Other organ involvement
Rt Response to steroid therapy

Every feature is classified into level 1 and level 2, depending on the specificity of the findings. A definitive diagnosis may be reached only in presence of histopathological confirmation of AIP, whereas in the absence of a clear histopathological confirmation, various diagnostic combinations of the criteria should be used for the diagnosis [10].

Histopathology

Lymphoplasmacytic sclerosing pancreatitis (LPSP) is pathognomonic of AIP. LPSP is diagnosed when at least three of the following four histologic criteria are present on a pancreatic core biopsy or resection specimen: (a) peri-ductal lymphoplasmacytic infiltrate without granulocytic infiltration; (b) obliterative phlebitis; (c) storiform fibrosis; (d) abundant (>10 cells/HPF) IgG4-positive cells.

As reported by many authors, a diffuse IgG4 infiltration may be seen in the pancreatic tissue of these patients. However, both an elevation of serum IgG4 and a positive tissue immunostaining for IgG4 are by themselves insufficient for the diagnosis. Many other benign and malignant diseases, such as primary sclerosing cholangitis, cholangiocarcinoma and pancreatic cancer, may have an elevated serum IgG4 and positive IgG4 immunostaining. Furthermore, a European multicenter study on resected AIP showed that only 79.4 % of the patients with AIP have high tissue levels of IgG4+ plasma cells [12]. The IgG4 infiltration is highly suggestive of AIP only if the ratio IgG4/IgG is >40 % or if their frequency is >10 cells/HPF [10].

Because of the complexity of the histological finding and the frequent small size of the tissue biopsies obtained by endoscopic ultrasound-guided core biopsy, an expert pathologist is required for the interpretation of the pathological specimens. The final diagnosis of AIP is frequently difficult on preoperative biopsies and the differential diagnosis with malignant diseases may remain.

Imaging

Computed tomography (CT) and Magnetic resonance (MRI) are the most commonly used imaging techniques when pancreatic and biliary diseases are suspected. The ICDC divided the finding into parenchymal and ductal changes [10]. The pancreatic parenchyma is more easily assessed by CT and MRI, while the ductal changes are more precisely evaluated by magnetic resonance cholangiopancreatography (MRCP) or by the more invasive endoscopic retrograde cholangiopancreatography (ERCP).

The most typical appearance of AIP is a diffuse enlargement of the pancreas, which is described in about 40 % of the patients. This particular finding is frequently highly suggestive of AIP. The diagnosis is more challenging if there is a focal enlargement with a mass-forming appearance of the pancreas, which is reported in 36 % of cases. Ruling out a malignancy may be extremely difficult in these cases. Around 30 % of patient with AIP have no enlargement of the pancreas [13].

Contrast CT scan is usually helpful in differentiating AIP from pancreatic malignancies. Most AIP patients show hypoattenuation during the arterial/pancreatic phase with a hyperattenuation during the venous/delayed phase. Pancreatic cancer usually shows hypoattenuation in the arterial phase but remains hypo-enhancing even in the venous phase. The presence of a capsule-like rim around the pancreas or around the affected area is described only in 35 % of the patients, but is reported to have a high specificity for AIP (see Fig. 5.1). The presence of a low density mass, main pancreatic duct dilation, or distal atrophy are more typical for pancreatic cancer.

On MRI, AIP appears as diffuse or focally enlarged pancreas which is hypointense on T1-weighted images, slightly hyperintense on T2-weighted images, and has heterogenously diminished enhancement in the late phase of contrast enhancement. Even on MRI a capsule-like rim may be identified; it usually appears as hypointense rim on both T1 and T2-weighted images [14].

The presence of ductal changes is frequently reported in AIP. The main techniques for investigating the ductal structures of the pancreas are MRCP and ERCP. ERCP has been reported as the technique with the highest sensitivity for visualizing the main pancreatic duct narrowing. The typical appearance of AIP on ERCP is the presence of single or multiple segmental strictures of the main pancreatic duct, without upstream dilation as seen in pancreatic cancers. The strictures are typically long unlike short strictures in pancreatic cancer.

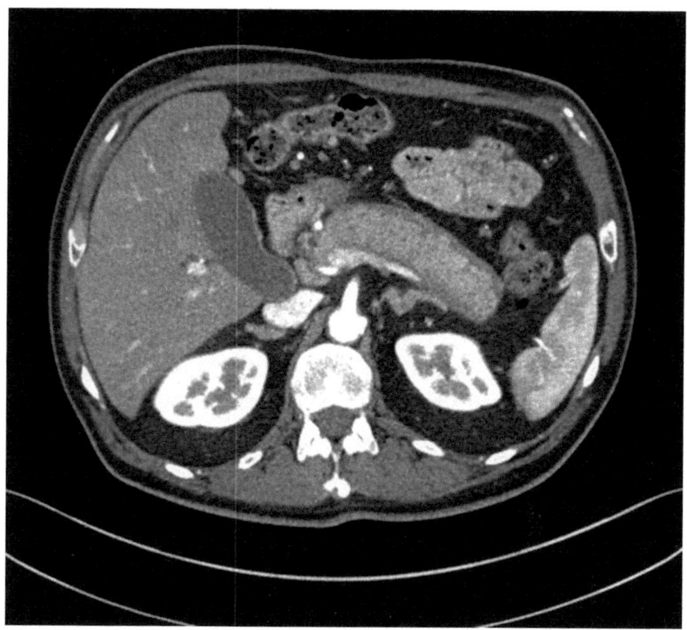

Fig. 5.1 Typical features of AIP type 1 at CT scan: diffuse enlargement of the pancreas with a peripheral capsule-like rim and dilation of the intra-hepatic bile duct

The use of secretin stimulation may be helpful in differentiating a stricture secondary to AIP because it frequently resolves after the secretin injection in AIP. While MRI is helpful in visualizing the pancreatic parenchyma and duct, MRCP should be interpreted with caution as ~25 % of normal subjects have non-visualization of portions of the pancreatic duct that could be mistaken for stricture without upstream dilation. MRCP is also useful for evaluating biliary involvement in the disease, especially the intrahepatic bile ducts [8, 14].

The role of endoscopic ultrasound (EUS) is particularly important for the diagnosis of AIP, especially in those cases in which serological and radiological criteria are not conclusive. It may be difficult to differentiate AIP from pancreatic cancer using conventional EUS imaging alone. Some authors described particular features frequently detected in AIP and not in cancer, such as diffuse hypoechoic areas, diffuse enlargement of the gland, bile duct wall thickening, and peri-hypoechoic margins. Some studies showed that the accuracy of the technique may increase using contrast-enhanced harmonic EUS (CEH-EUS) and EUS-elastography. These additional techniques may provide additional information on the vascular patterns and the stiffness of the tissue, with a better differentiation among benign and malignant solid pancreatic masses [15]. The advantage of EUS is the ability to obtain histological samples by core biopsies for tissue diagnosis.

Serology

IgG4 is considered a serological marker of AIP and checking the levels of IgG4 in the serum is increasingly becoming a common practice. Like any other serologic markers, it is far from being optimal, and an unrestricted use may lead to diagnostic mistakes. Serum IgG4 elevation is not pathognomonic of AIP and many benign and malignant conditions (e.g., allergies, primary sclerosing cholangitis, pancreatic cancer, cholangiocarcinoma) may also have an elevation of serum IgG4. IgG4 is typically the least abundant of the IgG subclasses, making up <5 % of total serum IgG in healthy adults. It is a unique immunoglobulin with peculiar characteristics. The production of IgG4 is increased by repeated or prolonged exposure to allergens. IgG4 interacts poorly with the complement and is a weak activator of the complement pathways due to its half-antibody exchange reaction, also referred to as fragment antigen-binding (Fab)-arm exchange. Therefore, patients with AIP generally do not have decreased complement levels. In addition, IgG4 has rheumatoid-factor activity and can bind the Fc portion of other IgG antibodies, particularly other IgG4 molecules. Similar to the IgG rheumatoid factors, IgG4 can mediate a direct damage to cellular structures [3].

Clinical Use

AIP is strongly associated with an elevation of serum IgG4 and tissue infiltration with IgG4+ plasma cells, neither of which is specific to AIP. Hence, the measurement of serum IgG4 should be limited to patients with suspicion of AIP. The mean age of patients with AIP is around 60 years, and the presentation with pancreatitis is rare (see AIP clinical presentation). Therefore, in young patients with acute or recurrent pancreatitis, a routine check of IgG4 should be avoided. There is high variability in IgG4 levels between different subjects. Therefore, an acute or recurrent pancreatitis with isolated elevation in serum IgG4 levels may be inappropriately diagnosed as AIP. A pancreatitis with elevation of IgG4 should not be considered as AIP in the absence of other criteria confirming the diagnosis (see AIP clinical presentation). Furthermore, there are many other conditions and diseases, which may present with elevated serum IgG4 levels. The differential diagnosis between AIP and cancer is crucial, especially in those patients, in which the clinical presentation is jaundice, with a mass/enlargement of the pancreas head on imaging. Unfortunately, up to 10 % of the pancreatic cancers present with high IgG4 levels. Therefore, detecting an elevation in serum IgG4 levels, does not exclude a neoplastic disease.

Primary sclerosing cholangitis may also present with jaundice and elevated IgG4 levels and the differential diagnosis with AIP with biliary involvement may be very difficult. In fact, according to the ICDC serum IgG4 should be considered only as one of the criteria for the diagnosis.

The specificity of the IgG4 in differentiating AIP from other diseases, especially from cancer, is higher when serum IgG4 levels are >2× upper limit of normal. But even high IgG4 level is diagnostic as a sole criterion; a combination with the other criteria is needed for the diagnosis [10].

Treatment

As described above, both AIP and IDCP show a dramatic response to steroids. The remission of the disease under steroids is reported in close to 100 % of cases in AIP. There is no complete consensus on the definition of remission, but at a minimum it should include resolution of inflammatory changes on imaging with normalization of the biochemical parameters (especially transaminase and cholestatic markers) and resolution of symptoms. The absence of response to steroids virtually excludes the diagnosis of AIP and requires more investigations to exclude other possible diseases, especially cancer. However, in advanced stages, the pancreas may be involved by severe fibrosis and atrophy, which are not reversible with the steroid treatment.

In a Japanese study [16], about 70 % of AIP patients improved spontaneously without any treatment. However, steroid therapy is strongly recommended for inducing the remission of the disease in symptomatic patients and in patients with extra-pancreatic lesions [17]. Furthermore, the response to steroids is useful for the confirmation of the diagnosis. However, the use of steroid trials for obtaining the diagnosis in patients with no collateral evidence of AIP should be limited to very select cases and should be considered only after a negative radiological and histological workup for malignancy. In patients with jaundice, some authors and the Japanese guidelines suggest endoscopic biliary drainage before starting steroid treatment. However, in AIP, a clinical and serological improvement of the jaundice is rapidly expected. Therefore, steroids alone without biliary drainage have been proposed in selected patients that not only avoid additional endoscopic procedures, but also facilitate the diagnosis using the fast improvement of the AIP-associated jaundice with steroid treatment.

Different strategies have been proposed for dosing steroids. The most accepted approach is a high-dosage of prednisone, 0.5–0.6 mg/kg/day or 40 mg/day for 2–4 weeks followed by tapering by 5 mg every 1–2 weeks over 3–4 months. The dose may be adjusted in old patients and in diabetics to reduce the steroid-related complications. After the first 4–6 weeks and at the end of the treatment, a clinical, radiological and biochemical reassessment should be performed to confirm response and complete remission of the disease, respectively [8]. If biliary stent has been placed prior to onset of treatment, it should be removed at the 4–6 week assessment. Lack of response and/or persistence of biliary stricture needing replacement of biliary stent strongly suggest an alternate diagnosis.

Relapse

AIP is characterized by a high relapse rate, reported in the literature between 20 and 60 %. A slow and prolonged tapering of the steroids and continuing a low dose therapy for 1–3 years or more may decrease the relapse rate [17]. Considering the high rate of steroid-induced complications, there is no international consensus on the indiscriminate administration of a long-term steroid therapy to all patients suffering from AIP.

Some risk factors have been identified to be associated with a higher rate of relapse. The involvement of extra-pancreatic organs, particularly the proximal common bile duct (intrahepatic bile duct and /or the supra-pancreatic portion of the extrahepatic bile duct), is probably related to the highest relapse rate. Other risk factors include the presence of a diffuse enlargement of the pancreas at the initial presentation and high serum IgG4 levels, especially after steroids treatment. Certain genetic predisposition, such as the substitution of aspartic acid at position 57 of the *DQB1* gene may be a predicting factor for relapse.

AIP relapses have been classified into clinical relapse (recurrence of symptoms), radiologic relapse (recurrence of radiologic abnormalities in the pancreas or in extra-pancreatic organs), serologic relapse (elevation of serum IgG4), and biochemical relapse (elevation of liver enzymes). The presence of a clinical relapse should be confirmed by imaging evidence of radiological relapse, which is a clear indication for treatment. Presence of nonspecific symptoms without radiological or biochemical relapse is not an indication for treatment. Similarly, an isolated elevation of the serum IgG4 levels is not an indication for treatment, even if it may be associated with a higher risk of future relapse. Marked (>2 fold) elevation of liver tests (transaminases, alkaline phosphatase), even without radiologic findings suggesting a relapse, is an indication for treatment, because it may represent an early relapse in the biliary three.

A relapse may occur during steroid taper or after withdrawal of steroids. If a relapse occurs while the patient is still on high dose (>20 mg/day) steroids, the diagnosis of AIP should be questioned. In relapses occur on low doses of steroid taper, increasing the dose of steroids and prolonging the taper is a reasonable approach; however, indefinitely exposing the patients to high-dose steroids should be avoided.

Many different strategies have been proposed for managing patients with disease relapse after a period of remission. The aim is to reinduce a complete remission and start a maintenance therapy to reduce the risk of relapses. These strategies include a second steroid treatment followed with slower steroids tapering, the combination use of steroids and immunosuppressive medications (ISs), or the use of biologic drugs (B-cell depletion therapy using monoclonal antibody) [8].

Typically, AIP relapse can be treated with the same regimen of high dose prednisone for 4 weeks followed by a prolonged taper. Some authors even keep the patient on a 2–3 years of low dose prednisone to reduce the relapse rate. A second strategy includes the combination use of steroids and ISs such as azathioprine, mycophenolate mofetil, and methotrexate as maintenance strategy. The patient should undergo a new cycle of steroids for reinducing remission. At the same time, the administration of ISs should be started and continued after steroid taper, since ISs have shown the ability to reduce the relapse rate. The third strategy is to use Rituximab (RTX), a monoclonal antibody that targeted against CD20 positive plasma cells which are mainly involved in the IgG4 production. It has been reported that RTX is able to induce and maintain remission in AIP and in other IgG4 related diseases [18]. Currently the use of RTX is limited only to patients in whom steroids therapy is contraindicated, who are intolerant to steroids or have side effects, or in those who failed immunosuppressive therapy. As RTX is the only alternative to steroids in inducing the remission, in the near future it may become the first strategy in select patients.

Idiopathic Duct-Centric Chronic Pancreatitis (IDCP)

Introduction

AIP and IDCP are two different diseases despite many similarities in their clinical course. Both share the same presentation symptoms, including jaundice, abdominal pain, weight loss, imaging features (enlargement of the pancreas), and rapid response to steroids. However, significant differences exist between them. While, AIP is a male predominant disease with the mean age of presentation in the seventh decade of life (60 and 65), IDCP patients lack significant gender differences and the age on presentation is generally one to two decades younger than that of AIP (45 years). The prevalence of these two subtypes is quite different. IDCP appears to be relatively common in the USA and Europe but rare in East Asia; nevertheless, patients with AIP outnumber those with IDCP even in Western countries.

Pathogenesis

As a consequence of the rarity of the disease, very little is known about the pathogenesis of IDCP. It is likely an immune-related entity due to the frequent association with inflammatory bowel disease and the response to steroid treatment [8].

Clinical Presentation

IDCP may present with obstructive jaundice with diffuse pancreatic enlargement on imaging studies. While the majority of patients with AIP present with obstructive jaundice (75%), patients with IDCP more frequently present with abdominal pain (68 %) and pancreatitis (34 %) as well as obstructive jaundice (47 %). On imaging studies, 40 % of AIP have diffuse pancreas swelling compared to only 25 % of IDCP; majority of IDCP present with focal enlargement. The elevation of serum IgG4 is seen only in 20 % of these patients in contrast to 70 % of AIP; there is also an absence of extra-pancreatic involvement in IDCP and lack of IgG4 positive plasma cells in affected tissues. Inflammatory bowel disease (predominantly ulcerative colitis) is seen up to 20–30 % in IDCP, while it is a rare association with AIP. No clear differences are reported in the literature in the radiological presentation between AIP and IDCP.

Histological Characteristics

Periductal lymphoplasmacytic infiltrate and inflammatory stroma are present in both AIP and IDCP. Granulocytic epithelial lesions (GEL) are pathognomonic of IDCP and are often found in medium and small ducts. It is characterized by neutrophilic infiltration of pancreatic ductal epithelial, which in severe cases can resemble microabscess and lead to obliteration of ductal lumen. Pancreatic involvement may be patchy and multiple areas may show a high concentration of neutrophils. IgG4 positive plasma cells are, if present, small in number and never exceed 40 % of IgG plasma cells. Obliterative phlebitis and storiform fibrosis are less prominent than in AIP.

Diagnosis

The diagnosis of IDCP is challenging. International consensus guideline has been developed to facilitate diagnosis of IDCP [10]. Because the elevations of serum IgG4 levels and other organ involvement are typically absent in IDCP, definitive diagnosis can only be made through demonstration of GEL on histology. A diagnosis of probable IDCP can be made when idiopathic pancreatitis is associated with IBD.

Treatment

Similar to AIP patients, all patients with IDCP respond rapidly to corticosteroid therapy using a similar prednisone regimen. Unlike in AIP, disease relapses are rare in IDCP. Despite that, a clinical, biochemical and radiological reassessment is mandatory after 1 month and at the end of the steroid therapy, confirming a complete regression of the radiologic abnormalities. The absence of a radiological response or the recurrence of symptoms, especially pancreatitis, should strongly support a reevaluation of the patient and different diagnosis should be considered.

Future Directions

AIP and IDCP are rare but more frequently recognized causes of pancreatitis that require high levels of suspicion to make a diagnosis. As the field expands, we will learn more about the true incidence of the disease; understand further the disease pathogenesis using AIP animal models and explore more easily administered medical treatment that may lower the relapse rate of this disease. For IDCP, currently the diagnosis is based on pathology. With a better understanding of this disease, hopefully, noninvasive techniques can be used for this purpose.

References

1. Yoshida K, Toki F, Takeuchi T, Watanabe S, Shiratori K, Hayashi N. Chronic pancreatitis caused by an autoimmune abnormality. Proposal of the concept of autoimmune pancreatitis. Dig Dis Sci. 1995;40(7):1561–8.
2. Hamano H, Kawa S, Horiuchi A, Unno H, Furuya N, Akamatsu T, et al. High serum IgG4 concentrations in patients with sclerosing pancreatitis. N Engl J Med. 2001;344(10):732–8.
3. Stone JH, Zen Y, Deshpande V. IgG4-related disease. N Engl J Med. 2012;366(6):539–51. doi:10.1056/NEJMra1104650.

4. Uchida K, Masamune A, Shimosegawa T, Okazaki K. Prevalence of IgG4-related disease in Japan based on nationwide survey in 2009.IntJRheumatol.2012;2012:358371.doi:10.1155/2012/358371. Epub 2012 Jul 31.

5. Umehara H, Okazaki K, Masaki Y, Kawano M, Yamamoto M, Saeki T, et al. Research Program for Intractable Disease by Ministry of Health, Labor and Welfare (MHLW) Japan G4 team. A novel clinical entity, IgG4-related disease (IgG4RD): general concept and details. Mod Rheumatol. 2012;22(1):1–14.

6. Ikeura T, Manfredi R, Zamboni G, Negrelli R, Capelli P, Amodio A, et al. Application of international consensus diagnostic criteria to an Italian series of autoimmune pancreatitis. United European Gastroenterol J.2013;1(4):276–84. doi:10.1177/2050640613495196.

7. Sah RP, Chari ST, Pannala R, Sugumar A, Clain JE, Levy MJ, et al. Differences in clinical profile and relapse rate of type 1 versus type 2 autoimmune pancreatitis. Gastroenterology. 2010;139(1):140–8; quiz e12-3. doi: 10.1053/j.gastro.2010.03.054. Epub 2010 Mar 27.

8. Hart PA, Zen Y, Chari ST. Recent advances in autoimmune pancreatitis. Gastroenterology. 2015;149(1):39–51. doi:10.1053/j.gastro.2015.03.010. Epub 2015 Mar 12.

9. Frulloni L, Lunardi C, Simone R, Dolcino M, Scattolini C, Falconi M, et al. Identification of a novel antibody associated with autoimmune pancreatitis. N Engl J Med. 2009;361(22):2135–42. doi:10.1056/NEJMoa0903068.

10. Shimosegawa T, Chari ST, Frulloni L, Kamisawa T, Kawa S, Mino-Kenudson M, et al. International consensus diagnostic criteria for autoimmune pancreatitis: guidelines of the International Association of Pancreatology. Pancreas. 2011;40(3):352–8. doi:10.1097/MPA.0b013e3182142fd2.

11. Kamisawa T, Chari ST, Lerch MM, Kim MH, Gress TM, Shimosegawa T. Recent advances in autoimmune pancreatitis: type 1 and type 2. Gut. 2013;62(9):1373–80. doi:10.1136/gutjnl-2012-304224. Epub 2013 Jun 8.

12. Zamboni G, Lüttges J, Capelli P, Frulloni L, Cavallini G, Pederzoli P, et al. Histopathological features of diagnostic and clinical relevance in autoimmune pancreatitis: a study on 53 resection specimens and 9 biopsy specimens. Virchows Arch. 2004;445(6):552–63. Epub 2004 Oct 27.

13. Suzuki K, Itoh S, Nagasaka T, Ogawa H, Ota T, Naganawa S. CT findings in autoimmune pancreatitis: assessment using multiphase contrast-enhanced multisection. Clin Radiol. 2010;65(9):735–43. doi:10.1016/j.crad.2010.06.002.

14. Manfredi R, Frulloni L, Mantovani W, Bonatti M, Graziani R, Pozzi MR. Autoimmune pancreatitis: pancreatic and extrapancreatic MR imaging-MR cholangiopancreatography findings at diagnosis, after steroid therapy, and at recurrence. Radiology. 2011;260(2):428–36. doi:10.1148/radiol.11101729. Epub 2011 May 25.
15. Moon SH, Kim MH. Autoimmune pancreatitis: role of endoscopy in diagnosis and treatment. Gastrointest Endosc Clin N Am. 2013;23(4):893–915. doi:10.1016/j.giec.2013.06.005. Epub 2013 Jul 5.
16. Kamisawa T, Shimosegawa T, Okazaki K, Nishino T, Watanabe H, Kanno A, et al. Standard steroid treatment for autoimmune pancreatitis. Gut. 2009;58(11):1504–7. doi:10.1136/gut.2008.172908. Epub 2009 Apr 26.
17. Okazaki K, Uchida K, Sumimoto K, Mitsuyama T, Ikeura T, Takaoka M. Autoimmune pancreatitis: pathogenesis, latest developments and clinical guidance. Ther Adv Chronic Dis. 2014;5(3):104–11. doi:10.1177/2040622314527120.
18. Hart PA, Topazian MD, Witzig TE, Clain JE, Gleeson FC, Klebig RR, et al. Treatment of relapsing autoimmune pancreatitis with immunomodulators and rituximab: the Mayo Clinic experience. Gut. 2013;62(11):1607–15. doi:10.1136/gutjnl-2012-302886. Epub 2012 Aug 30.

Part 2
Clinical Scenario: Painless Jaundice/ Unintentional Weight Loss

Chapter 6
Pancreas Adenocarcinoma and Ampullary Cancer

Chad Barnes, Kathleen K. Christians, Douglas B. Evans, and Susan Tsai

Introduction

Patients who present with painless jaundice represent a challenging diagnostic dilemma. The development of painless jaundice, particularly if associated with older age, weight loss, or worsening diabetes, may be due to a periampullary tumor, such as pancreatic ductal adenocarcinoma (PDAC), ampulla of Vater adenocarcinoma (AVAC), duodenal cancer, or distal cholangiocarcinoma. This chapter focuses on both PDAC and AVAC, as they are the most common malignancies arising in the periampullary region. PDAC is the most common periampullary tumor and is the tenth most common cancer in the USA [1]. In 2015, it was estimated that 46,420 people would be diagnosed with PDAC, and of those diagnosed, 39,590 were expected to die of this disease [2]. Importantly, it has been recognized that the majority of patients with PDAC may have distant metastases at the time of diagnosis, even in the absence of radiographic evidence of disease [3]. As such, the oncologic management of PDAC has evolved to emphasize

C. Barnes, M.D. • K.K. Christians, M.D. • D.B. Evans, M.D. • S. Tsai, M.D., M.H.S. (✉)
Department of Surgery, Medical College of Wisconsin,
9200 W Wisconsin Ave, Milwaukee, WI 53226, USA
e-mail: stsai@mcw.edu

© Springer International Publishing Switzerland 2016
K. Dua, R. Shaker (eds.), *Pancreas and Biliary Disease*,
DOI 10.1007/978-3-319-28089-9_6

the early administration of systemic therapy for virtually every stage of disease. In addition, multiple randomized clinical trials have demonstrated that even in earlier stage disease, patient survival is improved with multimodality therapy and that surgery by itself is rarely curative. In comparison to PDAC, AVACs are more common in men, present with small tumors, and in general are less biologically aggressive [4]. As a result, multimodality therapy is often administered selectively in AVAC based on the pathologic stage. Given the combined prevalence of these two malignancies, most health care providers will encounter patients with one of these diseases at some time throughout their practice in medicine. The goal of this chapter is to describe the clinical staging system and treatment options for patients with PDAC and highlight how the management of AVAC may differ from PDAC. This chapter also provides a background for primary care providers which may help to address concerns raised by patients and families impacted by these diseases.

Question 1: I Was Told that I Have Pancreatic Cancer. How Advanced is My Cancer?

Answer: Oncologists rely on staging systems to help communicate information regarding prognosis and to assist with appropriate treatment planning. Staging is particularly critical for PDAC, since operative interventions can be particularly complicated and require a significant postoperative recovery. As such, surgery should be reserved only for patients who will derive a significant benefit from the removal of the primary tumor. The clinical stage is determined by physical exam and radiographic imaging. The four clinical stages of PDAC from least to most advanced are: resectable, borderline resectable, locally advanced, and metastatic disease (Table 6.1). The former two stages are considered to represent operable disease, and therefore, may be amenable to multimodality therapy and surgical resection.

TABLE 6.1 Comparison of National Comprehensive Cancer Network clinical staging definitions and the Medical College of Wisconsin staging definition

Stage	MCW	NCCN
Resectable		
SMA, Celiac	No abutment	No abutment
Hepatic artery (HA)	No abutment	No abutment
SMV/PV	≤50 % narrowing of SMV, PV, SMV/PV	No abutment, distortion, tumor thrombus or encasement
Borderline resectable		
SMA, Celiac	≤180°	<180°
Hepatic artery (HA)	Short segment encasement*	1 GDA encasement up to the HA or 2 direct abutment of HA w/o extension to celiac axis
SMV/PV	>50 % narrowing of SMV, PV, SMV/PV*	1 Impingement and narrowing of the lumen 2 Encasement or short segment venous occlusion*
Other	CT scan findings suspicious but not diagnostic of metastatic disease	
Locally advanced		**Unresectable**
SMA, Celiac	>180°	>180°
SMV/PV	Occlusion w/o option for reconstruction	Unreconstructable SMV/PV
Metastatic		1 Aortic invasion or encasement
Extrapancreatic disease	Peritoneal or distant metastases	2 LN metastases beyond the field of resection

*Amenable to vascular reconstruction

The latter two stages are considered to be inoperable disease, and are best treated with chemotherapy with or without radiation therapy. If a patient undergoes surgery, pathologic stage can be further refined based on characteristics of the resected specimen. However, unlike other less aggressive solid tumors, in which pathologic staging is used to direct additional therapy after surgery (adjuvant therapy), pathologic staging for PDAC (Table 6.2) does not change the recommendation in favor of adjuvant therapy and therefore is of more limited utility.

Clinical stage is determined by the relationship between the tumor and adjacent vascular structures. The gold-standard diagnostic study used to define this relationship is a computed tomography (CT) scan with both late arterial and portal venous phases (dual phase). Dual phase CT imaging defines the relationship of the tumor to major venous (superior mesenteric vein [SMV]/portal vein [PV]) and arterial (superior mesenteric artery [SMA], celiac artery [CA]) structures and may identify the presence of metastatic disease. As a rule, patients with a new diagnosis of PDAC should be presented in a multidisciplinary conference to gain the input of dedicated abdominal radiologists, surgeons, medical oncologists, and radiation oncologists, in order to accurately determine clinical stage, consider available clinical trials, and develop the best overall treatment plan.

Initial Evaluation of a Patient with PDAC

The diagnostic evaluation of a patient with suspected PDAC begins with a detailed history and physical examination. Symptoms associated with PDAC may vary depending on tumor location, with tumors located in the head of the pancreas causing painless jaundice, as compared to tumors located in the body and tail of the pancreas, which may cause back pain. Other common signs and symptoms include weight loss (51 %), abdominal pain (39 %), nausea/vomiting (13 %), and pruritus (11 %) [6]. Risk factors for PDAC include advanced age, smoking, chronic pancreatitis, diabetes

TABLE 6.2 AJCC PDAC Staging [5]

Primary tumor (T)	
Tx	Primary tumor cannot be assessed
T0	No evidence of primary tumor
Tis	Carcinoma in situ
T1	Tumor limited to pancreas, 2 cm or less in greatest dimension
T2	Tumor limited to the pancreas, more than 2 cm in greatest dimension
T3	Tumor extends beyond the pancreas, but without involvement of the celiac axis or superior mesenteric artery
T4	Tumor involves the celiac axis or the superior mesenteric artery (unresectable primary tumor)
Regional lymph nodes (N)	
Nx	Regional lymph nodes cannot be assessed
N0	No regional lymph node metastasis
N1	Regional lymph node metastasis
Distant metastasis (M)	
M0	No distant metastasis
M1	Distant metastasis

Anatomic stage/prognostic groups

Stage 0	Tis	N0	M0
Stage IA	T1	N0	M0
Stage IB	T2	N0	M0

(continued)

Table 6.2 (continued)

Stage IIA	T3	N0	M0
Stage IIB	T1	N1	M0
	T2	N1	M0
	T3	N1	M0
Stage III	T4	Any N	M0
Stage IV	Any T	Any N	M1

mellitus, and obesity. In particular, a patient who presents with weight loss <u>and</u> worsening diabetes is at high risk for having an undiagnosed PDAC; such patients should undergo abdominal imaging and have a referral to a pancreatic cancer specialist. In addition, a careful family history should be obtained, as approximately 10 % of patients may have a genetic predisposition for PDAC. Patients who are considered to be at high risk for PDAC (lifetime risk $\geq 10\%$) are those with two first-degree family members with PDAC or three any-degree family members with PDAC [7].

A comprehensive physical examination should be performed on all patients being evaluated for PDAC. However, with the exception of jaundice, the physical exam is often unremarkable. Patients with advanced disease may have a palpable abdominal mass at the umbilicus (Sister Mary Joseph node) or supraclavicular lymphadenopathy (Virchow's node) on exam, suggestive of metastatic disease. One third of patients with periampullary tumors will have a palpable gallbladder (Courvoisier's sign) due to biliary obstruction resulting in gallbladder ectasia. Other relevant findings may include ascites, signs of cachexia, and venous thrombophlebitis.

The initial laboratory evaluation should include a baseline complete blood count, basic metabolic panel, and hepatic function tests. Tumor markers such as carbohydrate antigen 19-9 (CA19-9) should also be obtained. CA19-9 is a sialylated

Lewis antigen, which is an epitope found on mucins secreted by PDAC cells. Several studies have demonstrated that CA 19-9 is associated with tumor stage, resectability, and risk of recurrence [8, 9]. Very high CA 19-9 (>2000 U/mL) levels have been associated with an increased risk of having metastatic disease [10]. One of its limitations as a biomarker is that CA19-9 is not produced in approximately 10–15 % of the general population [11]. Additionally, in the setting of biliary obstruction, CA19-9 levels are commonly falsely elevated, limiting its prognostic relevance when the total serum bilirubin is greater than 2 mg/dL [12].

Imaging is essential for the clinical staging of PDAC and in the absence of palpable metastatic disease, clinical staging is impossible without high quality abdominal imaging. For this reason, it is imperative that the correct imaging modality is utilized and reviewed by an experienced radiologist, with particular emphasis on the relationship of the tumor to adjacent vascular structures. Currently, the preferred imaging modality is the multi-detector CT with IV contrast obtained in both the late arterial and portal venous phases with thin (3 mm or less) slices and with three dimensional (3D) reconstructions. The separate arterial and venous phase images are essential to defining the relationship of the pancreatic tumor to the surrounding arterial (CA and SMA) and venous (SMV and PV) structures [13].

Defining the Clinical Stage

The utilization of abdominal imaging is essential, as the pancreas is a retroperitoneal organ which is located near several critical vascular structures. Importantly, the relationship of the tumor to these vascular structures greatly impacts oncologic prognosis and the ability to be able to achieve a negative resection margin [14, 15]. Therefore, the clinical stage of disease is defined by the relationship between the primary tumor and the arterial structures (common hepatic artery, celiac artery, and SMA) and the venous structures (SMV/PV) (Table 6.1). In general, staging separates patients into two

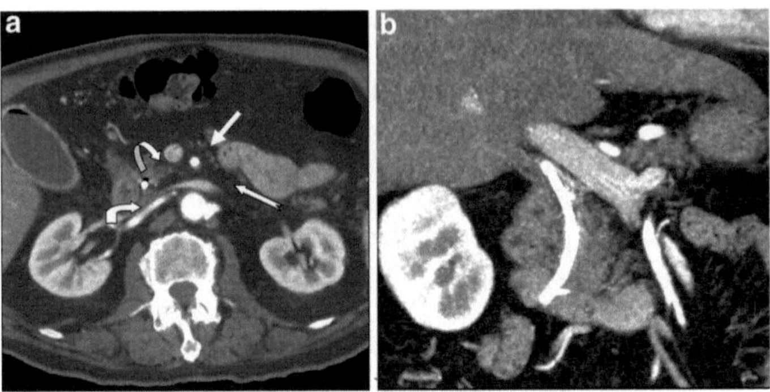

Fig. 6.1 Resectable Pancreatic Cancer, (**a**) well defined fat plane between tumor and SMA, (**b**) SMV/PV narrowing less than 50 %

categories, those with potentially localized disease (resectable or borderline resectable PDAC) or those with advanced disease (locally advanced or metastatic PDAC).

Resectable PDAC (Fig. 6.1) is defined by an absence of tumor extension to major vascular structures, including the SMA, CA, hepatic artery, or SMV/PV. Contact of a vessel with the tumor, which is characterized by the absence of normal soft tissue planes between the tumor and vessel, is defined as abutment if the contact involves ≤ 180° of the vessel circumference, and encasement if the contact involves > 180°. At some institutions, the definition of resectable PDAC has been expanded to include those patients who may have SMV/PV abutment or encasement that results in less than 50 % narrowing of the vessel lumen. Historically, encasement of the SMV/PV was considered a contraindication for surgery and surgical resection was limited to patients without encasement of the SMV/PV and no abutment of the SMA. However, with evolving surgical experience, high volume pancreatic programs have reported that patients with PDAC who receive preoperative (neoadjuvant) therapy and undergo pancreatectomy with vascular resection and reconstruction experience equivalent surgical morbidity and mortality, as well as long term survival, as compared to patients who underwent standard pancreatectomy [16]. As such, at select centers, tumors which involve the SMV/

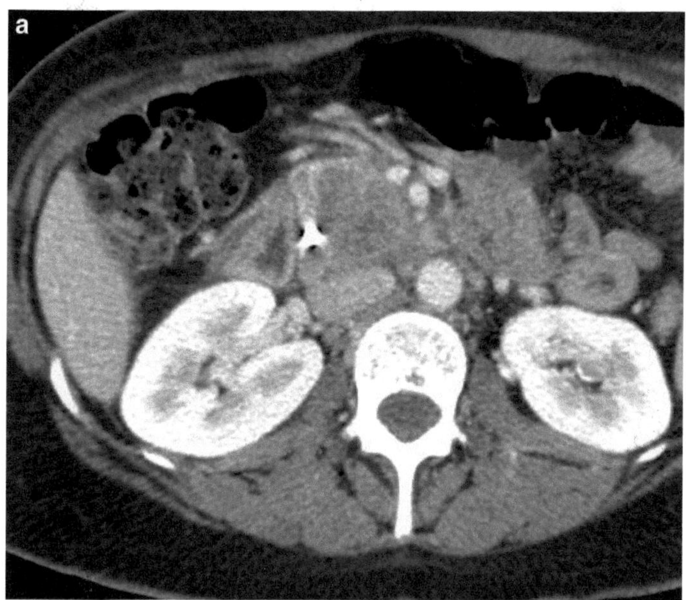

FIG. 6.2 Borderline Resectable Pancreatic Cancer. (**a**) abutment of < 180° SMA

PV without significant narrowing are considered resectable. The primary anatomic criterion which distinguished borderline resectable PDAC from resectable PDAC is the presence of tumor abutment of ≤ 180° of the SMA or CA. The borderline resectable category also includes tumor abutment/encasement of a short segment of the hepatic artery—usually at the origin of the GDA, or an occluded SMV/PV—amenable to reconstruction.

The degree of tumor–artery relationship also defines borderline resectable (Fig. 6.2) and locally advanced PDAC (Fig. 6.3). The degree of arterial abutment/encasement is critical because of the clinical observation that induction therapy may sterilize at least the periphery of the tumor thereby facilitating a complete resection, especially in patients whose tumor–artery relationship is limited to abutment. In contrast, with arterial encasement the likelihood of a margin

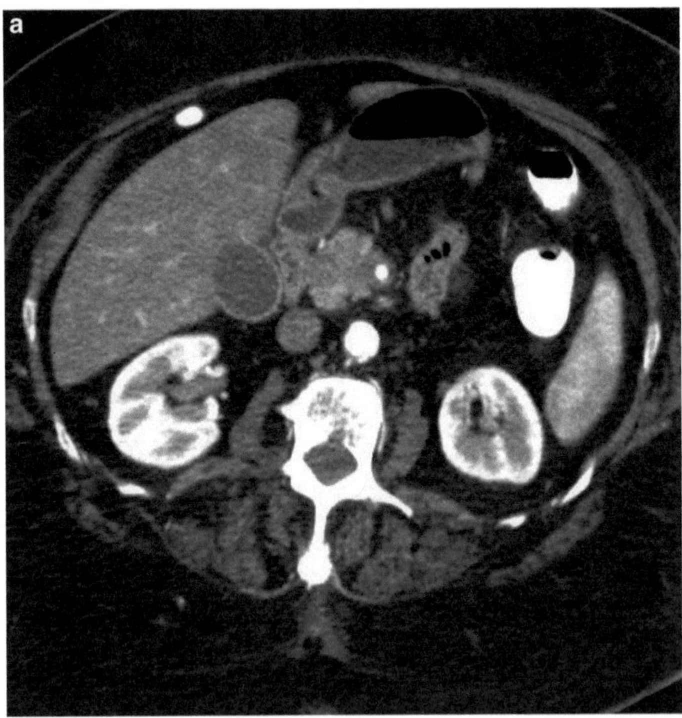

Fɪɢ. 6.3 Locally Advanced Pancreatic Cancer. (**a**) >180° involvement of the SMA

negative resection is very low, and attempted arterial resection and reconstruction in patients with large, locally advanced tumors have been associated with increased perioperative morbidity and mortality [17]. Therefore, locally advanced tumors are usually considered inoperable. In addition, the locally advanced category also includes patients with SMV/PV occlusion with no technical option for reconstruction. Since the tumor–vessel relationships are critical to staging and treatment planning, all PDAC patients, especially those without obvious metastatic disease, should have their cases presented in a multidisciplinary tumor board with dedicated abdominal imaging radiologists, surgical oncologists, medical oncologists, and radiation oncologists all present. Finally, metastatic disease is defined by the presence of extrapancreatic metastases on radiographic imaging [18]. Importantly, a select proportion of patients may have radiographic lesions which are indeterminate for metastases (usually too small to accurately characterize or biopsy), even in the absence of SMA abutment or venous narrowing. These patients are considered by some institutions to have BLR PC, and are offered neoadjuvant therapy with the reasoning that true unequivocal metastatic disease (if present) may be detected at subsequent restaging evaluations [19].

Question 2: What Is the Difference Between Neoadjuvant Therapy and Adjuvant Therapy for PDAC?

Answer: Oncologic therapy delivered before an anticipated operation to remove the primary tumor is called "neoadjuvant" therapy, as compared to therapy which is delivered after the primary tumor is surgically excised, which is referred to as "adjuvant" therapy. Historically, patients with resectable PDAC have been treated with surgery followed by adjuvant therapy. Patients with borderline resectable PDAC are recommended to receive neoadjuvant therapy prior to surgery. However, as the understanding of PDAC tumor biology improves, neoadjuvant therapy is increasingly being adopted in the management of patients with resectable PDAC as well. It is important to emphasize that surgery alone will not be curative in the vast majority of operated patients.

Treatment of PDAC

As with other solid tumors, the treatment for PDAC is determined by the clinical stage. Simply stated, patients with metastatic disease should receive systemic therapy, while patients with localized disease may benefit from surgery if the tumor can be completely removed. One unique aspect of PDAC biology is that the majority of patients who are diagnosed with PDAC will have metastatic disease (subclinical) regardless of radiographic findings [3]. Even among patients who appear to have resectable disease, the median survival rate with surgery followed by adjuvant therapy is only 24 months, suggesting a high prevalence of occult metastases [20, 21]. Multiple randomized controlled trials have demonstrated a survival benefit of adjuvant therapy after surgical resection for all patients regardless of pathologic stage, suggesting that there is no stage of disease that will not benefit from systemic therapy [22, 23]. While the need for systemic therapy in the management of PDAC is universally accepted, current controversies have centered on the sequencing of systemic therapy in the context of multimodality therapy. Recognizing the high risk for the development of metastatic disease, the management of every stage of PDAC has evolved to emphasize the early administration of systemic therapy prior to any locoregional therapy and is currently supported by consensus guidelines for the management of patients with borderline resectable and locally advanced PDAC [24, 25]. Arguably this rationale may be extended to patients with resectable PDAC as well.

Limitations of Adjuvant Therapy

The treatment sequencing for patients with resectable PDAC remains controversial, in particular, whether patients should receive surgery followed by adjuvant therapy (surgery-first approach) or neoadjuvant therapy followed by surgery (neoadjuvant approach). The impact of the magnitude and the complexity of a pancreatic operation on a patient's physiology should not be underestimated. Perioperative mortality associated with surgical resections of the pancreatic head (pancreaticoduodenectomy or Whipple procedure) were once reported to be as high as 30 % but with improvements in surgical technique and perioperative management, they are currently reported to be associated with a 90-day mortality of approximately 4 %, when performed at high volume centers [26]. Significant postoperative complications occur in approximately 30 % of patients, including pancreatic fistulas, delayed gastric emptying, and infections [21]. The prolonged recovery from surgical resection is not uncommon and can be an impediment to the successful administration of planned adjuvant therapy. Analysis of the Surveillance, Epidemiologic, and End Results (SEER) database suggests that 50 % of patients who are treated with a surgery-first approach fail to receive adjuvant therapy [27]. Given the high risk of developing metastatic disease even among patients with localized PDAC, a reliance on adjuvant therapy to treat micrometastatic disease is unrealistic as it can only be successfully administered to half of the patients.

Rationale for Neoadjuvant Therapy

To address the limitations of adjuvant therapy, a growing interest has emerged in alternative treatment sequencing. Neoadjuvant therapy for PDAC has several theoretical advantages over adjuvant therapy (summarized in Table 6.2). In contrast to an adjuvant approach, neoadjuvant therapy ensures the delivery of all components of multimodality treatment to all patients who undergo a potentially curative pancreatectomy. Importantly, since neoadjuvant therapy offers an "induction" phase lasting approximately 2–3 months, individuals with unfavorable tumor biology who develop early metastatic disease are identified prior to surgery. Importantly, in the subset of patients (up to 20–30 %) who are found to have disease progression after neoadjuvant therapy (before surgery), the morbidity of an operation is avoided. For those patients who are found to have disease progression after neoadjuvant therapy, at the time of preoperative restaging, a major operation is avoided; an operation which, in retrospect, would have resulted in early disease recurrence if a surgery first treatment approach had been used. Such patients benefit greatly from their accurate identification as a subset having accelerated tumor growth not responsive to a local therapy such as surgery. When chemoradiation is utilized as part of neoadjuvant therapy, the delivery of chemoradiation in a well-oxygenated environment improves the efficacy of radiation and decreases the toxicity to adjacent normal tissue [28, 29]. The addition of radiation has important pathologic implications with several series reporting decreased rates of positive margins and node positive disease [30–32].

Experience with neoadjuvant chemoradiation for patients with resectable PDAC suggests a survival benefit for those who complete neoadjuvant therapy and undergo successful resection of the primary tumor as compared to patients treated with a surgery first strategy who receive postoperative adjuvant therapy [33, 34]. Two clinical trials involving patients with resectable PDAC who received neoadjuvant chemoradiation and pancreaticoduodenectomy reported median survivals approaching 3 years as compared to approximately 2 years for those who complete adjuvant therapy after a surgery first approach, and less than 2 years for those who fail to receive adjuvant therapy after pancreaticoduodenectomy [20, 21, 33, 34]. In part, the survival advantage observed in the patients who were treated with a neoadjuvant approach is due to the identification of those patients with disease progression (aggressive tumor biology) after induction therapy and before surgery which removes them from consideration of pancreaticoduodenectomy. In addition, theoretical advantages of neoadjuvant treatment sequencing include the treatment of micrometastases when they are radiographically occult and perhaps more sensitive to systemic therapy, and at a time when host defenses and innate immune surveillance have not been impaired by the stress of a major operation (as systemic therapy/chemoradiation is delivered prior to surgery).

At the author's institution, outside of a clinical trial, patients with resectable PDAC are recommended to receive neoadjuvant chemoradiation based on the report of Evans and colleagues [33]. Radiosensitizing chemotherapy is given concurrently with external beam radiation over a course of 28 fractions (lasting approximately 5.5 weeks). Restaging imaging and labs are obtained approximately 4 weeks after the last radiation dose, and in the absence of disease progression, patients are offered surgical resection. Since patients with borderline resectable PDAC are at higher risk for harboring radiographically occult distant metastases, a longer period of induction therapy is recommended for these patients. At the author's institution, patients with borderline resectable PDAC receive 2 months of chemotherapy followed by chemoradiation. Restaging imaging and labs are obtained after 2 months of induction chemotherapy and again following the completion of chemoradiation.

Importantly, multidisciplinary care is crucial in the coordinated management of PDAC. The scope of the multidisciplinary team is vast and includes medical, surgical, and radiation oncologists, diagnostic radiologists, advanced endoscopists, genetic counselors, dietitians, and endocrine specialists, all of whom play an important role in minimizing the toxicities associated with the treatment and with care coordination. All patients with PDAC undergoing neoadjuvant therapy should be reviewed at each restaging in a multidisciplinary conference to assure timely coordination of care, accurate staging, and optimal treatment planning.

Question 3: What Is Ampullary Cancer and How Is It Different from PDAC?

Answer: Ampullary cancers, or ampulla of Vater adenocarcinomas (AVAC) are neoplasms arising from within the epithelium of the ampulla of Vater. It is the second most common cancer in the periampullary region, after PDAC. Though the surgical management of ampullary and PDAC is the same (pancreaticoduodenectomy), patients with ampullary cancer who undergo a curative surgical resection have a much better prognosis.

Ampulla of Vater Adenocarcinoma

AVACs are relatively uncommon, accounting for less than 1 % of gastrointestinal cancers. Although most AVAC are sporadic, patients with familial adenomatous polyposis (FAP) have an incidence of AVAC which has been reported to range from 3 to 12 %, and the genotype of the adenomatous polyposis gene mutation can predict the clinical risk of AVAC [35]. AVACs have a higher incidence among men and due to the anatomic location, patients will often develop symptoms with small tumors, allowing for earlier detection than in the case of PDAC [4]. In addition, patients with AVAC may have a more favorable disease prognosis than patients with PDAC due both to earlier diagnosis and more favorable tumor biology. For patients with ampullary cancer who undergo a curative surgical resection, single institutional data would suggest a 5-year survival rate as high as 68 %, compared to a 20 % 5-year survival rate in patients with PDAC who undergo multimodality therapy to include a curative surgical resection [20, 36].

Initial Evaluation of a Patient with PDAC

The clinical presentation of AVAC is quite similar to that seen in PDAC [37]. Symptoms that are highly predictive of malignancy include dark urine, pruritus, and jaundice [37]. Other symptoms include nausea and vomiting, abdominal pain, pruritus, and occult gastrointestinal bleeding. The diagnostic work up should include the following laboratory studies: CBC, BMP, hepatic function panel, CA19-9, and carcinoembryonic antigen (CEA). As with PDAC, a dual phase CT scan is essential in the diagnosis and staging of AVAC. Unlike PDAC, AVAC are generally small, may not involve the adjacent pancreatic head, and can frequently be missed by CT imaging alone [38]. Additionally, endoscopic retrograde cholangiopancreatography (ERCP) is very helpful in the diagnosis of AVAC. ERCP allows for direct visualization of the tumor site, which helps to distinguish AVAC from PDAC, and enables tissue biopsy of the papilla and ampullary segments of the pancreatic duct and common bile duct [39]. In addition, endoscopic ultrasound (EUS) has significantly improved diagnostic accuracy as compared to a dual phase CT scan, with reported 100 % positive predictive value and 61 % negative predictive value [40].

The staging system for ampullary cancer is based on the criteria developed by American Joint Cancer Committee (AJCC), and is summarized in Table 6.3. As compared to PDAC, in which the tumor stage is defined by tumor size and tumor extension to vascular structures, the tumor stage for AVAC is defined by the extent of tumor growth into the duodenum, pancreas, or peripancreatic soft tissues (Table 6.3). As expected, pathologic stage is correlated with survival; negative prognostic factors include greater tumor stage (T3-T4) and node positive disease (N1) [41]. In a recent analysis of the SEER database, which included 421 patients with T1 AVAC, only 163 patients had nodes removed for staging, and of these patients, 33 (22 %) had lymph node metastases, suggesting that even small AVACs have a high risk of nodal metastases [42].

Treatment of AVAC

Due to the rarity of the tumor, the management of AVACs has been most frequently reported as retrospective single-institution case reports. Consensus guidelines do not exist to guide the management of AVAC, which has largely been extrapolated from the management of duodenal and pancreaticobiliary cancers. While endoscopic techniques have been described for the management of small benign ampullary adenomas, for AVAC, surgical resection remains the locoregional therapy of choice for patients with localized disease. Surgical resection with a pancreaticoduodenectomy ensures negative margins and adequate lymph node sampling for optimal adequate staging [37, 42].

TABLE 6.3 AJCC AVAC Staging [5]

Primary tumor (T)			
Tx		Primary tumor cannot be assessed	
T0		No evidence of primary tumor	
Tis		Carcinoma in situ	
T1		Tumor confined in the ampulla of Vater or sphincter of Oddi	
T2		Tumor involves the duodenal wall	
T3		Tumor invades pancreas	
T4		Tumor invades peripancreatic soft tissue or other organs	
Regional lymph nodes (N)			
Nx		Regional lymph nodes cannot be assessed	
N0		No regional lymph node metastasis	
N1		Regional lymph node metastasis	
Distant metastasis (M)			
M0		No distant metastasis	
M1		Distant metastasis	
Anatomic stage/prognostic groups			
Stage 0	Tis	N0	M0
Stage IA	T1	N0	M0
Stage IB	T2	N0	M0
Stage IIA	T3	N0	M0
Stage IIB	T1	N1	M0
	T2	N1	M0
	T3	N1	M0
Stage III	T4	Any N	M0
Stage IV	Any T	Any N	M1

Recurrence rates following surgical resection have been reported to range from 15 to 38 % for locoregional recurrences and 15–40 % for metastatic progression [36, 43, 44]. No prospective study has been performed which has evaluated the benefit of adjuvant therapy for AVAC, although some studies have included AVAC in evaluating the role of adjuvant therapy in periampullary tumors. The largest study, European Study Group for Pancreatic Cancer (ESPAC 3), contained the largest proportion of patients with AVAC of any prospective randomized study (with ~70 % of patients enrolled having AVAC); 192 patients with AVAC received adjuvant chemotherapy and 105 patients were observed [45]. Of all patients on the trial, approximately 50 % had T3 or T4 tumors and 60 % had lymph node metastases. The overall median survival of all patients who received no adjuvant therapy was 35.2 months, as compared to 43.1 months for patients in the chemotherapy arms, but this did not reach statistical significance ($p = 0.25$). However, after adjusting for other prognostic factors, the authors concluded that there was a modest benefit of adjuvant therapy for periampullary cancers. Importantly, the median survival for patients with AVAC in this trial was 53.1 months. Other large single-institution studies have demonstrated 5-year survival rates for patients with AVAC of approximately 40 % following pancreaticoduodenectomy [46, 47]. The role of adjuvant chemotherapy and radiation therapy in the management of patients with AVAC remains controversial and to date there are no published guidelines regarding the use of adjuvant therapy. However, based on collective single-institution experiences, adjuvant therapy should be considered in patients with node positive disease or T3/T4 tumors [48, 49].

One important observation from the ESPAC-3 trial was the demonstration of the challenges in administering adjuvant therapy after major pancreatic resection. Of the 289 patients randomized to receive adjuvant chemotherapy, 44 (15 %) never received any adjuvant therapy and only 140 (48 %) received all of the six planned cycles of chemotherapy. As with PDAC, the benefits of neoadjuvant treatment sequencing may be beneficial for patients with AVAC, particularly if at diagnosis, the patients have large (T3/T4) tumors (for example, evidence of pancreatic invasion on CT or EUS) or evidence of lymph node metastases.

Conclusions

Management of patients with PDAC and AVAC starts with careful staging evaluation and the coordinated treatment planning of a multidisciplinary team. Given the magnitude of surgical interventions, adjuvant therapy may not be feasible in many patients. Therefore, consideration of neoadjuvant therapy has practical appeal and oncologic advantages, and allows patients to most effectively receive stage appropriate therapies while minimizing the toxicities of unnecessary surgery.

References

1. Jemal A, Bray F, Center MM, Ferlay J, Ward E, Forman D. Global cancer statistics. CA Cancer J Clin. 2011;61(2):69–90.
2. Pancreatic Adenocarcinoma 2015 [updated Version 2.2015. Available from: http://www.nccn.org/professionals/physician_gls/pdf/pancreatic.pdf.
3. Sohal DP, Walsh RM, Ramanathan RK, Khorana AA. Pancreatic adenocarcinoma: treating a systemic disease with systemic therapy. J Natl Cancer Inst. 2014;106(3):dju011.
4. Goodman MT, Yamamoto J. Descriptive study of gallbladder, extrahepatic bile duct, and ampullary cancers in the United States, 1997–2002. Cancer Causes Control. 2007;18(4):415–22.
5. AJCC Cancer Staging Manual. 7th ed. In: Edge S, Byrd DR, Compton CC, Fritz AG, Greene FL, Trotti A, editors. New York: Springer-Verlag; 2010. p. 648.
6. McIntyre CA, Winter JM. Diagnostic evaluation and staging of pancreatic ductal adenocarcinoma. Semin Oncol. 2015;42(1):19–27.
7. Canto MI, Harinck F, Hruban RH, Offerhaus GJ, Poley JW, Kamel I, et al. International Cancer of the Pancreas Screening (CAPS) Consortium summit on the management of patients

with increased risk for familial pancreatic cancer. Gut. 2013; 62(3):339–47.

8. Ferrone CR, Finkelstein DM, Thayer SP, Muzikansky A, Fernandez-delCastillo C, Warshaw AL. Perioperative CA19-9 levels can predict stage and survival in patients with resectable pancreatic adenocarcinoma. J Clin Oncol. 2006;24(18): 2897–902.

9. Barton JG, Bois JP, Sarr MG, Wood CM, Qin R, Thomsen KM, et al. Predictive and prognostic value of CA 19–9 in resected pancreatic adenocarcinoma. J Gastrointest Surg. 2009;13(11): 2050–8.

10. Hartwig W, Strobel O, Hinz U, Fritz S, Hackert T, Roth C, et al. CA19-9 in potentially resectable pancreatic cancer: perspective to adjust surgical and perioperative therapy. Ann Surg Oncol. 2013;20(7):2188–96.

11. Tempero MA, Uchida E, Takasaki H, Burnett DA, Steplewski Z, Pour PM. Relationship of carbohydrate antigen 19–9 and Lewis antigens in pancreatic cancer. Cancer Res. 1987;47(20):5501–3.

12. Mann DV, Edwards R, Ho S, Lau WY, Glazer G. Elevated tumour marker CA19-9: clinical interpretation and influence of obstructive jaundice. Eur J Surg Oncol. 2000;26(5):474–9.

13. Raman SP, Horton KM, Fishman EK. Multimodality imaging of pancreatic cancer-computed tomography, magnetic resonance imaging, and positron emission tomography. Cancer J. 2012; 18(6):511–22.

14. Tran Cao HS, Balachandran A, Wang H, Nogueras-Gonzalez GM, Bailey CE, Lee JE, et al. Radiographic tumor-vein interface as a predictor of intraoperative, pathologic, and oncologic outcomes in resectable and borderline resectable pancreatic cancer. J Gastrointest Surg. 2014;18(2):269–78. discussion 78.

15. Chun YS, Milestone BN, Watson JC, Cohen SJ, Burtness B, Engstrom PF, et al. Defining venous involvement in borderline resectable pancreatic cancer. Ann Surg Oncol. 2010;17(11): 2832–8.

16. Tseng JF, Raut CP, Lee JE, Pisters PW, Vauthey JN, Abdalla EK, et al. Pancreaticoduodenectomy with vascular resection: margin status and survival duration. J Gastrointest Surg. 2004;8(8):935– 49. discussion 49–50.

17. Nakao A, Takeda S, Inoue S, Nomoto S, Kanazumi N, Sugimoto H, et al. Indications and techniques of extended resection for pancreatic cancer. World J Surg. 2006;30(6):976–82. discussion 83–4.

18. Pancreatic adenocarcinoma. NCCN Clinical Practice Guidelines in Oncology (NCCN guidelines) 2012; http://www.nccn.org/professionals/physician_gls/pdf/pancreatic.pdf.

19. Katz MH, Pisters PW, Evans DB, Sun CC, Lee JE, Fleming JB, et al. Borderline resectable pancreatic cancer: the importance of this emerging stage of disease. J Am Coll Surg. 2008;206(5):833–46. discussion 46–8.

20. Winter JM, Brennan MF, Tang LH, D'Angelica MI, Dematteo RP, Fong Y, et al. Survival after resection of pancreatic adenocarcinoma: results from a single institution over three decades. Ann Surg Oncol. 2012;19(1):169–75.

21. Winter JM, Cameron JL, Campbell KA, Arnold MA, Chang DC, Coleman J, et al. 1423 pancreaticoduodenectomies for pancreatic cancer: A single-institution experience. J Gastrointest Surg. 2006;10(9):1199–210. discussion 210–1.

22. Oettle H, Neuhaus P, Hochhaus A, Hartmann JT, Gellert K, Ridwelski K, et al. Adjuvant chemotherapy with gemcitabine and long-term outcomes among patients with resected pancreatic cancer: the CONKO-001 randomized trial. JAMA. 2013;310(14):1473–81.

23. Klinkenbijl JH, Jeekel J, Sahmoud T, van Pel R, Couvreur ML, Veenhof CH, et al. Adjuvant radiotherapy and 5-fluorouracil after curative resection of cancer of the pancreas and periampullary region: phase III trial of the EORTC gastrointestinal tract cancer cooperative group. Ann Surg. 1999;230(6):776–82. discussion 82–4.

24. Evans DB, Farnell MB, Lillemoe KD, Vollmer Jr C, Strasberg SM, Schulick RD. Surgical treatment of resectable and borderline resectable pancreas cancer: expert consensus statement. Ann Surg Oncol. 2009;16(7):1736–44.

25. Tempero MA, Arnoletti JP, Behrman S, Ben-Josef E, Benson 3rd AB, Berlin JD, et al. Pancreatic adenocarcinoma. J Natl Compr Cancer Netw. 2010;8(9):972–1017.

26. Swanson RS, Pezzi CM, Mallin K, Loomis AM, Winchester DP. The 90-Day Mortality After Pancreatectomy for Cancer Is Double the 30-Day Mortality: More than 20,000 Resections From the National Cancer Data Base. Annals of surgical oncology. 2014.

27. Mayo SC, Gilson MM, Herman JM, Cameron JL, Nathan H, Edil BH, et al. Management of patients with pancreatic adenocarcinoma: national trends in patient selection, operative management, and use of adjuvant therapy. J Am Coll Surg. 2012;214(1):33–45.

28. Evans DB, Rich TA, Byrd DR, Cleary KR, Connelly JH, Levin B, et al. Preoperative chemoradiation and pancreaticoduodenectomy for adenocarcinoma of the pancreas. Arch Surg. 1992;127(11):1335–9.
29. Pilepich MV, Miller HH. Preoperative irradiation in carcinoma of the pancreas. Cancer. 1980;46(9):1945–9.
30. Takahashi H, Ogawa H, Ohigashi H, Gotoh K, Yamada T, Ohue M, et al. Preoperative chemoradiation reduces the risk of pancreatic fistula after distal pancreatectomy for pancreatic adenocarcinoma. Surgery. 2011;150(3):547–56.
31. Raut CP, Evans DB, Crane CH, Pisters PW, Wolff RA. Neoadjuvant therapy for resectable pancreatic cancer. Surg Oncol Clin N Am. 2004;13(4):639–61. ix.
32. Willett CG, Lewandrowski K, Warshaw AL, Efird J, Compton CC. Resection margins in carcinoma of the head of the pancreas. Implications for radiation therapy. Ann Surg. 1993;217(2): 144–8.
33. Evans DB, Varadhachary GR, Crane CH, Sun CC, Lee JE, Pisters PW, et al. Preoperative gemcitabine-based chemoradiation for patients with resectable adenocarcinoma of the pancreatic head. J Clin Oncol. 2008;26(21):3496–502.
34. Varadhachary GR, Wolff RA, Crane CH, Sun CC, Lee JE, Pisters PW, et al. Preoperative gemcitabine and cisplatin followed by gemcitabine-based chemoradiation for resectable adenocarcinoma of the pancreatic head. J Clin Oncol. 2008; 26(21):3487–95.
35. Bjork J, Akerbrant H, Iselius L, Bergman A, Engwall Y, Wahlstrom J, et al. Periampullary adenomas and adenocarcinomas in familial adenomatous polyposis: cumulative risks and APC gene mutations. Gastroenterology. 2001;121(5):1127–35.
36. Showalter TN, Zhan T, Anne PR, Chervoneva I, Mitchell EP, Yeo CJ, et al. The influence of prognostic factors and adjuvant chemoradiation on survival after pancreaticoduodenectomy for ampullary carcinoma. J Gastrointest Surg. 2011;15(8):1411–6.
37. Hornick JR, Johnston FM, Simon PO, Younkin M, Chamberlin M, Mitchem JB, et al. A single-institution review of 157 patients presenting with benign and malignant tumors of the ampulla of Vater: management and outcomes. Surgery. 2011;150(2):169–76.
38. Raman SP, Fishman EK. Abnormalities of the distal common bile duct and ampulla: diagnostic approach and differential diagnosis using multiplanar reformations and 3D imaging. AJR Am J Roentgenol. 2014;203(1):17–28.

39. Panzeri F, Crippa S, Castelli P, Aleotti F, Pucci A, Partelli S, et al. Management of ampullary neoplasms: a tailored approach between endoscopy and surgery. World J Gastroenterol. 2015;21(26):7970–87.
40. Tran TC, Vitale GC. Ampullary tumors: endoscopic versus operative management. Surg Innov. 2004;11(4):255–63.
41. Sessa F, Furlan D, Zampatti C, Carnevali I, Franzi F, Capella C. Prognostic factors for ampullary adenocarcinomas: tumor stage, tumor histology, tumor location, immunohistochemistry and microsatellite instability. Virchows Arch. 2007;451(3):649–57.
42. Amini A, Miura JT, Jayakrishnan TT, Johnston FM, Tsai S, Christians KK, et al. Is local resection adequate for T1 stage ampullary cancer? HPB. 2015;17(1):66–71.
43. Jabbour SK, Mulvihill D. Defining the role of adjuvant therapy: ampullary and duodenal adenocarcinoma. Semin Radiat Oncol. 2014;24(2):85–93.
44. Woo SM, Ryu JK, Lee SH, Yoo JW, Park JK, Kim YT, et al. Recurrence and prognostic factors of ampullary carcinoma after radical resection: comparison with distal extrahepatic cholangiocarcinoma. Ann Surg Oncol. 2007;14(11):3195–201.
45. Neoptolemos JP, Moore MJ, Cox TF, Valle JW, Palmer DH, McDonald AC, et al. Effect of adjuvant chemotherapy with fluorouracil plus folinic acid or gemcitabine vs observation on survival in patients with resected periampullary adenocarcinoma: the ESPAC-3 periampullary cancer randomized trial. JAMA. 2012;308(2):147–56.
46. Winter JM, Cameron JL, Olino K, Herman JM, de Jong MC, Hruban RH, et al. Clinicopathologic analysis of ampullary neoplasms in 450 patients: implications for surgical strategy and long-term prognosis. J Gastrointest Surg. 2010;14(2):379–87.
47. Hsu HP, Yang TM, Hsieh YH, Shan YS, Lin PW. Predictors for patterns of failure after pancreaticoduodenectomy in ampullary cancer. Ann Surg Oncol. 2007;14(1):50–60.
48. Zhou J, Hsu CC, Winter JM, Pawlik TM, Laheru D, Hughes MA, et al. Adjuvant chemoradiation versus surgery alone for adenocarcinoma of the ampulla of Vater. Radiother Oncol. 2009;92(2):244–8.
49. Krishnan S, Rana V, Evans DB, Varadhachary G, Das P, Bhatia S, et al. Role of adjuvant chemoradiation therapy in adenocarcinomas of the ampulla of vater. Int J Radiat Oncol Biol Phys. 2008;70(3):735–43.

Part 3
Clinical Scenario: Incidental Finding on CT/Dizziness/Secretary Diarrhea/Skin Rash

Chapter 7
Neuroendocrine Tumors of the Pancreas

George Younan, Susan Tsai, Douglas B. Evans, and Kathleen K. Christians

What Are Pancreatic Neuroendocrine Tumors (PNETs) and Are They Cancer?

Suggested Response to the Patient

Pancreatic tumors are classified by the pancreatic cell of origin from which the tumor arose [1]. The pancreas contains multiple nests of endocrine cells known as the islet cells of Langerhans. These islets are found scattered throughout the pancreas. Individual cell types secrete specific hormones; for example, beta cells produce insulin whereas alpha cells produce glucagon. Tumors originating from those endocrine cells, once termed "islet cell tumors", are now referred to as neuroendocrine tumors of the pancreas (or pancreatic neuroendocrine tumors [PNET]).

While all adenocarcinomas of the pancreas are considered malignant (cancer is a synonym for malignant), in order to consider a PNET malignant, it must demonstrate metastatic

G. Younan • S. Tsai, M.D., M.H.S. • D.B. Evans, M.D.
K.K. Christians, M.D. (✉)
Department of Surgery, Division of Surgical Oncology,
Medical College of Wisconsin, 9200 W Wisconsin Ave.,
Milwaukee, WI 53226, USA
e-mail: kchristi@mcw.edu

© Springer International Publishing Switzerland 2016
K. Dua, R. Shaker (eds.), *Pancreas and Biliary Disease*,
DOI 10.1007/978-3-319-28089-9_7

spread to regional lymph nodes or distant sites. Except for sporadic insulinomas which are isolated to the pancreas at the time of diagnosis (and are uniformly benign with no ability to metastasize), all other PNETs, if given enough time, will likely demonstrate malignant behavior. However, non-metastatic PNETs can be graded in terms of their biological aggressiveness (potential for metastatic behavior) [2]. PNETs have a wide range of clinical behaviors and the prognosis can be multifactorial, relating to the site of origin, functional status and specific tumor characteristics [3]. Due to this variability, a uniform pathologic classification was published by the World Health Organization in 2010 (Table 7.1). It was based on tumor characteristics including grade and Ki-67 value of the primary tumor; the latter being a measure of tumor proliferation [3–5]. Tumors were classified into three broad categories based on their malignant potential/prognosis: benign/uncertain, low, and high malignant potential. Such a classification is commonly referred to as well-differentiated endocrine tumors, well-differentiated endocrine carcinomas, and poorly differentiated endocrine carcinomas [4]. Risk factors of aggressiveness include size, degree of cell proliferation, whether or not the tumor has invaded surrounding structures or blood vessels and the presence of tumor spread to distant organs [5, 6].

Brief Review of the Literature

Approximately 49,000 people were diagnosed with pancreas cancer in the USA in 2014. However, only 2–4 % of those had

TABLE 7.1   THE WORLD HEALTH ORGANIZATION CLASSIFICATION OF PNETS

Differentiation	Grade	Mitotic count	Ki-67 index (%)
Well differentiated	Low grade (G1)	<2 per 10 HPF	<3
Well differentiated	Intermediate grade (G2)	2–20 per 10 HPF	3–20
Poorly differentiated	High grade (G3)	>20 per 10 HPF	>20

a PNET, for an incidence of 1–2/100,000 people [7, 8]. PNETs may be sporadic in inheritance or less commonly, run in families. Multiple Endocrine Neoplasia type 1 (MEN1) is a genetic syndrome that results in tumors of the pituitary gland, parathyroids, and the pancreas. PNETs can also occur in (1) Von Hippel–Lindau (VHL) syndrome which also includes tumors of the central nervous system, the kidneys and the adrenals, (2) Tuberous Sclerosis Complex (TSC), a disease which also includes tumors in the brain, kidneys, skin, and eyes, and (3) Neurofibromatosis type 1 (NF-1), a condition where tumors grow along the nerves in the skin, brain, and internal organs.

PNETs are classified according to their ability to secrete hormones and, if they do, the type of hormone that is produced. Tumors that do not produce hormones (nonfunctional) are the most common type and constitute 70–80 % of PNETs. Most of the symptoms that nonfunctional PNETs cause are due to the local effects of the tumor itself [9]. In contrast, functional tumors, which make up 20–30 % of PNETs, overproduce specific hormones [1]. For example, endocrine cells of the pancreas produce insulin and glucagon, two hormones involved in regulating blood sugar, in addition to many other digestive and metabolic properties. Gastrin, somatostatin, and vasoactive intestinal peptide (VIP) are three other hormones also produced by endocrine cells of the pancreas. Tumors originating from these cells are called insulinoma, glucagonoma, gastrinoma, somatostatinoma, and VIPoma, respectively (Table 7.2) [7].

How Are PNETs Diagnosed?

Diagnosis of PNETs includes two general objectives: a biochemical evaluation and localization of the tumor. Neuroendocrine tumors of the pancreas have a broad range of clinical presentations. Functional tumors usually present with signs and symptoms of overproduction of a specific hormone. Nonfunctional tumors are either found incidentally on imaging studies done for other reasons or cause local symptoms due to compression/obstruction of other organs or blood vessels. Patient history and physical examination are the first and one of the most important parts of the initial patient encounter. Nonspecific symptoms of abdominal pain, fatigue and weakness may be present but usually the patient is asymptomatic or has just recently become symptomatic. A high index of suspicion for familial syndromes is imperative in all patients diagnosed with a PNET and in patients with a positive family history, evaluation for the associated tumor constellation should be undertaken.

Brief Review of the Literature

Functional Tumors

The most common functional PNET is an *insulinom a* which is usually sporadic in inheritance and benign (90 %). Rarely, insulinomas are part of the MEN-1 syndrome (pancreas, pituitary, parathyroid) in which case they are usually multifocal within the pancreas. Patients usually present with signs and symptoms of hypoglycemia caused by high insulin levels. These "neuroglycopenic" symptoms may include weakness, excessive perspiration, palpitations, altered mental status, seizures, and in severe cases, coma [10]. A 72-h controlled fast measuring blood glucose and insulin levels drawn at regular intervals is often diagnostic for insulinomas. One has to always exclude the rare circumstance where a patient has factitiously low blood glucose levels due to administration of exogenous insulin or diabetes medications of the sulfonylurea class [11]. Insulin is synthesized as a larger molecule called proinsulin. The latter is cleaved and processed inside beta cells into insulin and C-peptide. A high level of insulin and absence of C-peptide on blood tests is consistent with factitious hypoglycemia, usually found in health care workers who have access to insulin. Insulinomas are usually hypervascular, well-circumscribed, solitary masses on axial imaging and can be found in any part of the pancreas. They are usually

TABLE 7.2   FUNCTIONAL CLASSIFICATION OF PNETs

Tumor name	Pancreas cell	Hormone	Malignancy %	Location	Size
Insulinoma	Alpha	Insulin	10–15	Pancreas any part	<2 cm in 90 %
Glucagonoma	Beta	Glucagon	60	Pancreas body, tail	Large
Gastrinoma	G-cell	Gastrin	60–75	Gastrinoma triangle (mostly duodenum)	<3 cm
Somatostatinoma	D-cell	Somatostatin	50–70	Pancreas head	Large
VIPoma	D2-cell	VIP	50–80	Pancreas tail	Large
Nonfunctioning	D1-cell	None	60–90	Pancreas, (mostly head)	Variable

small in size and are less than 2 cm in the majority of the cases [12, 13]. They can be multifocal in MEN-1 syndrome, thus the importance of examining the pancreas for other smaller lesions at the time of initial diagnostic imaging (and the importance of knowing whether the patient does or does not have MEN1 before operation).

Gastrinoma is the second most common PNET and the most common PNET found in MEN-1 patients; one third of gastrinoma patients have a hereditary endocrinopathy. High blood levels of gastrin are seen in Zollinger–Ellison Syndrome, in which patients present with intractable ulcers. Excessive stimulation of parietal cells in the body of the stomach by gastrin leads to high levels of acid secretion. These ulcers tend to be hard to treat, occur in young patients and arise in unusual locations (jejunal) [14]. Associated symptoms include abdominal pain, nausea and diarrhea, and weight loss. Gastrinomas can be diagnosed by measuring serum levels of gastrin with and without stimulation by the hormone secretin. Secretin, under normal circumstances, suppresses gastrin secretion; however, in gastrinoma patients, it stimulates gastrin production to very high levels. Gastrinomas are historically known to be found in an area referred to as the "gastrinoma triangle," especially when unifocal and sporadic in nature. The gastrinoma triangle is anatomically defined by the junction of the cystic and common hepatic ducts superiorly, the junction of the neck and body of the pancreas medially, and the area between the second and third portion of the duodenum inferiorly [15].

Glucagonomas secrete high levels of glucagon. Typical clinical manifestations include new onset diabetes, diarrhea, deep vein or arterial thrombosis, weight loss, abdominal pain, depression, and dermatitis. Approximately 70 % of glucagonoma patients have a characteristic rash referred to as "necrolytic migratory erythema," an eruption that occurs in areas of friction on the body such as buttocks, groin and feet [16]. Patients with glucagonoma present with elevated blood glucose and glucagon levels, anemia, and low protein levels as these proteins are used to make glucose. Most glucagonomas are found in the body and tail of the pancreas and tend to be large in size.

Somatostatinomas are rare PNETs and are usually malignant. Somatostatin is known to be the universal inhibitor hormone. It inhibits actions of insulin and gastrin, and pancreatic exocrine enzymes, leading to high blood sugar levels, gallstones, and malabsorption of ingested food leading to diarrhea [17]. Somatostatinomas tend to be large and are located mainly in the pancreatic head [12].

VIP tumors are also rare PNETs which are mostly benign and solitary. Excess VIP hormone secretion is associated with a cluster of symptoms that have been named Verner–Morrison syndrome. This syndrome includes diarrhea, low serum potassium and low gastric acid secretion [18]. The majority of VIPomas are found in the tail of the pancreas [12].

Nonfunctional Tumors

Nonfunctional PNETs do not produce clinically active hormones; however, they are known to secrete peptides such as pancreatic polypeptide, neurotensin, chromogranin A, and neuron-specific enolase. Chromogranin A, in particular, can be clinically helpful as a tumor marker to guide treatment and signal recurrence and disease progression; it is present in 60–100 % of nonfunctioning PNETs [19–21]. Any PNET can cause signs and symptoms of local tumor compression of adjacent organs depending on the size and the location of the primary tumor. Tumors of the head of the pancreas can cause obstruction of the common bile duct which can lead to jaundice, pruritus, acholic stools, and dark urine. Tumors of the body and tail of the pancreas often grow to reach large sizes before causing local symptoms.

Tumor localization and extent of disease are key to the diagnosis and treatment of patients with PNETs. Localized, unifocal disease is treated differently than multifocal and metastatic disease. Traditional imaging techniques using ultrasound (US), computed tomography (CT), magnetic resonance imaging (MRI), positron emission tomography (PET), or radiolabeled octreotide scans have been the mainstay for localizing PNETs. New endoscopic and nuclear imaging technologies are also now part of the available armamentarium. Upper endoscopy is augmented by the use of an ultrasound probe on the tip of the endoscope, otherwise termed an "endoscopic ultrasound" (EUS). This can provide improved visualization of the tumor and surrounding lymph nodes compared to transabdominal ultrasound. EUS is especially useful for detection of small tumors and/or multiple tumors in patients with MEN1. Additionally, when indicated, EUS can be utilized to perform a fine needle aspiration (FNA). The aspirate (EUS-FNA biopsy) is considered a biopsy of the tumor and has a high sensitivity for diagnosing a PNET [22, 23]. Transabdominal ultrasound (U/S) detects PNETs only 40 % of the time as it is not very sensitive for detecting small tumors or regional lymph node metastases, but it is highly specific for PNETs if found [12]. PNETs appear as a well-defined circular mass that is darker than the surrounding pancreas and is well vascularized when Doppler mode is used [24].

Computed tomography (CT) and magnetic resonance imaging (MRI) are comparable and identify at least 70–75 % of pancreatic neuroendocrine tumors; a number which is increasing with improved technology. They have the advantage of detecting extrapancreatic lesions (liver metastases) with an 85–90 % detection rate. Neuroendocrine tumors are hypervascular and therefore best detected during the early arterial phase of a dual phase CT scan, when the tumor-to-pancreas contrast is greatest [12, 23, 25]. Nuclear medicine imaging, such as octreotide scans, play a key role in detection of neuroendocrine tumors due to a distinct feature that up to 80 % of these tumors express somatostatin receptors [12, 26]. Figures 7.1 and 7.2 contain classic images of a PNET by CT, MRI, and Octreotide scan of a patient treated at our institution for a pancreas body neuroendocrine tumor.

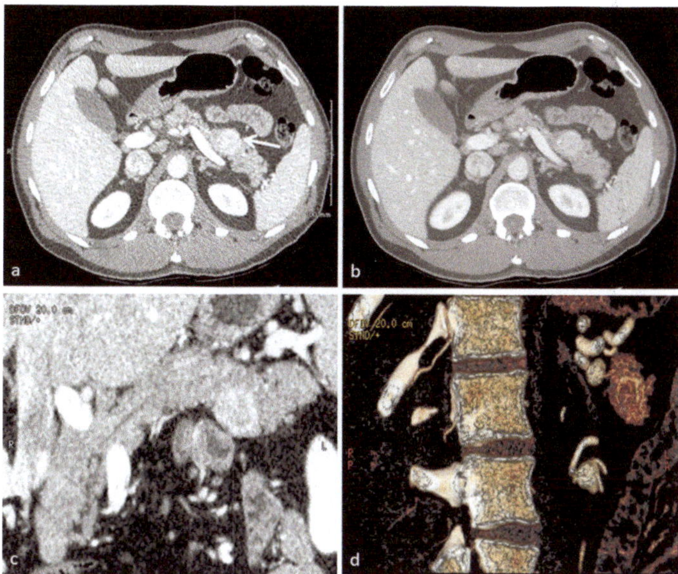

FIG. 7.1 Axial sections of CT scan of a pancreas body neuroendocrine tumor (*white arrow*) seen enhancing in early arterial phase in (**a**), with faded enhancement in the venous phase in (**b**). The same tumor is seen in a coronal section of the arterial phase in (**c**), angiographic 3D reconstruction of the well vascularized tumor seen in (**d**)

How Long Will I Survive? Will I Need Chemotherapy?

Prognosis and Treatment Options for Pancreatic Neuroendocrine Tumors

Suggested Response to the Patient

There has been a tremendous expansion in the available therapies for PNETs over the past decade, in parallel with an increase in the incidental radiological detection of these tumors in younger patients [27, 28]. Relative to pancreatic adenocarcinoma, patients with PNETs are usually long-lived (5-year overall survival of 80 %) [29]. The goal, after initial

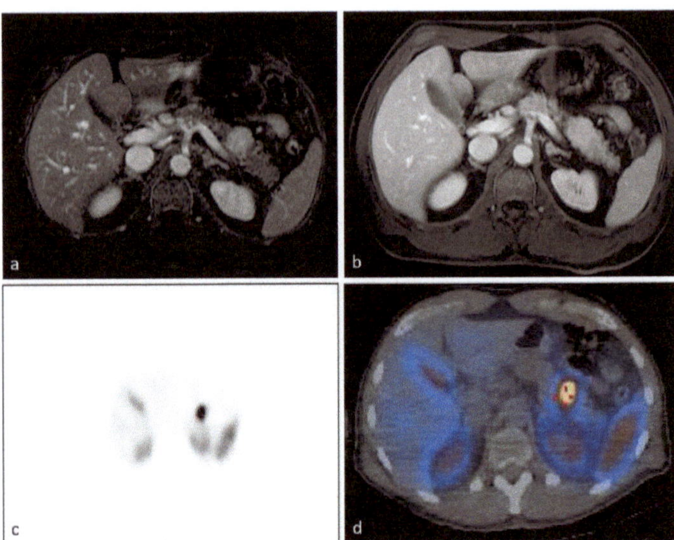

Fɪɢ. 7.2 Axial MRI sections of the same tumor seen in Fig. 7.1, showing increased signal intensity in T2-weighted images in (**a**), and T1-weighted images in (**b**). Octreotide scan images are seen alone (**c**) or fused (**d**), with CT scan that clearly show tumor radiolabel uptake

diagnosis, is to classify and stage each patient's tumor in order to assign the optimal treatment strategy. These cases are usually discussed at multidisciplinary conferences where physicians from multiple disciplines establish the appropriate personalized treatment. Disciplines include surgery, gastro-enterology, radiology, medical and radiation oncology, and transplantation.

Brief Review of the Literature

Symptom Control

In patients with functional PNETs, treatment usually begins by alleviating symptoms due to excess hormone production. Insulinoma treatment includes avoiding episodes of serious hypoglycemia; this can be done with serial glucose monitoring during the day, consumption of multiple small meals, and the use of anti-insulin medications such as Diazoxide, Verapamil, or Dilantin [13]. Medical treatment of gastrinomas is geared toward suppression of gastric acid secretion, and this is successfully done with high dose proton-pump inhibitors. For patients with VIPoma or glucagonomas, diarrhea, elevated glucose levels, and electrolyte abnormalities are treated with supportive care that typically includes insulin, repletion of fluid and electrolyte abnormalities, and close monitoring of nutritional status. Somatostatin analogues (SSA) such as Octreotide have been the mainstay of symptom control for patients with PNETs. Octreotide not only inhibits hormone secretion from these tumors, but also has a tumoristatic effect [30, 31]. Recent trials proved the effectiveness of SSAs for treatment of locally advanced and metastatic PNETs and this has been incorporated into national and international guidelines [32–34]. Local mass effect caused by PNETs in the pancreatic head may cause biliary obstruction, resulting in jaundice and pruritus. Symptomatic relief of these symptoms can be achieved by stenting the obstruction open using endoscopic or percutaneously placed stents [35–37].

Treatment

There has been a rapid expansion in the armamentarium of treatment modalities that can be offered to PNET patients in the last decade. Medical, interventional, and surgical options are available; however, consensus is still lacking on proper treatment sequencing [28]. The key step is to determine the clinical and biological information of the primary tumor and personalize treatment accordingly [38]. Workup is usually started by ruling out metastatic disease. EUS with fine needle aspiration biopsy of the tumor is done to assess for tumor grade and Ki-67 status. The Ki-67 status of the tumor is critically important for the determination of proper treatment.

Since surgery is the only known curative treatment, the next step in management is determining surgical resectability of the tumor. In solitary, low grade tumors, confined to the pancreas, minimally invasive surgery is the current state-of-the-art approach. Laparoscopic and robotic-assisted approaches are now commonly used supported by multiple studies which have proved safety and efficacy [39]. The goal of treatment is to remove the tumor while preserving as much of the pancreas as possible; otherwise known as a "parenchymal preservation" strategy. This allows preservation of endocrine and exocrine function of the pancreas when possible [40–42]. Depending on the location of the tumor and the status of the rest of the pancreas, surgical options may include enucleation, central pancreatectomy, distal pancreatectomy, pancreaticoduodenectomy (Whipple procedure), or total pancreatectomy. Complete surgical resection is also associated with prolonged survival even in the setting of metastatic disease (when the primary and distant sites can all be surgically excised) [29, 43–46]. Unfortunately, a high percentage of patients present with extensive, unresectable tumors and the role of surgery is often limited to symptom control; in such patients, systemic therapy and sandostatin analogue therapy are often the initial choice of treatment [47–51]. Liver transplantation for PNETs is used infrequently, and is controversial [52].

Up to 85 % of patients with PNETs present with synchronous liver metastases or develop metachronous disease to the liver years after the primary tumor was removed [53]. In patients with unresectable, liver dominant disease, several other treatment modalities confer positive outcomes with modest side effects [54]. Liver metastases can be treated with trans-arterial embolization or chemo-embolization (TAE, TACE), radio-embolization, ablation, or in limited cases, external beam radiation [53–59]. TAE or TACE are based on the knowledge that these tumors are supplied by branches of the hepatic artery (rather than the portal venous system). Selective embolization of branches of the hepatic artery with small spheres, with or without chemotherapy is the basis of such procedures. Ablation techniques involve heat (radiofrequency or microwaves) or cold (cryotherapy) [48, 60–63]. Radiation can either be delivered transarterial (yttrium 90) or by external beam. The latter is usually reserved for isolated, unresectable tumors, in anatomically difficult locations that are not amenable to other techniques [64]. One interesting treatment option that is not yet available in the USA includes the use of radiolabeled somatostatin analogues. Radioactive molecules are attached to a somatostatin analogue which binds tumor cells and cytotoxicity is by means of radiation selectively delivered to those cells. This method avoids radiation to normal cells. This technique is referred to as peptide receptor radionuclide therapy (PRRT) [65, 66].

In patients with advanced PNETs, whether metastatic, unresectable, or high grade and poorly differentiated, several systemic therapies have been used. Conventional chemotherapy that included streptozocin (STZ), 5-fluorouracil (5-FU), and doxorubicin used to be the mainstay of treatment in this category of patients. These agents promote tumor cell death through interference with DNA synthesis. Although initially shown to be quite effective, response rates have not been as favorable in more recent reports [33, 34, 67]. New chemotherapeutic agents such as capecitabine and temozolomide have shown more promise with a radiological response rate of up to 70 %, and such agents have even been used to downstage metastatic dsisease for surgical resection [28, 68]. Capecitabine is processed in the liver to produce fluorouracil, a compound that inhibits DNA synthesis in tumor cells. Temozolomide is another cytotoxic agent that gets cleaved into an active metabolite causing tumor cell death through a process of DNA alkylation. In general, chemotherapy is reserved for inoperable disease or to downstage borderline resectable disease thereby facilitating a less difficult operation [67, 69].

Recently, several trials investigated and proved the efficacy of targeted therapies in patients with advanced PNETs. New agents target specific proteins made by PNETs. Of those, everolimus, which belongs to a class of drugs called inhibitors of the mammalian target of Rapamycin (mTOR), has been shown to slow disease progression [70–73]. Sunitinib has been shown to prolong survival by inhibiting vascular endothelial growth factor (VEGF) receptors [74, 75].

Conclusion

The incidence of neuroendocrine tumors of the pancreas is on the rise. PNETs have a wide variety of clinical presentations and biological behaviors. Whereas significant progress has been made in the understanding and classification of these tumors, consensus protocols for treatment sequencing are still somewhat poorly defined. Surgery is the only potentially curative therapy, however, most of these patients present with metastatic disease, and may require a combination of multiple modalities that include cytotoxic chemotherapeutic agents, targeted biological agents, and radio/chemo-embolization.

References

1. Klimstra DS. Nonductal neoplasms of the pancreas. Mod Pathol. 2007;20 Suppl 1:S94–112.
2. Kunz PL, Reidy-Lagunes D, Anthony LB, Bertino EM, Brendtro K, Chan JA, et al. Consensus guidelines for the management and treatment of neuroendocrine tumors. Pancreas. 2013;42(4):557–77. Pubmed Central PMCID: 4304762.
3. Klimstra DS, Modlin IR, Coppola D, Lloyd RV, Suster S. The pathologic classification of neuroendocrine tumors: a review of nomenclature, grading, and staging systems. Pancreas. 2010;39(6):707–12.
4. Kloppel G. Tumour biology and histopathology of neuroendocrine tumours. Best Pract Res Clin Endocrinol Metab. 2007;21(1):15–31.
5. Imamura M. Recent standardization of treatment strategy for pancreatic neuroendocrine tumors. World J Gastroenterol. 2010;16(36):4519–25. Pubmed Central PMCID: 2945482.
6. Kloppel G, Rindi G, Perren A, Komminoth P, Klimstra DS. The ENETS and AJCC/UICC TNM classifications of the neuroendocrine tumors of the gastrointestinal tract and the pancreas: a statement. Virchows Arch. 2010;456(6):595–7.
7. Yao JC, Eisner MP, Leary C, Dagohoy C, Phan A, Rashid A, et al. Population-based study of islet cell carcinoma. Ann Surg Oncol. 2007;14(12):3492–500. Pubmed Central PMCID: 2077912.
8. Yao JC, Hassan M, Phan A, Dagohoy C, Leary C, Mares JE, et al. One hundred years after "carcinoid": epidemiology of and

prognostic factors for neuroendocrine tumors in 35,825 cases in the United States. J Clin Oncol. 2008;26(18):3063–72.

9. Franko J, Feng W, Yip L, Genovese E, Moser AJ. Non-functional neuroendocrine carcinoma of the pancreas: incidence, tumor biology, and outcomes in 2,158 patients. J Gastrointest Surg. 2010;14(3):541–8.

10. Iglesias P, Lafuente C, Martin Almendra MA, Lopez Guzman A, Castro JC, Diez JJ. Insulinoma: a multicenter, retrospective analysis of three decades of experience (1983–2014). Endocrinol Nutr. 2015;62:306–13.

11. Service FJ, Natt N. The prolonged fast. J Clin Endocrinol Metab. 2000;85(11):3973–4.

12. Balachandran A, Tamm EP, Bhosale PR, Patnana M, Vikram R, Fleming JB, et al. Pancreatic neuroendocrine neoplasms: diagnosis and management. Abdom Imaging. 2013;38(2):342–57.

13. Okabayashi T, Shima Y, Sumiyoshi T, Kozuki A, Ito S, Ogawa Y, et al. Diagnosis and management of insulinoma. World J Gastroenterol. 2013;19(6):829–37. Pubmed Central PMCID: 3574879.

14. Jensen RT, Niederle B, Mitry E, Ramage JK, Steinmuller T, Lewington V, et al. Gastrinoma (duodenal and pancreatic). Neuroendocrinology. 2006;84(3):173–82.

15. Stabile BE, Morrow DJ, Passaro Jr E. The gastrinoma triangle: operative implications. Am J Surg. 1984;147(1):25–31.

16. Kovacs RK, Korom I, Dobozy A, Farkas G, Ormos J, Kemeny L. Necrolytic migratory erythema. J Cutan Pathol. 2006;33(3):242–5.

17. Epelboym I, Mazeh H. Zollinger-Ellison syndrome: classical considerations and current controversies. Oncologist. 2014;19(1):44–50. Pubmed Central PMCID: 3903066.

18. Verner JV, Morrison AB. Islet cell tumor and a syndrome of refractory watery diarrhea and hypokalemia. Am J Med. 1958;25(3):374–80.

19. Krampitz GW, Norton JA. Current management of the zollinger-ellison syndrome. Adv Surg. 2013;47(1):59–79.

20. Krampitz GW, Norton JA. Pancreatic neuroendocrine tumors. Curr Probl Surg. 2013;50(11):509–45.

21. Massironi S, Conte D, Sciola V, Spampatti MP, Ciafardini C, Valenti L, et al. Plasma chromogranin A response to octreotide test: prognostic value for clinical outcome in endocrine digestive tumors. Am J Gastroenterol. 2010;105(9):2072–8.

22. Bernstein J, Ustun B, Alomari A, Bao F, Aslanian HR, Siddiqui U, et al. Performance of endoscopic ultrasound-guided fine needle aspiration in diagnosing pancreatic neuroendocrine tumors. Cytojournal. 2013;10:10. Pubmed Central PMCID: 3709383.
23. Mallorca Consensus Conference participants, European Neuroendocrine Tumor Society, Sundin A, Vullierme MP, Kaltsas G, Plockinger U. ENETS consensus guidelines for the standards of care in neuroendocrine tumors: radiological examinations. Neuroendocrinology. 2009;90(2):167–83.
24. Oshikawa O, Tanaka S, Ioka T, Nakaizumi A, Hamada Y, Mitani T. Dynamic sonography of pancreatic tumors: comparison with dynamic CT. AJR Am J Roentgenol. 2002;178(5):1133–7.
25. Rockall AG, Planche K, Power N, Nowosinska E, Monson JP, Grossman AB, et al. Detection of neuroendocrine liver metastases with MnDPDP-enhanced MRI. Neuroendocrinology. 2009;89(3):288–95.
26. Kwekkeboom DJ, Krenning EP. Somatostatin receptor imaging. Semin Nucl Med. 2002;32(2):84–91.
27. Boudreaux JP, Klimstra DS, Hassan MM, Woltering EA, Jensen RT, Goldsmith SJ, et al. The NANETS consensus guideline for the diagnosis and management of neuroendocrine tumors: well-differentiated neuroendocrine tumors of the Jejunum, Ileum, Appendix, and Cecum. Pancreas. 2010;39(6):753–66.
28. Strosberg J. Advances in the treatment of pancreatic neuroendocrine tumors (pNETs). Gastrointest Cancer Res. 2013;6(4 Suppl 1):S10–2. Pubmed Central PMCID: 3849907.
29. Chen H, Hardacre JM, Uzar A, Cameron JL, Choti MA. Isolated liver metastases from neuroendocrine tumors: does resection prolong survival? J Am Coll Surg. 1998;187(1): 88–92. discussion -3.
30. Rinke A, Muller HH, Schade-Brittinger C, Klose KJ, Barth P, Wied M, et al. Placebo-controlled, double-blind, prospective, randomized study on the effect of octreotide LAR in the control of tumor growth in patients with metastatic neuroendocrine midgut tumors: a report from the PROMID Study Group. J Clin Oncol. 2009;27(28):4656–63.
31. Arnold R, Wied M, Behr TH. Somatostatin analogues in the treatment of endocrine tumors of the gastrointestinal tract. Expert Opin Pharmacother. 2002;3(6):643–56.
32. Miljkovic MD, Girotra M, Abraham RR, Erlich RB. Novel medical therapies of recurrent and metastatic gastroenteropancreatic neuroendocrine tumors. Dig Dis Sci. 2012;57(1):9–18.

33. Pavel M, Baudin E, Couvelard A, Krenning E, Oberg K, Steinmuller T, et al. ENETS Consensus Guidelines for the management of patients with liver and other distant metastases from neuroendocrine neoplasms of foregut, midgut, hindgut, and unknown primary. Neuroendocrinology. 2012;95(2):157–76.

34. Kulke MH, Anthony LB, Bushnell DL, de Herder WW, Goldsmith SJ, Klimstra DS, et al. NANETS treatment guidelines: well-differentiated neuroendocrine tumors of the stomach and pancreas. Pancreas. 2010;39(6):735–52. Pubmed Central PMCID: 3100728.

35. van der Gaag NA, Rauws EA, van Eijck CH, Bruno MJ, van der Harst E, Kubben FJ, et al. Preoperative biliary drainage for cancer of the head of the pancreas. N Engl J Med. 2010;362(2):129–37.

36. Aadam AA, Evans DB, Khan A, Oh Y, Dua K. Efficacy and safety of self-expandable metal stents for biliary decompression in patients receiving neoadjuvant therapy for pancreatic cancer: a prospective study. Gastrointest Endosc. 2012;76(1):67–75.

37. Wasan SM, Ross WA, Staerkel GA, Lee JH. Use of expandable metallic biliary stents in resectable pancreatic cancer. Am J Gastroenterol. 2005;100(9):2056–61.

38. Raymond E, Garcia-Carbonero R, Wiedenmann B, Grande E, Pavel M. Systemic therapeutic strategies for GEP-NETS: what can we expect in the future? Cancer Metastasis Rev. 2014;33(1):367–72.

39. Shakir M, Boone BA, Polanco PM, Zenati MS, Hogg ME, Tsung A, et al. The learning curve for robotic distal pancreatectomy: an analysis of outcomes of the first 100 consecutive cases at a high-volume pancreatic centre. HPB (Oxford). 2015;17(7):580–6. Pubmed Central PMCID: 4474504.

40. Jensen RT, Cadiot G, Brandi ML, de Herder WW, Kaltsas G, Komminoth P, et al. ENETS Consensus Guidelines for the management of patients with digestive neuroendocrine neoplasms: functional pancreatic endocrine tumor syndromes. Neuroendocrinology. 2012;95(2):98–119. Pubmed Central PMCID: 3701449.

41. Cherif R, Gaujoux S, Couvelard A, Dokmak S, Vuillerme MP, Ruszniewski P, et al. Parenchyma-sparing resections for pancreatic neuroendocrine tumors. J Gastrointest Surg. 2012;16(11):2045–55.

42. Daouadi M, Zureikat AH, Zenati MS, Choudry H, Tsung A, Bartlett DL, et al. Robot-assisted minimally invasive distal

pancreatectomy is superior to the laparoscopic technique. Ann Surg. 2013;257(1):128–32.
43. Hill JS, McPhee JT, McDade TP, Zhou Z, Sullivan ME, Whalen GF, et al. Pancreatic neuroendocrine tumors: the impact of surgical resection on survival. Cancer. 2009;115(4):741–51.
44. Martin RC, Kooby DA, Weber SM, Merchant NB, Parikh AA, Cho CS, et al. Analysis of 6,747 pancreatic neuroendocrine tumors for a proposed staging system. J Gastrointest Surg. 2011;15(1):175–83.
45. Norton JA, Kivlen M, Li M, Schneider D, Chuter T, Jensen RT. Morbidity and mortality of aggressive resection in patients with advanced neuroendocrine tumors. Arch Surg. 2003;138(8):859–66.
46. Norton JA, Warren RS, Kelly MG, Zuraek MB, Jensen RT. Aggressive surgery for metastatic liver neuroendocrine tumors. Surgery. 2003;134(6):1057–63. discussion 63–5.
47. Sarmiento JM, Heywood G, Rubin J, Ilstrup DM, Nagorney DM, Que FG. Surgical treatment of neuroendocrine metastases to the liver: a plea for resection to increase survival. J Am Coll Surg. 2003;197(1):29–37.
48. Nazario J, Gupta S. Transarterial liver-directed therapies of neuroendocrine hepatic metastases. Semin Oncol. 2010;37(2):118–26.
49. Osborne DA, Zervos EE, Strosberg J, Boe BA, Malafa M, Rosemurgy AS, et al. Improved outcome with cytoreduction versus embolization for symptomatic hepatic metastases of carcinoid and neuroendocrine tumors. Ann Surg Oncol. 2006;13(4):572–81.
50. Coan KE, Gray RJ, Schlinkert RT, Pockaj BA, Wasif N. Metastatic carcinoid tumors--are we making the cut? Am J Surg. 2013;205(6):642–6.
51. Touzios JG, Kiely JM, Pitt SC, Rilling WS, Quebbeman EJ, Wilson SD, et al. Neuroendocrine hepatic metastases: does aggressive management improve survival? Ann Surg. 2005;241(5):776–83. Pubmed Central PMCID: 1357132, discussion 83–5.
52. Mazzaferro V, Pulvirenti A, Coppa J. Neuroendocrine tumors metastatic to the liver: how to select patients for liver transplantation? J Hepatol. 2007;47(4):460–6.
53. Del Prete M, Fiore F, Modica R, Marotta V, Marciello F, Ramundo V, et al. Hepatic arterial embolization in patients with

neuroendocrine tumors. J Exp Clin Cancer Res. 2014;33:43. Pubmed Central PMCID: 4038067.

54. De Jong MC, Farnell MB, Sclabas G, Cunningham SC, Cameron JL, Geschwind JF, et al. Liver-directed therapy for hepatic metastases in patients undergoing pancreaticoduodenectomy: a dual-center analysis. Ann Surg. 2010;252(1):142–8.

55. Memon K, Lewandowski RJ, Mulcahy MF, Riaz A, Ryu RK, Sato KT, et al. Radioembolization for neuroendocrine liver metastases: safety, imaging, and long-term outcomes. Int J Radiat Oncol Biol Phys. 2012;83(3):887–94. Pubmed Central PMCID: 3297703.

56. Yao KA, Talamonti MS, Nemcek A, Angelos P, Chrisman H, Skarda J, et al. Indications and results of liver resection and hepatic chemoembolization for metastatic gastrointestinal neuroendocrine tumors. Surgery. 2001;130(4):677–82. discussion 82–5.

57. Gupta S, Johnson MM, Murthy R, Ahrar K, Wallace MJ, Madoff DC, et al. Hepatic arterial embolization and chemoembolization for the treatment of patients with metastatic neuroendocrine tumors: variables affecting response rates and survival. Cancer. 2005;104(8):1590–602.

58. Hur S, Chung JW, Kim HC, Oh DY, Lee SH, Bang YJ, et al. Survival outcomes and prognostic factors of transcatheter arterial chemoembolization for hepatic neuroendocrine metastases. J Vasc Interv Radiol. 2013;24(7):947–56. quiz 57.

59. Pitt SC, Knuth J, Keily JM, McDermott JC, Weber SM, Chen H, et al. Hepatic neuroendocrine metastases: chemo- or bland embolization? J Gastrointest Surg. 2008;12(11):1951–60. Pubmed Central PMCID: 3342849.

60. Rhee TK, Lewandowski RJ, Liu DM, Mulcahy MF, Takahashi G, Hansen PD, et al. 90Y Radioembolization for metastatic neuro-endocrine liver tumors: preliminary results from a multi-institutional experience. Ann Surg. 2008;247(6):1029–35.

61. Kennedy AS, Dezarn WA, McNeillie P, Coldwell D, Nutting C, Carter D, et al. Radioembolization for unresectable neuroendocrine hepatic metastases using resin 90Y-microspheres: early results in 148 patients. Am J Clin Oncol. 2008;31(3):271–9.

62. Bhagat N, Reyes DK, Lin M, Kamel I, Pawlik TM, Frangakis C, et al. Phase II study of chemoembolization with drug-eluting beads in patients with hepatic neuroendocrine metastases: high incidence of biliary injury. Cardiovasc Intervent Radiol. 2013;36(2):449–59. Pubmed Central PMCID: 3596485.

63. Groeschl RT, Pilgrim CH, Hanna EM, Simo KA, Swan RZ, Sindram D, et al. Microwave ablation for hepatic malignancies: a multiinstitutional analysis. Ann Surg. 2014;259(6):1195–200.
64. Kvols LK, Turaga KK, Strosberg J, Choi J. Role of interventional radiology in the treatment of patients with neuroendocrine metastases in the liver. J Natl Compr Canc Netw. 2009;7(7):765–72.
65. Bushnell Jr DL, O'Dorisio TM, O'Dorisio MS, Menda Y, Hicks RJ, Van Cutsem E, et al. 90Y-edotreotide for metastatic carcinoid refractory to octreotide. J Clin Oncol. 2010;28(10):1652–9.
66. Valkema R, Pauwels S, Kvols LK, Barone R, Jamar F, Bakker WH, et al. Survival and response after peptide receptor radionuclide therapy with [90Y-DOTA0, Tyr3]octreotide in patients with advanced gastroenteropancreatic neuroendocrine tumors. Semin Nucl Med. 2006;36(2):147–56.
67. Kouvaraki MA, Ajani JA, Hoff P, Wolff R, Evans DB, Lozano R, et al. Fluorouracil, doxorubicin, and streptozocin in the treatment of patients with locally advanced and metastatic pancreatic endocrine carcinomas. J Clin Oncol. 2004;22(23):4762–71.
68. Strosberg JR, Fine RL, Choi J, Nasir A, Coppola D, Chen DT, et al. First-line chemotherapy with capecitabine and temozolomide in patients with metastatic pancreatic endocrine carcinomas. Cancer. 2011;117(2):268–75.
69. Kos-Kudla B, O'Toole D, Falconi M, Gross D, Kloppel G, Sundin A, et al. ENETS consensus guidelines for the management of bone and lung metastases from neuroendocrine tumors. Neuroendocrinology. 2010;91(4):341–50.
70. Yao JC, Shah MH, Ito T, Bohas CL, Wolin EM, Van Cutsem E, et al. Everolimus for advanced pancreatic neuroendocrine tumors. N Engl J Med. 2011;364(6):514–23. Pubmed Central PMCID: 4208619.
71. Pavel ME, Hainsworth JD, Baudin E, Peeters M, Horsch D, Winkler RE, et al. Everolimus plus octreotide long-acting repeatable for the treatment of advanced neuroendocrine tumours associated with carcinoid syndrome (RADIANT-2): a randomised, placebo-controlled, phase 3 study. Lancet. 2011;378(9808):2005–12.
72. Capozzi M, Caterina I, De Divitiis C, von Arx C, Maiolino P, Tatangelo F et al. Everolimus and pancreatic neuroendocrine tumors (PNETs): activity, resistance and how to overcome it. Int J Surg. 2015;21(Suppl 1):S89–94.

73. Yao JC, Phan AT, Chang DZ, Wolff RA, Hess K, Gupta S, et al. Efficacy of RAD001 (everolimus) and octreotide LAR in advanced low- to intermediate-grade neuroendocrine tumors: results of a phase II study. J Clin Oncol. 2008;26(26):4311–8. Pubmed Central PMCID: 2653122.
74. Raymond E, Dahan L, Raoul JL, Bang YJ, Borbath I, Lombard-Bohas C, et al. Sunitinib malate for the treatment of pancreatic neuroendocrine tumors. N Engl J Med. 2011;364(6):501–13.
75. Chan JA, Kulke MH. New treatment options for patients with advanced neuroendocrine tumors. Curr Treat Options Oncol. 2011;12(2):136–48.

Part 4
Clinical Scenario: Incidental Finding on CT

Chapter 8
Cystic Lesions of the Pancreas

Omer Basar and William R. Brugge

Abbreviations

BD-IPMN	Branch-duct intraductal papillary mucinous neoplasm
CEA	Serum carcinoembryonic antigen
CLE	Confocal laser endomicroscopy
CPEN	Cystic pancreatic endocrine neoplasms
CT	Computed tomography
ERCP	Endoscopic retrograde cholangiopancreatography
EUS	Endoscopic ultrasonography
EUS-FNA	Endoscopic ultrasound guided fine needle aspiration
FNA	Fine-needle aspiration

O. Basar, M.D.
Pancreas Biliary Center, Gastrointestinal Unit, Massachusetts
General Hospital, 55 Fruit St., Boston, MA 02114, USA
Department of Gastroenterology, University of Hacettepe,
Ankara, Turkey
e-mail: obasar@mgh.harvard.edu

W.R. Brugge, M.D. (✉)
Pancreas Biliary Center, Gastrointestinal Unit, Massachusetts
General Hospital, 55 Fruit St., Boston, MA 02114, USA
e-mail: wbrugge@partners.org

© Springer International Publishing Switzerland 2016
K. Dua, R. Shaker (eds.), *Pancreas and Biliary Disease*,
DOI 10.1007/978-3-319-28089-9_8

IPMN	Intraductal papillary mucinous neoplasm
MCN	Mucinous cystic neoplasm
MDCT	Multidetector CT
MD-IPMN	Main-duct intraductal papillary mucinous neoplasm
MR	Magnetic resonance
MRCP	Magnetic resonance cholangiopancreatography
PCL	Pancreatic cystic lesions
PCN	Pancreatic cystic neoplasms
RFA	Radiofrequency ablation
SCN	Serous cystic neoplasm
SPN	Solid pseudopapillary neoplasm
US	Ultrasonography
VHL	von Hippel–Lindau disease

Question 1: I Was Told that I Have a Cyst in My Pancreas. Is It Cancer? How Did I Get It?

With increasing use of high resolution imaging techniques, pancreatic cysts are now being discovered with increasing frequency. It is important to determine whether a pancreatic cyst is benign (usually no treatment is needed) or pre-neoplastic (benign cyst having a potential to become cancerous) or neoplastic (must be resected). Non-neoplastic cysts of the pancreas account for 80 % of all pancreatic cysts and the most common is the pancreatic pseudocyst, which is mostly a local complication of acute pancreatitis. The prevalence of neoplastic cysts increases with age and can be associated with genetic abnormalities. Neoplastic cysts usually include a serous or mucinous epithelium, which shows its neoplastic potential: serous cysts are typically benign and mucinous have at least some malignant potential.

Question 2: Can My Cyst Be Treated Without Surgery?

The most common non-neoplastic cyst, pseudocysts, mostly resolves over time without any treatment. In cases that cysts cause symptoms or become infected drainage, is required.

Today, endoscopic drainage is the preferred technique for treatment and surgery is reserved for those who failed endoscopic approach.

The most common mucinous neoplastic cyst is IPMN and all IPMNs have a potential for malignancy progression over time. For the subtype main duct-IPMN, international consensus guidelines recommend resection for all patients, since the incidence of invasive carcinoma is high and its 5-year survival rates are low. For the subtype branch duct IPMN, given the low risk of low malignant progression, most of the BD-IPMN patients without symptoms or risk factors should be followed up. An alternative treatment is EUS-guided cyst ablation and ethanol and/or paclitaxel injection. Radio-frequency ablation is still under investigation.

MCNs are the other group of mucinous cyst and current consensus guidelines recommend surgical resection. For patients refusing surgery, EUS-guided cyst ablation therapies may be considered.

Serous cystic neoplasm has an excellent prognosis; surgery is recommended only for patients with symptoms.

Question 3: What If I Don't Do Anything; Will the Cyst Become a Cancer?

Pseudocyts will not become a cancer.

The mean frequency of developing malignancy in MD-IPMN is 61.6 %. The prognosis of SCN is excellent and these patients are commonly managed conservatively.

Introduction

Pancreatic cystic lesions (PCL) are relatively rare and in recent years they are being increasingly recognized with the improvement and widespread use of cross-sectional imaging tools [1, 2]. The vast majority of PCL are recognized incidentally in asymptomatic patients and the others are discovered in patients with symptoms such as abdominal pain and jaundice.

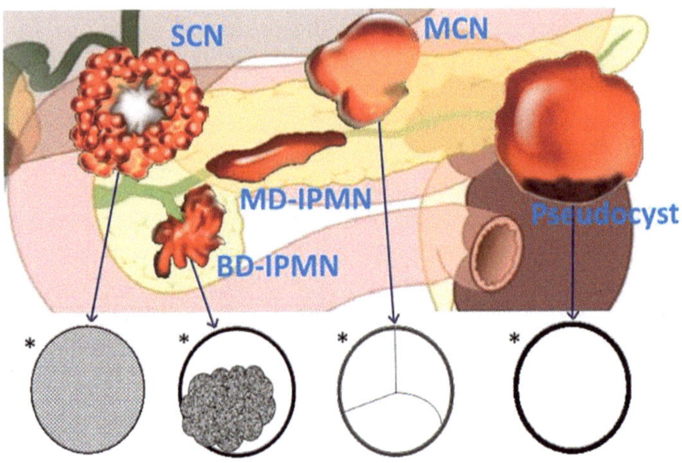

FIG. 8.1 Illustrations of the common pancreatic cysts. (*) The schematization of the morphology of cysts

In the past, most of the pancreatic cysts were believed to be pseudocysts, and the others were believed to be extremely rare. However, PCL are now recognized to be an extensive group of pancreatic tumors showing different histological, demographical, morphological, and clinical characteristics. The prevalence of pancreatic cystic lesions is reported to be ranging from 1.2 to 19 % in image-based studies (Fig. 8.1), [1–4]. A study evaluated 24,039 CT or MRI scans and reported that 290 patients (1.2 %) had pancreatic cysts, and a majority of the patients had no history of pancreatitis [5]. In an autopsy series on 300 patients, cystic lesions were found in 73 cases (24.3 %) [6]. The prevalence of cysts increases with age [3].

A number of systems have been used to classify pancreatic cysts. PCL may be broadly categorized as either non-neoplastic or neoplastic cysts (Table 8.1). Today, neoplastic cysts of pancreas are defined more commonly as pancreatic cystic neoplasms (PCN). PCN are frequently found to have a mucinous or serous epithelial lining. Serous cystic neoplasms are considered typically benign and cause symptoms

TABLE 8.1 Pancreatic cystic lesions

Non-neoplastic cysts

- *Epithelial*

  Lymphoepithelial cyst
  Mucinous non-neoplastic cysts
  Squamoid cysts
  Enterogenous cysts
  Endometrial cyst
  Para-ampullary duodenal wall cyst

- *Non-epithelial*

  Pseudocyst
  Infection-related cyst
  Simple cyst
  Retention cyst

Neoplastic cysts (pancreatic cystic neoplasms)

- *Mucinous cystic lesions*

  Intraductal papillary mucinous neoplasm

  Mucinous cystic neoplasm

- *Non-mucinous cystic lesions*

  Serous cystic neoplasm

  Solid pseudopapillary neoplasm

  Cystic pancreatic endocrine neoplasm

  Acinar-cell cystic neoplasm

- *Other neoplastic cystic lesions*

  Ductal adenocarcinoma with cystic degeneration

secondary to space occupying mass effect. Mucinous cysts, including mucinous cystic neoplasm and intraductal papillary mucinous neoplasm, have a malignant potential. Thus, it is important to distinguish a non-neoplastic cyst from neoplastic or non-mucinous from mucinous cyst because the latter are considered being premalignant lesions. Non-neoplastic cysts of pancreas account up to 80 % of all PCL, however, the prevalence of PCN increase with age [1, 2, 5]. Because many of these lesions are indistinguishable from each other preoperatively, many of them were resected unknowingly. In recent years, diagnostic methods, management algorithms and treatment options of PCL have been gradually changed. Accurate diagnosis is mandatory for PCL to choose the optimal management, which includes either follow-up conservatively or resect surgically. In this chapter, the major types of PCL are reviewed based on the recent advances in the diagnosis and management of these lesions.

Non-neoplastic Cysts

Non-neoplastic cysts of pancreas are benign lesions, which can be further classified as epithelial and non-epithelial cysts. Epithelial, non-neoplastic cysts of pancreas are categorized as lymphoepithelial cyst, mucinous non-neoplastic cysts, squamoid cysts, enterogenous cysts, endometrial cysts and para-ampullary duodenal wall cyst [7–9]. These lesions can be either congenital or acquired. Imaging studies are not usually sufficient enough to distinguish epithelial cysts from their mucinous complements. Although these entities are benign, because they often mimic mucinous neoplastic cysts, definite diagnosis is usually challenging until they are resected. Non-epithelial, non-neoplastic pancreatic cysts include pancreatitis-associated pseudocysts, the most common cyst of the pancreas, retention cysts, and infection related cysts including parasitic cysts [10]. On the other hand, cystic transformation of pancreas is observed in autosomal dominant polycystic renal disease [11], medullary cystic kidneys [12], congenital syndromes and cystic fibrosis [13].

Lymphoepithelial cysts are often thought to arise from the pancreas but they are characteristically round and well-bordered peri-pancreatic cysts. On cross-sectional imaging, they appear classically cystic and endoscopic ultrasonography (EUS) reveals a solid appearing cystic lesion filled with uniform, homogenous, hypo-echoic material. Pathological examination of a resected cyst shows an outer border of benign lymphoid tissue with an inner lining of squamous epithelium ("lympho"+"epithelial"). Aspirated fluid with EUS guided fine needle aspiration (EUS-FNA) is a viscous, thick, pasty material. Cytology of the aspirated fluid reveals anucleated squamous cells, keratinaceous debris, lymphocytes, and histiocytes. Since lymphoepithelial cysts are benign, surgical resection is only advised for patients with symptoms due to mass affect.

Although there is an uncertainty whether congenital, simple, benign cysts occur in pancreas, these cysts are generally classified as a subgroup of non-neoplastic cysts. Non-solid simple cysts are seen in patients with cystic fibrosis within a diffusely atrophic fatty parenchyma. Simple cysts, which are of no clinical significance, are also demonstrated in patients with polycystic renal disease.

Pancreatic Pseudocysts

Pancreatic pseudocysts are the most common cystic lesions of pancreas and are inflammatory fluid collections associated with pancreatitis. These lesions mainly effect adult men and are local complications of acute pancreatitis due to different etiologies such as chronic alcoholism, biliary or traumatic pancreatitis [14]. The most common local complication of acute and chronic pancreatitis is peri-pancreatic and sometimes

TABLE 8.2 Fluid collections of acute pancreatitis

Type of pancreatitis	Fluid collection	Time
Interstitial edematous pancreatitis	Acute pancreatic fluid collection	<4 weeks after onset
Interstitial edematous pancreatitis	Pancreatic **Pseudocyst**	>4 weeks after onset
Necrotizing pancreatitis	Acute necrotic collection	<4 weeks after onset
Necrotizing pancreatitis	Walled-off necrosis	>4 weeks after onset

intra-pancreatic fluid collections. According to the revised Atlanta classification, local complications of acute pancreatitis are acute peri-pancreatic fluid collections, pancreatic pseudocyst, acute necrotic collections and walled-off necrosis [15]. Considering the absence or presence of pancreatic necrosis, acute fluid collections within 4 weeks from onset of acute pancreatitis, are named acute pancreatic fluid collection and acute necrotic collection. After the development of an enhancing capsule, a persistent acute pancreatic fluid collection is further termed a pancreatic pseudocyst and an acute necrotic collection is referred to as a walled-off necrosis. All of these entities can be either infected or sterile (Table 8.2). Pseudocyst occurs in 10–20 % of acute pancreatitis [16]. The definition "pseudocyst" applies to a peri-pancreatic cystic lesion, which has no epithelial lining and therefore is not a true cyst [17]. The development of a well-defined wall composed of granulation or fibrous tissue distinguishes a pseudocyst from an acute fluid collection. Pancreatic pseudocysts are thought to arise from disruption of main pancreatic duct or its branches in the absence of identifiable pancreatic necrosis [15]. Without an antecedent episode of acute pancreatitis, pseudocyst may also arise insidiously in patients with chronic pancreatitis [18]. Rarely, pseudocysts may also arise in acute necrotizing pancreatitis patients, which is called "disconnected duct syndrome". In this syndrome, a still viable distal pancreatic remnant is separated by parenchymal necrosis of the neck and body of pancreas [19]. Additionally, after surgical necrosectomy, a pseudocyst may develop due to necrosis and subsequent leakage of pancreatic secretions from disconnected ducts into necrosectomy cavity [19]. Pseudocysts are round or oval, well circumscribed homogenous fluid collections, with a well-defined enhancing wall, which essentially contain no solid material inside. Rarely, pseudocysts may be multilocular and irregular in shape. Pseudocysts are usually single but may be multiple in 10 % of cases. Pseudocysts contain fluid, which is usually rich in amylase and lipase due to the constant communication with pancreatic ducts, and pseudocysts are usually sterile [17].

In contrast, small pancreatic pseudocysts are usually surrounded by a thin wall and are usually closely associated with the pancreas. Pseudocysts may sometimes be large, which occupy spaces adjacent to the stomach and pancreas or remote areas, including the chest. Pseudocysts can be localized in the liver, usually in the left lobe [20, 21], in the spleen [22, 23], and rarely in the kidney [24]. Histologically, the walls of pseudocysts consist of fibrosis and inflammatory tissue without epithelial lining, and are similar in all types of pseudocysts. The size of pseudocysts varies from 2 to 20 cm [14, 17, 18].

Clinical manifestations of pseudocysts are related with a local mass effect. The common symptoms associated with chronic pancreatic pseudocysts are usually mild recurrent abdominal pain, nausea and vomiting, early satiety, and weight loss. Generally, the size and the duration of cysts are the most important predictors for symptoms related to a pseudocyst [25]. Physical examination is rarely diagnostic for pseudocysts; a palpable, smooth, firm, non-tender mass in epigastric region, usually moving with breathing, may be a physical finding of large pseudocysts. Weight loss, which is observed in 20 % of patients due to gastric compression, results in poor intake as well as maldigestion. Jaundice is noted in 10 % of patients, who usually progresses slowly, and arises as a result of bile duct compression by the pseudocyst or the inflamed pancreas itself. Fever and chills are unusual in chronic, uncomplicated pseudocysts and presence of fever in these patients should raise the suspicion of pseudocyst infection [26].

Diagnosis

A pancreatic pseudocyst is clinically suspected when the episode of acute pancreatitis does not resolve, in the presence of continuous abdominal pain after clinical resolution of acute pancreatitis, persistent high levels of amylase and an onset of a palpable epigastric mass after an episode of acute pancreatitis. In some cases the episode of acute pancreatitis may not be clinically overt or patients might have had mild pancreatitis. Transabdominal ultrasonography (US) is usually the initial diagnostic procedure for a pseudocyst. An echoic structure associated with distal acoustic enhancement is the usual appearance on US. Abdominal computed tomography (CT) is superior to US with a sensitivity of 90–100 % to detect a pseudocyst. A patient with a history of pancreatitis and abdominal CT revealing a round or oval well circumscribed fluid filled lesion surrounded by a thick, dense wall adjacent to pancreas is almost diagnostic for a pancreatic pseudocyst [14] (Fig. 8.2). CT may also show clues of acute or chronic pancreatitis, when evaluating the adjacent pancreatic tissue. Big pseudocysts may be seen in the mediastinum, pelvis or may involve the mesentery, as well. Although pseudocysts are

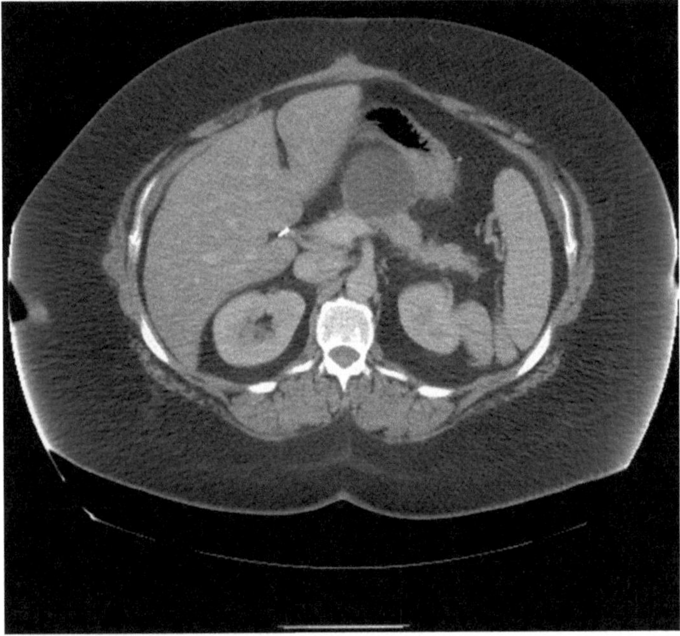

FIG. 8.2 CT showing a 3 cm pseudocyst in the body of pancreas indenting the stomach

most commonly unilocular, fibrotic strands within the cavity may cause multiple septations, which is frequently encountered in patients with post-pancreatitis complex fluid collections. Since pancreatic mucinous cysts can also be septated, it may be difficult to distinguish pseudocysts from pancreatic mucinous cysts without analyzing the cystic fluid. A pseudocyst may also contain debris, blood, or it may sometimes be infected, which is observed as high-attenuation areas within the fluid-filled cavity. When a pseudocyst is infected, the liquid becomes purulent, but does not contain solid material. CT scans can also provide more detailed information regarding the surrounding anatomy and can demonstrate additional pathologies. Persistent communication of a pseudocyst with pancreatic duct can be shown by contrast enhanced CT, which may help determine the management of the disease. On the other hand, magnetic resonance cholangiography (CP) is superior to CT in demonstrating this communication [27, 28], but usually magnetic resonance imaging (MRI) and MRCP do not add any extra information over CT [29]. Although CT is more popular, MRI may be more helpful before therapeutic interventions of complex fluid collection [30]. ERCP is not essential for diagnosis of pseudocysts but it can be helpful for treatment in some cases.

To further evaluate a pancreatic cysts EUS can be used, which is superior to distinguishing pseudocysts from other PCL [31]. In the EUS examination pseudocysts are seen as anechoic, fluid-filled lesions adjacent to the upper GI tract and pancreas (Fig. 8.3). A thick, hyperechoic rim often surrounds pseudocysts. Calcifications in a cyst wall are highly suggestive of a mucinous cystadenoma, rather than a pseudocyst. Debris may be observed in the cystic cavity and may represent blood, infection, or necrotic material. Color Doppler of the wall will often reveal multiple, prominent vessels, including para-gastric varices.

In cases where CT demonstrates gas within the pseudocyst, an infected pseudocyst should be suspected. In the absence of gas, fine-needle aspiration (FNA) with Gram staining and culture for bacteria may help diagnose the infection.

EUS guided FNA, including cystic fluid analysis, discriminates pseudocysts from neoplastic cysts in more than 90 % of the patients [26]. A high amylase activity in the aspirated cyst is a strong predictor of a communication with the pancreatic duct, which helps confirm the diagnosis of a pseudocyst. On the other hand, relatively low levels of CEA in the cystic fluid may distinguish a pseudocyst from Intraductal papillary mucinous neoplasm (IPMN) and mucinous cystic neoplasm (MCN) [32]. Cytological analysis of a pseudocyst for histiocytes, inflammatory cells and degenerative debris and more importantly, to rule out a mucinous lesion is also needed. Epithelial cells should raise the suspicion of a cystic neoplasm rather than a pseudocyst [32]; presence of granulocytes suggests an acute infection.

Treatment

Spontaneous resolution is observed in the majority of acute peri-pancreatic fluid collections. A small percentage of fluid

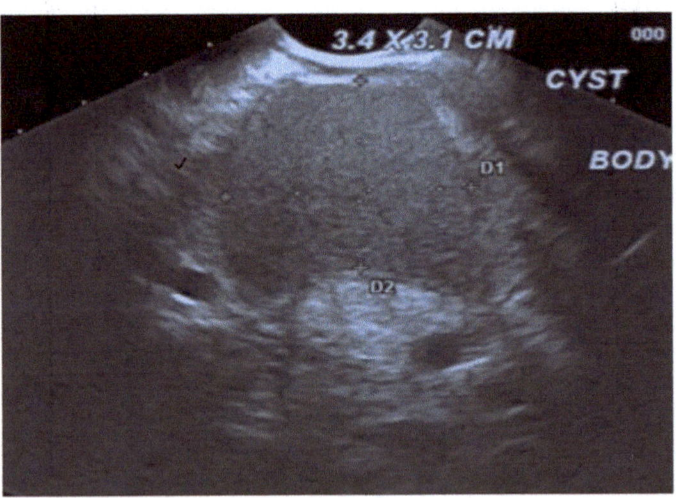

FIG. 8.3 EUS revealing a pseudocyst 3.4×3.1 cm in diameter in the body of pancreas

collections mature into pseudocysts. Most of these pseudocysts also resolve over time without any treatment. Small pseudocysts, which are less than 4 cm in diameter, often disappear without any complications; however, bigger pseudocysts are more likely to cause symptoms or complications. Approximately 25 % of pseudocysts cause symptoms, or become infected and require drainage, less than 10 % of cases experience a complication [30, 33]. Spontaneous resolution of pseudocysts takes place through fistulation into the GI tract or the pancreatic duct. The indications for interventions to drain are symptomatic persistent pseudocyst or cysts with complications such as bleeding, infection, biliary obstruction or gastric outlet syndrome. Forty percent of pseudocysts that are smaller than 6 cm in diameter requires drainage [34]. For large or symptomatic cysts, after excluding infection or necrotic material, drainage is usually satisfactory. In cases when CT demonstrates gas inside the fluid collection, infection is clinically suspected, but FNA is usually required to rule out the infection. Surgical drainage is not the first preferred method for infected pseudocyst today.

Several types of procedures may be used for draining a pseudocyst [35]. Under the guidance of US/CT, percutaneous drainage with percutaneous catheter placement is a simple way. This simple percutaneous drainage procedure has a high short term success, but high risk of complications with significant discomfort to the patient exits [14]. Percutaneous drainage with retroperitoneal approach through the lateral flank, which avoids perforation of bowel and solid organs, is generally more preferable than anterior approach through the peritoneal cavity [36]. The overall success rate of surgical drainage performed by providing a large anastomosis between the pseudocyst cavity and the stomach or small bowel is very high; however, this invasive technique has high complication rates. Surgery should be reserved for those who cannot tolerate or failed endoscopic drainage [37].

Presently, endoscopic drainage is the preferred technique for the treatment of pancreatic pseudocysts [38]. Endoscopic retrograde cholangiopancreatography (ERCP) guided

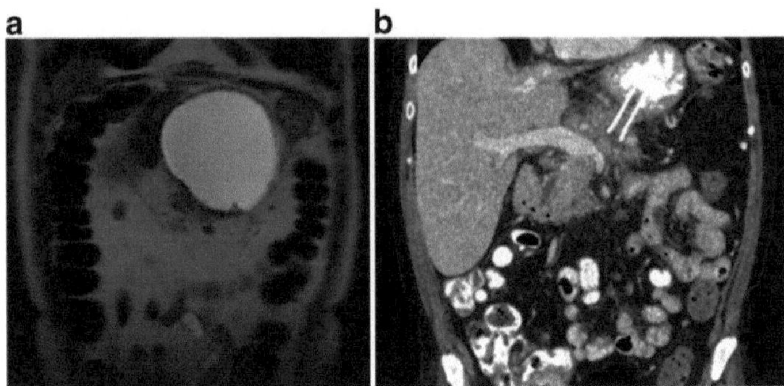

FIG. 8.4 (**a**) MRI showing a large pseudocyst in a patient with alcoholic pancreatitis. EUS guided cystogastrostomy was performed and two metallic stents were placed. (**b**) CT showing almost complete resolution of the pseudocyst

drainage through ampulla of Vater should be preferred when a communication between pancreatic duct and pseudocyst is suspected. The trans-papillary approach of drainage has also been found to be useful when pseudocysts are associated with strictures or are as a result of leakage from the main pancreatic duct [39].

Trans-gastric or trans-duodenal approaches are preferred for pseudocysts that are in proximity to gastroduodenal wall (Fig. 8.4). EUS is helpful to determine the size, location, and thickness of the pseudocyst wall. Endoscopic drainage is relatively contraindicated in cysts having a wall thickness greater than 1 cm or when large intervening vessels or varices are evident with EUS. In the absence of a visible bulge in the stomach, EUS guidance is required for drainage. Furthermore, necrotic pancreatic tissue can be removed through an endoscopic cystogastrostomy or duodenostomy via balloon dilation of the fistula tract. Overall, endoscopic drainage is successful in more than 90 % of the cases, with a complication rate of 13 %, and recurrence rates of less than 10 % [26].

Pancreatic Cystic Neoplasms

IPMN, MCN, serous cystic neoplasm (SCN), solid pseudopapillary neoplasm (SPN), and Cystic pancreatic endocrine neoplasms (CPEN) are the main types of PCN (Table 8.1). Population based studies showed that SCN account for 32–39 %, MCN for 10–45 %, IPMN for 21–33 %, and SPN for less than 10 % of all PCN in Western Hemisphere. A nationwide survey from Korea reported that IPMN account for 41 %, MCN for 25.2 %, SPN for 18.3 %, SCN for 15.2 %, and others for 0.3 % of PCN [1, 40]. Since the diagnosis and management varies in each type of PCN, differentiating one from another is important.

Intraductal Papillary Mucinous Neoplasms

IPMNs were first described in 1982 and they were initially thought as rare neoplasms. Prior to The World Health Organization classification of IPMN in 1996, they were named as papillary carcinoma, mucinous ductal ectasia or villous adenoma and many of these mucinous lesions were misclassified. IPMNs have become a major clinical focus in recent years because of the increased use of cross-sectional imaging in clinical practice and increased identification of asymptomatic PCLs.

IPMNs originate from pancreatic ductal cells and may involve pancreatic ducts diffusely or in a multifocal manner. IPMNs are mucinous cystic lesions of the pancreas characterized by mucin-secreting, papillary projections from the pancreatic ductal surface [41]. Hence IPMN is an intraductal proliferation of neoplastic mucin-producing columnar epithelium rising from the main pancreatic duct or its side branches. Intraluminal growth causes dilatation of the involved duct and its proximal segment. The most common site of involvement is the head of the pancreas as a solitary cystic lesion, but may be multifocal in 20–30 % of the cases.

Although the exact incidence of IPMNs is unknown, it is believed that 20–50 % of all PCNs are IPMNs [1, 41, 42]. In a recent surgical series IPMNs accounted up to 36 % of all resected cysts of pancreas [43]. Radiographically and histopathologically, based on the involvement of pancreatic ductal system, IPMN are classified into either main-duct IPMN (MD-IPMN) or branch-duct (BD-IPMN) or mixed-IPMN (both dilation of the main and side branch ducts). The main pancreatic duct is segmentally or diffusely involved in MD-IPMN and is usually >10 mm in diameter. In 5–10 % of cases, the main pancreatic duct is diffusely involved [41, 42]. Carcinoma-in-situ is observed in up to 60 % and invasive adenocarcinoma in up to 45 % of cases. Hence patients with MD-IPMN in general should undergo resection [44–47]. A non-dilated main duct communicates with one or more side branch ducts in BD-IPMN and multifocal involvement is seen in up to 40 % of cases [48, 49]. In patients with BD-IPMN who had undergone resection, 40 % malignancy is reported [45, 46, 48, 49]. When side branch dilation is associated with main duct dilation, it is called mixed-IPMN and malignancy rate is reported to be in between those of MD-IPMN and BD-IPMN, who had undergone resection.

Currently, most of the investigators and clinicians believe that IPMNs represents a field defect [50]. IPMN covers a spectrum of precursor lesions from adenoma to intraductal carcinoma to invasive cancer. Recent reports state that IPMN, as a dysplastic premalignant lesion, has a potential to progress from low-grade dysplasia to invasive carcinoma [51, 52]. According to degree of dysplasia WHO classified IPMNs into subgroups; (1) IPMNs with low- or intermediate-grade dysplasia, (2) IPMNs with high-grade dysplasia (carcinoma in situ), and (3) IPMNs with an associated invasive carcinoma. Currently, dysplasia is classified as low, moderate or high by most histopathological assessments. Detailed histological studies further classified IPMN into subtypes including gastric foveolar type, intestinal, pancreatobiliary, and intraductal oncocytic papillary subtype. Gastric foveolar type epithelium is predominantly seen in BD-IPMN, which are usually low-grade lesions [53]. On the other hand, intestinal type is mostly present in MD-IPMN and has an intermediate to high-grade dysplasia. Colloid type adenocarcinoma usually develops in association with intestinal type IPMN and it indicates better prognosis [54]. Invasive cancers developing from pancreatobiliary IPMN are usually tubular-type adenocarcinoma, which tend to have worse prognosis than colloid adenocarcinoma. Intraductal oncocytic papillary cancers are very rare and cancers developing from them show different oncocytic cytology and they are suggested to be identical with ductal adenocarcinoma [55, 56]. Patients with gastric-type IPMN have the best prognosis, whereas those with intestinal and pancreatobiliary type have worse prognosis. The types of mucin expressed by subtypes of IPMN are summarized in Table 8.3.

Diagnosis

IPMNs are usually detected in asymptomatic patients incidentally discovered on cross-sectional imaging performed for another reasons. Some patients may present with recurrent non-specific symptoms including abdominal pain and discomfort, malaise, nausea and vomiting [41]. Patients with an associated invasive carcinoma may present with jaundice, weight loss and diabetes mellitus. IPMNs presents predominantly in men with a mean age of 65. Laboratory tests including complete blood count, liver enzymes, pancreatic enzymes, are usually within normal limits. Serum carcinoembryonic antigen (CEA) and CA 19-9 are generally not of diagnostic

TABLE 8.3 Types of mucin expressed by different subtypes of IPMN

Subtype	Mucin
Gastric foveolar type	Overexpression of MUC5AC, MUC6
Intestinal type	Overexpression of MUC5AC, MUC2 and weak expression of MUC6
Pancreatobiliary type	MUC1, MUC5AC

TABLE 8.4 Genetics of IPMN

Genetic abnormality	Frequency
KRAS mutation	38–100 % [57, 58]
Loss of p16	78 % [59]
p53 mutation	50 % [60]
SMAD4/DPC4 expression	In almost all of noninvasive IPMN [59]
Loss of SMAD4/DPC4 expression	10 % of colloid cancer [59]
PIK3CA mutation	11 % [61]
GNAS mutation	66 % [62]
STK11/LKB1 gene inactivation	25 % [63]

value [1]. Genetic abnormalities in IPMNs are summarized in Table 8.4.

The diagnosis of IPMN is classically established by imaging [64]. The aim of imaging studies in patients with IPMN includes detecting and differentiating them from the other types of PCL, differentiating the type of IPMN (MD-IPMN or BD-IPMN) and evaluating it for resectability.

Although it was a standard procedure in the past, endoscopy and ERCP have a limited role for the evaluation of IPMN today [64]. The finding of a dilated main pancreatic duct (usually >10 mm) with filling defects, in the absence of imaging features of acute pancreatitis and obstructing lesions is highly suggestive of MD-IPMN. In some cases, during endoscopy or ERCP, the pancreatic orifice is patulous, and mucin that is emanating from the ampulla can be visualized ("fish-mouth" papilla). However, absence of this endoscopic feature in no way excludes the diagnosis. In the absence of pancreatitis features, cystic dilations of side branch ducts (multiple parenchymal cysts on imaging), especially if these are communicating with the main pancreatic duct, are generally considered indicative of BD-IPMN. The other types of PCN are very rarely multifocal and it should be kept in mind that multiple benign cysts may be seen in cystic fibrosis and polycystic renal disease. Moreover, in some occasions, due to mucus plugging, the cystic side branch ducts cannot be filled with contrast. Since ERCP is an invasive procedure with complications, one of the limited usages of ERCP is that ERCP identifies the intraductal papillary outgrowths of IPMN and may also identify a communication with a cyst and the main pancreatic duct. In addition, visualization of the entire pancreatic ductal system is not always possible due to copious amount of mucin during ERCP.

In clinical practice, most of the PCL are usually discovered by conventional imaging modalities (US, CT and MRI) which are usually performed for other reasons [65, 66]. Conventional imaging differentiates the types of PCL by evaluating the location, number, size, calcification, septations and pancreatic duct dilation. High quality cross sectional imaging is crucial for assessing PCL. Currently, multidetector CT (MDCT), which allows pancreatic thin sections, has become the most common method for evaluating PCL. Besides providing excellent visualization of mural nodules, calcifications and septations, MDCT also evaluates the pancreatic parenchyma. MDCT predicts the malignant features of pancreatic cyst with an accuracy of 56–85 % [67] and, the presence of thick septations, mural nodules and cyst wall thickness are signs of high-grade dysplasia and invasive carcinoma. When discriminating an aggressive type IPMN from non-aggressive IPMN, MRI with MRCP can be similar to MDCT in their diagnostic yield [68, 69] (Fig. 8.5). The sensitivity of MRCP may be better in showing a communication between the main duct and the cystic lesion [69]. On the other hand, it is reported that a combination of MDCT with MRI may be more helpful to obtain a specific diagnosis rather than either tool alone. In addition, both CT and MRI are accurate enough to detect metastasis in cases with IPMN associated invasive carcinoma.

EUS has become the more valuable procedure for the diagnosis of IPMNs as it has high resolution capacity and better imaging characteristics compared with cross-sectional imaging [70]. Moderate to marked dilation of the main pancreatic duct (either segmentally or diffusely) is the main EUS finding of IPMN. Pancreatic duct dilation is often associated

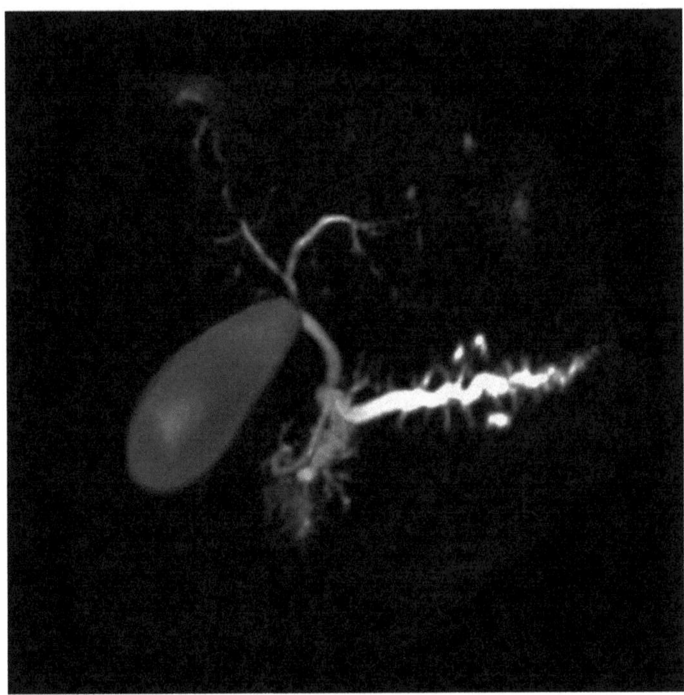

FIG. 8.5 MRCP revealing a diffusely dilated main pancreatic duct with its side branches consisted with a MD-IPMN

with intraductal mural nodules in patients with MD-IPMN. On the other hand, main pancreatic duct obstruction with mucus may result in parenchymal changes, which are similar with changes in pancreatitis. These parenchymal changes are enlargement of the pancreas or parenchymal atrophy, which makes it difficult to distinguish IPMN from chronic pancreatitis. The main duct is normal sized or mildly dilated in patients with BD-IPMN and the presence of multiple cysts, ranging from 5 to 20 mm in diameter reveals an appearance of a "cluster of grapes" (Fig. 8.6). Excellent visualization of internal septations, cyst wall thickening, debris in the cyst, mural nodule and papillary projections can be provided by

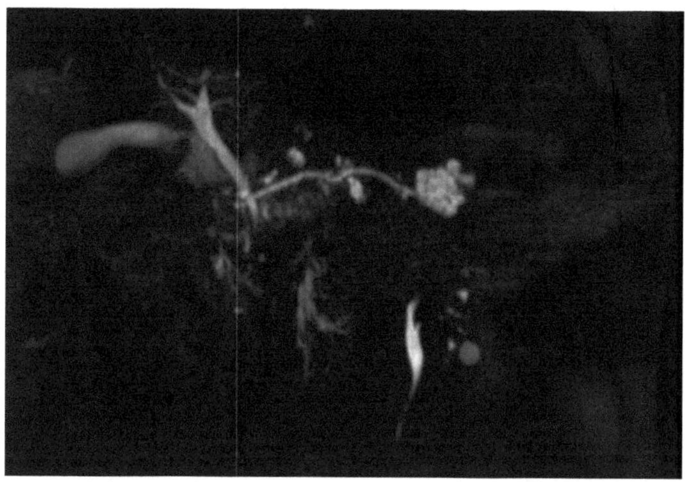

Fig. 8.6 Complex septated cystic lesion in the tail of pancreas consisted with cluster of grapes appearance of BD-IPMN on MRCP

EUS. EUS also allows visualization of lymph node metastases and vascular invasion [1, 31, 41, 70].

EUS criteria for malignancy in patients with MD-IPMN include marked dilatation of the main pancreatic duct (>10 mm), and large tumors (>40 mm) with irregular septa in patients with BD-IPMN. A mural nodule greater than 10 mm in size is a feature of malignancy in both MD-IPMN and BD-IPMN [71]. The accuracy of EUS to differentiate a benign cyst from malignant IPMN varies from 40 to 90 % in several studies which is superior to US, ERCP and cross-sectional imaging tools [72]. In contrast, EUS has a low accuracy in differentiating malignancy from areas of focal parenchymal inflammation, which mimic malignancy.

EUS guided FNA can be performed and the aspirated fluid sent for biochemical, cytological and DNA analysis [73, 74] (Fig. 8.7). Macroscopically observed highly viscous, gelatinous fluid is suggestive of either IPMN or MCN. High levels of CEA in cystic fluid, which is detected both in patients with IPMN and MCN, reflects the presence of a mucinous epithelium.

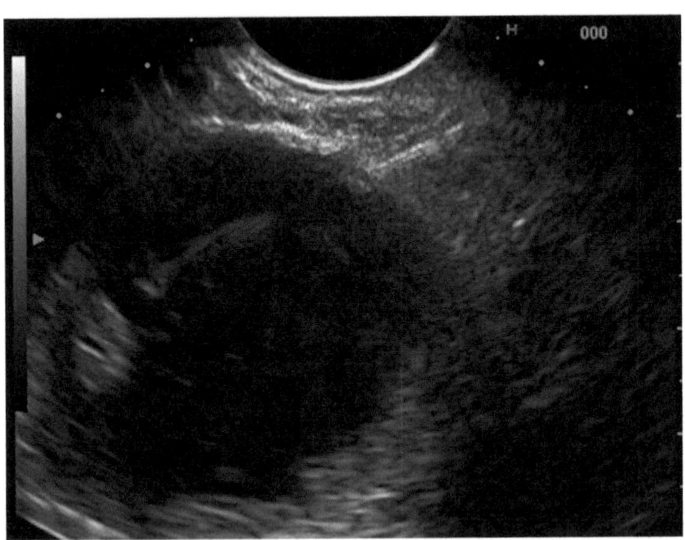

Fig. 8.7 EUS-FNA of a BD-IPMN with a mural nodule

Rather than predicting IPMN associated invasive cancer or differentiating IPMN from MCN, cystic fluid CEA levels better distinguishes non-mucinous cyst from mucinous ones. In a prospective study of patients with PCL, a cut-off CEA level of 192 ng/mL was found to be the best predictor of a mucinous cyst with a sensitivity of 73 %, specificity of 84 %, and accuracy of 79 % [75]. When compared with CA19.9, CA125, CA72-4 and CA15-3, CEA provided the best accuracy for the diagnosis of cystic mucinous neoplasms. IPMN may also have elevated cyst fluid amylase levels since it usually communicates with main pancreatic duct as against MCN and SCN [32, 76].

In a recent study, the amounts for glucose and kynurenine were significantly lower in mucinous cysts compared with non-mucinous cysts, however, neither of them could discriminate a malignant cyst from a premalignant one [77]. The clinical utility of these biomarkers needs to be further studied. Aspirated pancreatic cyst fluid involves exfoliated epithelial cells to be analyzed for cytology, whether the cyst is mucinous or non-mucinous. Unfortunately, cytology of the aspirated material is usually non-diagnostic because of the low cellularity and limited volume. A positive cytology is typically 100 % specific for detecting malignancy in patients with mucinous cysts [78]. Additionally, the accuracy of cyst fluid analysis for detecting high-grade dysplasia is 80 % to predict malignancy [79].

Finally, markers of dysplasia including KRAS mutation, p53 mutation and loss of p16 and SMAD4 were investigated. In the initial studies, KRAS mutation alone was found to be highly specific for mucinous neoplasms. Further studies demonstrated KRAS mutation followed by allelic loss could be a predictor for malignant cysts. However, the sensitivity of KRAS mutation for detecting mucinous cysts was very low [80]. Although, KRAS being an early oncogenic mutation in adenoma-carcinoma sequence, it does not differentiate benign cysts from malignant ones. Additional studies reported that the assessment for GNAS mutations might help differentiate IPMN from mucinous cyst, but it cannot predict malignancy [81]. The detection of GNAS mutations seems to be specific for IPMN.

Confocal laser endomicroscopy (CLE), which uses low power laser, is a novel imaging technology. It shows in vivo histology of the gastrointestinal mucosa and a recent CLE miniprobe has been developed to to visualize the cyst wall and epithelium directly by passing it through a 19-gauge FNA needle during EUS-FNA., which is able. Preliminary studies reported that CLE has 59 % sensitivity and 100 % specificity to show the epithelial villous structures associated with IPMN [82].

Management

The mean frequency of malignancy in MD-IPMN is 61.6 % and that of invasive caner, 43.1 %. Studies revealed that patients with non-invasive IPMN tend to be 5 years older than those with invasive IPMN [69, 76]. The finding of low-grade dysplasia and invasive carcinoma coexisting in the same cyst suggests that all IPMNs have a potential for progression to malignancy over time. Since the incidence of invasive carcinoma is high and its 5-year survival rates are low (31–54 %), international consensus guidelines recommend resection for all patients with MD-IPMN. In cases when surgical margin is positive for high-grade dysplasia, additional resection should be tried to obtain at least moderate-grade dysplastic margin. In the same guideline, 5–9 mm dilation of main pancreatic duct is considered as a "worrisome feature", and the patients are recommended for follow-up but not immediate resection. Worrisome features for IPMN include a cyst size greater than 3 cm, thickened/enhancing cyst walls, presence of lymphadenopathies, non-enhancing mural nodule, main pancreatic duct size of 5–9 mm and sudden change in caliber of pancreatic duct with distal pancreatic atrophy. Besides, high-risk stigmata include obstructive jaundice in a patient with cystic lesion at the head of pancreas, enhancing solid component within the cyst and main pancreatic duct size greater than 10 mm in diameter [71].

The mean frequency of malignancy in resected BD-IPMN is 25.5 % and the mean frequency of invasive cancer is 17.7 %. BD-IPMN mostly occurs in the elderly patients. Patients with non-invasive BD-IPMN have similar ages with invasive BD-IPMN [83]. The annual malignancy rate is only 2–3 %. At the time of initial diagnosis, given the low risk to malignant progression, most of the BD-IPMN patients without symptoms should be followed up [69]. Risk factors suggesting progression to malignancy are rapidly increasing cyst size, mural nodule and cytology showing high-grade dysplasia. Size, however by itself, does not appear to correlate with risk of malignancy and data is not enough for immediate resection in patients with BD-IPMN >3 cm in the absence of "high-risk stigmata" and "worrisome features" [71].

The need for long-term follow-up of patients with BD-IPMN who are younger (<65 years) increases the cumulative risk of malignancy and cost of management is the main challenge. Some patients may refuse surgery or surgery may be contraindicated in some high-risk patients. As an alternative treatment, EUS-guided cyst ablation has been tried [84]. During this procedure, ablation of the cyst epithelium is achieved with injecting cytotoxic agents such as ethanol and saline. For complete ablation, ethanol lavage was found superior to saline. Better results were obtained with the combination of paclitaxel injection and ethanol lavage. Combining ethanol with paclitaxel eliminated cysts in 62 % of patients with a median follow-up period of 21.7 months [84, 85]. In a pilot study, six patients with PCN underwent radiofrequency ablation (RFA) and the patients were followed up for 3–6 months. Complete resolution was observed in two of them [86].

The recurrence after surgical resection vary from 7 to 30 %. Annual monitoring with either CT or MRI for noninvasive IPMN and monitoring every 6 months for invasive IPMN is recommended [71]. For patients with BD-IPMN who did not undergo surgery and have cysts >2 cm without "worrisome features", performing EUS for every 3–6 months is recommended. MRI is also recommended as an alternative of EUS. Annual monitoring with cross-sectional modalities are suggested for BD-IPMN that are 2–3 cm in diameter, and 2–3 years intervals are suggested for BD-IPMN that are below 1 cm. Detecting malignant transformation of a benign cyst are the goal of follow-up in these patients [87].

Mucinous Cystic Neoplasms

MCN are reported to account for 23 % of all resected PCN [88]. They are more common in females, the mean age at diagnosis is younger, most commonly located in the pancreatic body or tail and are almost always solitary. The typical presentation is a female in her 50s with a solitary cyst in the tail of pancreas. In contrast, patients with IPMN usually present in an elderly male with a multifocal cysts identified in the head of pancreas.

MCN is defined as cyst-forming epithelial neoplasm that compromises a mucin-producing columnar ductal epithelium with an underlying ovarian-type stroma, not communicating with the main pancreatic duct [1, 89]. A thick layer of spindle cells containing receptors for progesterone and estrogen surrounds the MCN. This pathognomonic densely cellular "ovarian like tissue" simulates an ovarian hamartoma; even a sarcoma. The histological characteristics of the stroma and its tendency for luteinization suggest that the ovarian tissue possibly derivate the stromal component of MCN. It has been hypothesized that, during embryogenesis, the ectopic ovarian stroma in pancreas may release hormones and growth factors which results in proliferation of the nearby epithelium to proliferate and to form cystic tumors. The ovarian type mucosa of MCN stain variably for progesterone and estrogen receptors and human chorionic gonadotropin may help differentiate MCN from BD-IPMN. Interestingly, this stroma is also observed in postmenopausal females and even in male patients and it is crucial for diagnosis. Furthermore, mucinous transitional epithelium is the source of almost all MCN associated malignancies. MCN are classified as (1) mucinous cystadenoma (benign), (2) mucinous cystic tumor (borderline), and (3) mucinous cystadenocarcinoma (malignant) [90, 91].

The frequencies of KRAS mutations are reported to increase as the stage of dysplasia increase. In contrast, p53 mutations are frequently found only in cases with severe dysplasia or cancer [92, 93].

MCN is a single spherical cyst containing a thick mucin or a compound of mucin, blood and necrotic material; and it may be unilocular or multilocular. Except for a fistula formation, MCN do not communicate with pancreatic duct. On the other hand, a multicenter study from Japan reported a communication rate of 18 % in patients with MCN [94].

Up to one-third of MCN are reported to harbor an invasive carcinoma and risk factors for malignancy include large cyst size, advanced age, mural nodules and an associated mass. Lesions may be asymptomatic in 30 % of patients or may present with abdominal pain, discomfort, dyspepsia, anorexia, weight loss, fatigue, jaundice or palpable mass [95]. Routine laboratory tests are usually nonspecific, however in cases when the bile duct is obstructed, serum levels of cholestatic liver enzymes and bilirubin are elevated [45].

CT findings of MCN include a macrocyst with thin septae, which is best shown after intravenous contrast administration. Peripheral calcifications may be seen, which are named, "eggshell calcifications". They are lamellated and they contrast the central stellate calcifications of SCN. The cysts are seen bright (high signal intensity) on T2-weighted images on MRI. The wall of the cyst and septa are better shown on T1-weighted images after intravenous gadolinium administration. The presence of wall thickening, peripheral calcification, and thick septations can be suggestive of a malignant mucinous cystic neoplasm. In a study of 52 patients with MCN, the presence of these three findings predicted a 95 % risk of malignancy [96] (Fig. 8.8).

EUS findings of MCN include large, septated, thin-walled, fluid-filled cyst [4]. Usually, a communication with ductal system cannot be demonstrated. Thickening and irregularity of cyst wall, large size and visualization of intracystic solid components or adjacent solid mass are suggestive of malignancy. CEA levels in the aspirated fluid are elevated and generally amylase level is low. Cyst fluid cytology does not help distinguish MCN from IPMN. ERCP is not indicated, since MCN rarely communicate with pancreatic duct.

Because MCN can progress to cancer, current consensus guideline recommend surgical resection of all MCN [71]. Because of their location, MCN < 4 cm without mural nodules are recommended for laparoscopic resection (distal pancreatectomy) with splenic preservation. Patients with noninvasive MCN have excellent outcomes [97] and do not require follow-up after surgery since they are not at risk of recurrence and there is no cancer risk in the pancreatic remnant. In contrast, patients with invasive MCN are at risk of distant recurrences, and after resection the 2-year survival is 67 % and 5-year survival 50 % [1]. For patients who are not a good

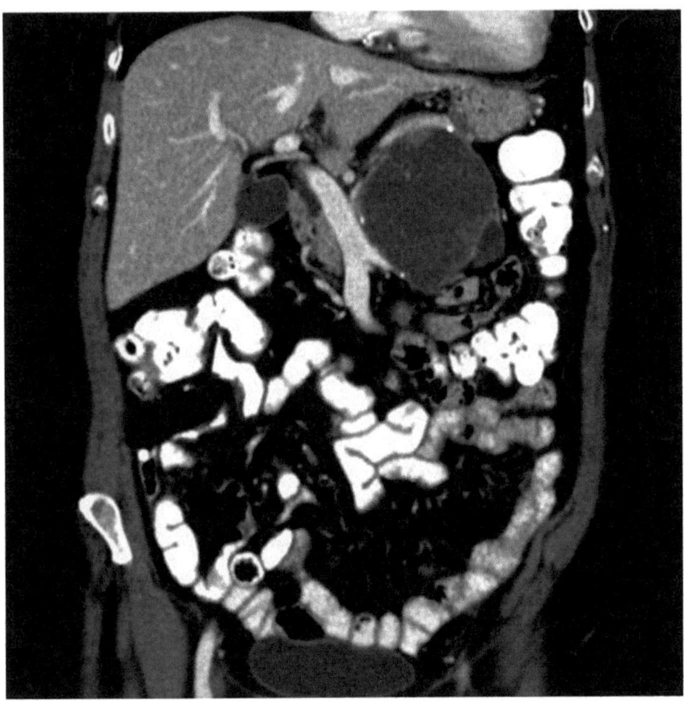

FIG. 8.8 Malignant MCN rising from the body of pancreas on CT

candidate for surgery or who refuse surgery, EUS-guided cyst ablation therapies may be considered. Patients having small lesions without a solid component may be followed up.

Serous Cystic Neoplasms

SCN are cystic neoplasms that arise from centroacinar cells and are thin walled cystic collections lined by a cuboidal epithelium. This cuboidal epithelium is typically PAS positive on staining (stain with glycogen) and the cyst typically consists of serous fluid. They are classified according to the degree of dysplasia as either serous cystadenoma or serous cystadenocarcinoma. More than 80 % of SCN occur in women at mean age of late 50s or early 60s. The most common site of involvement is pancreatic body or tail, SCN are mostly considered as benign lesions and tend to grow slowly and may achieve large diameters [98].

SCN is reported to develop in 90 % of patients with von Hippel–Lindau (VHL) syndrome, and a mutation in the VHL gene is seen in 70 % of serous cystadenoma patients [99]. KRAS mutations are rare in patients with SCN. SCN are characteristically benign lesions; to date only 25 malignant cases have been reported in the literature [1]. SCN are usually single, round lesions, which are sometimes >20 cm in diameter. The usual appearance of SCN is a cluster of numerous tiny microcysts, surrounding a more solid spongiform central core, which is termed a scar. The scar is usually stellate shaped and is usually located in the center of the lesion. A single layer of cuboidal epithelial cells lines SCN and they do not communicate with the pancreatic duct. The lesions are rich in vascular epithelial growth factor receptors, and a complex vascular structure supports the lesion. Four variants of serous cystadenoma are described: (1) macrocystic serous cystadenoma, which compromise previous serous oligocystic and ill-demarcated serous adenoma, (2) solid serous adenoma, which are well-circumscribed solid lesions that share the similar immune-histological and cytological features of classic SCN, (3) VHL-associated SCN that occur in patients with VHL syndrome having multiple serous cystadenomas and macrocystic variants, and (4) mixed serous neuroendocrine neoplasm. SCN typically involve the pancreas diffusely or in a patchy fashion in patients with VHL [100]. The rare entity, mixed serous neuroendocrine neoplasm is associated with pancreatic neuroendocrine neoplasms and is highly suggestive of VHL syndrome.

Most of these cysts are discovered incidentally during imaging studies. Patients are usually free of symptoms. Symptomatic patients with SCN present with abdominal pain, anorexia, palpable mass, fatigue, malaise, and weight loss. SCN may lead to biliary or pancreatic duct obstruction and may cause GI bleeding in cases when they erode into the adjacent bowel [91].

The classical appearance of SCN on CT and MRI is microcystic or less commonly oligocystic appearance. Multiple small cysts with a central fibrous scar are pathognomonic for microcystic-type lesions. A solid component, which is because of dense fibrous feature of this lesion, often appears on CT (Fig. 8.9).

The oligocystic (unilocular) SCN is often difficult to differentiate from BD-IPMN and MCN on CT/MRI, which have similar morphology [101]. SCN should be suspected in patients when a lobulated, unilocular cystic lesion without wall enhancement located in the pancreatic head [91]. The cystic fluid reveals lower signal intensity on T1-weighted fat-suppressed MRI when compared with fibrous matrix. In contrast, the fluid becomes bright on T2-weighted images. The classical findings of SCN on EUS are multiple small, anechoic cysts with thin septa. EUS with Doppler or contrast enhanced imaging tools may demonstrate the central region, which are typically hypervascular. The hypervascular nature can result in a bloody aspirate during EUS-FNA and show hemosiderin-laden macrophages. Low amylase levels, low CEA concentrations (usually <0.5 ng/mL) and rarely, the finding of PAS-positive stained cuboidal cells are the typical characteristics of the aspirated fluid [102]. Eighteen cases with SCN were included in a recent study and a superficial vascular network sign, which corresponds to the dense subepithelial capillary vascularization, was demonstrated by nCLE with 63 % sensitivity and 100 % specificity.

The prognosis of SCN is excellent. They are most commonly managed conservatively, reserving surgery for the rare symptomatic patients. Instead, some institutions prefer surgical resection. Studies suggest long-term survival after resection, even in rare cases with cystadenocarcinoma. Currently; the universally recommended indications for surgery are presence of symptoms, cyst size >4 cm and when the diagnosis is uncertain. Although increase in size is not a predictor of malignant transformation, large SCN are reported to grow faster and they are more likely to cause symptoms [98, 100].

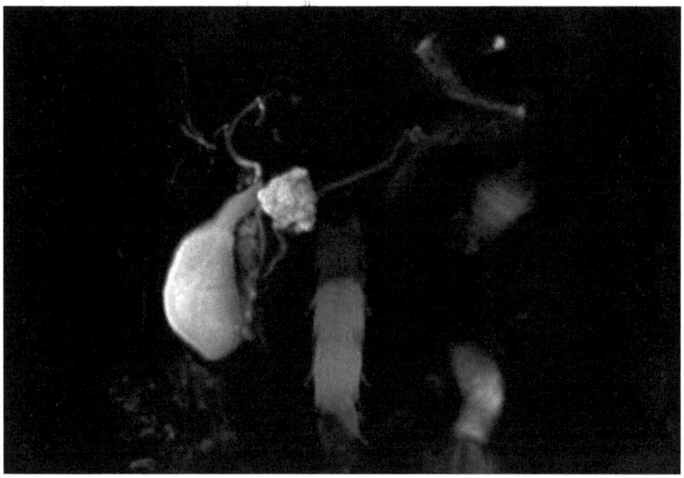

Fig. 8.9 Macrocystic lesion in the neck of pancreas consisted with SCN on MRCP

Solid Pseudopapillary Neoplasms

SPN were previously referred to solid and cystic pseudopapillary tumors or solid and cystic tumors. SPN are low-grade malignant neoplasms that consist of epithelial cells forming solid and pseudopapillary structures. Microscopically, they have solid (solid pseudopapillary) and cystic (hemorrhagic-necrotic pseudocystic) components. Poorly cohesive monomorphic cells and myxoid stromal bands having thin-walled blood vessels form the solid part. Eventually, the poorly cohesive neoplastic cells migrate and form a pseudopapilla with the residual neoplastic cells. Mucin is lacking, and glycogen is not conspicuous. SPN are single, large, well demarcated, round and often fluctuant masses. SPN commonly undergo hemorrhagic cystic degeneration [103].

SPN are classified as low-grade malignant neoplasms because they do not represent the histologic criteria of malignant behavior including vessel and perineural invasion, or parenchymal infiltration and metastasis [104]. SPN probably accounts for 5 % of PCN and predominantly found in young women at her 20s or 30s at diagnosis. Symptoms are usually related with mass effect such as pain, anorexia, nausea, vomiting, jaundice, and weight loss. SPN might also be an incidental finding.

CT reveals SPN as a well-circumscribed, encapsulated mass with varying areas of soft tissue and necrotic foci without septa. The capsule of SPN is frequently thick and enhancing and in one third of the patients, peripheral calcifications is visualized. SPN are well-defined lesions on MRI (Fig. 8.10). On T1-weighted images, high signal intensity reflects areas filled with blood and on T2-weighted images, these areas show low or inhomogeneous signal intensity [105].

On EUS, SPN demonstrates well-defined, hypoechoic mass, which include solid and cystic areas. In some patients, internal calcifications can be seen. Based on cytology and immunohistochemistry, the reported diagnostic accuracy of EUS-FNA for SPN is 65 %. Aspirated cyst fluid is typically highly cellular, sometimes may display necrotic debris. CEA

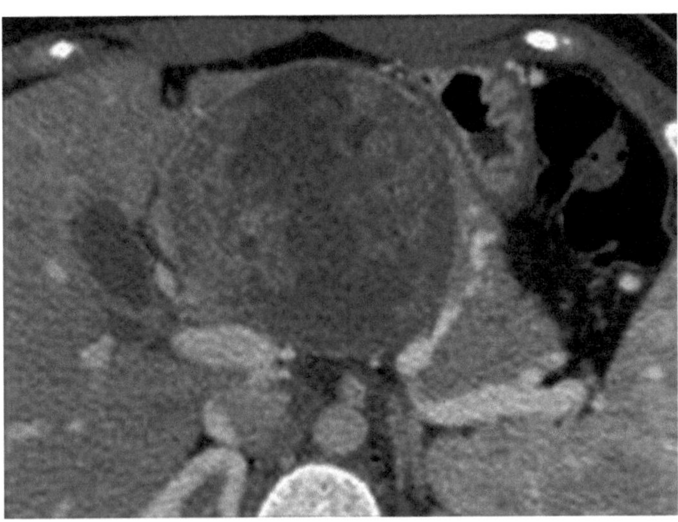

Fig. 8.10 MRI showing a large complex cystic SPN

levels of the cyst fluid are low, reflecting a nonmucinous epithelium [106].

Surgical resection is the main therapy. It is curative and recurrence after surgery is rare [1]. Long-term survival have been documented even in cases with local invasion, recurrences, or metastases [107]. To date, no definite biological or morphologic predictors of outcome have been documented. Older age of onset and SPN with an aneuploidy DNA content, are the suggested indicators of poor outcome.

Table 8.5 summarizes the general features of common pancreatic cysts.

Cystic Pancreatic Endocrine Neoplasms

CPEN are very rare and macroscopically they have an irregularly thickened wall. In the presence of a significant solid compartment, CT shows a mural enhancement, diagnostic feature of CPEN. FNA of the fluid is usually hemorrhagic and after aspiration, the residual lesion resembles a typical solid pancreatic endocrine neoplasm, which is a well-bordered hypoechoic mass (Fig. 8.11). Fine needle aspiration of the remnant cystic fluid shows cells with round, uniform nuclei that are stained with chromogranin and synaptophysin. CPENs are usually asymptomatic, incidentally diagnosed and hormonal related symptoms are very rare. Although current literature does not definitely describe the malignant behavior of CPEN, surgical resection is often suggested. Patients with comorbidities and elderly patients should be followed up with cross-sectional imaging.

General Approach to Diagnosis and Management

Various associations and multidisciplinary physician groups have recommended algorithms for the management of PCL (Fig. 8.12) [34, 108]. The aims of these guidelines are to estimate the behavior of PCL and the risk of missing a chance to treat an early malignancy, and to evaluate the risks of surgical

TABLE 8.5 Common features of some pancreatic cysts

Parameters	Pseudocyst	IPMN (MD and BD)	MCN	SCN
Demographics	Variable aged (adult) men, history of alcoholic, biliary or traumatic pancreatitis	Men in his 60s–70s	Women in her 40s–50s	Women in her 60s–80s
Gross features	Often in pancreatic tail, solitary small to very large size, fibrous-thick walled capsule	Often in head of pancreas, may be incidental and multifocal, multilocular	Often in body and tail, incidental, single, large, thick-walled	Entire pancreas, Numerous of small cysts or oligo/macrocystic
Microscopic features	Absence of epithelial lining, degenerative debris, inflammatory cells, histiocytes,	Mucin producing epithelium with papilla ± atypia, colloid-like mucin, positive mucin staining	Tall columnar mucin producing epithelium ± atypia, colloid-like mucin, positive mucin staining 'ovarian-like mucosa'	Often acellular and non-diagnostic, small cluster of cells with bland cuboidal morphology, positive glycogen staining, negative mucin staining
CT/MRI	Usually unilocular cyst, often pancreatic parenchymal inflammatory findings	MD; diffuse or limited involvement of MPD, BD; single cyst or cluster of cysts, communication to pancreatic duct, may be multifocal	Macrocysts with thick septa, peripheral eggshell calcification, wall thickening	Microcystic, multiple small cysts, central fibrous scar with calcification, occasionally oligocystic

EUS	Thick-walled, anechoic, unilocular cystic lesion, Findings of chronic pancreatitis	MD; dilated MPD, hyperechoic nodules arising from ductal wall. BD; small-cluster of grape-like dilations of BD, mural nodules	Large cystic lesion, few septa, no ductal dilation, occasionally focal, peripheral calcifications, atypical papillary projections	Multiple, anechoic, small, cystic areas, 'honeycomb' appearance, sometimes central fibrosis or calcifications
Cystic fluid characteristics	Low viscosity, clear or colored in brown to green, non-mucinous, sometimes hemorrhagic CEA ↓↓, amylase ↑, lipase ↑	High viscosity, viscous mucus, CEA usually ↑, Amylase ↑ (%60) KRAS mutation (+) (%80)	High viscosity, viscous mucus, CEA usually ↑, KRAS mutation (+) (%14) GNAS mutation (−)	Low viscosity, clear fluid, sometimes hemorrhagic, CEA ↓↓, amylase ↓↓
Confocal endomicroscopy	Not described	Epithelial villous structures, no vascular networking	Epithelial villous structures, no vascular networking	Thickened cyst wall, unilocular vascular networking, fibrous bands

MPD main pancreatic duct, *MD* main duct, *BD* branch duct

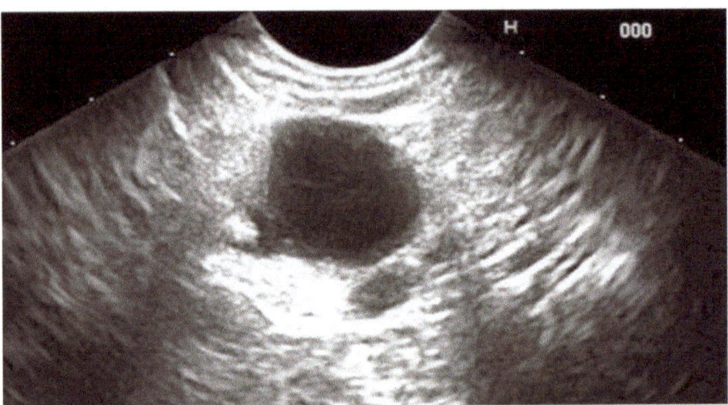

Fig. 8.11 EUS showing an anechoic 19×20 mm cystic lesion in the body of pancreas. The outer wall was irregular and thick with calcifications. After distal pancreatectomy, pathology revealed well-differentiated CPEN

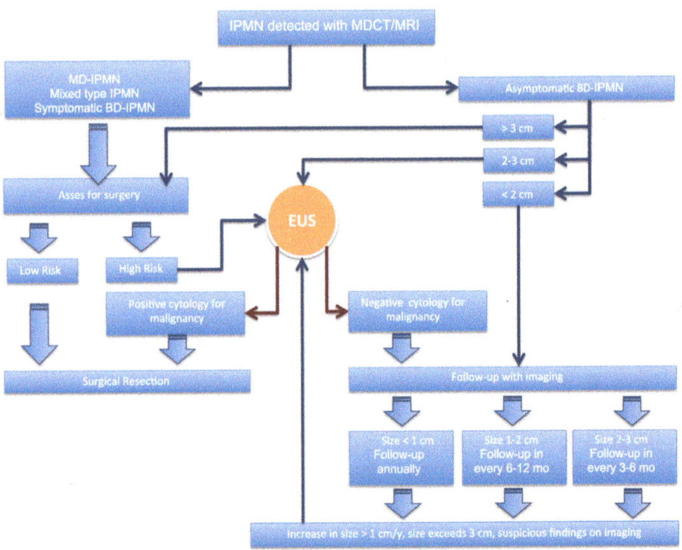

Fig. 8.12 A suggestive algorithm in patients with IPMN

resection or alternative therapies. Most of these guidelines highlight the size and morphology of the cyst as the most important issues. In general, the first step is to differentiate a pseudocyst from a PCN. The diagnosis of pseudocysts is mainly based on a pancreatitis history, biochemical and imaging findings. However, some patients with a pseudocyst may have mild pancreatitis or may not have a clinically recognized pancreatitis. On the other hand, some patients with PCN may present with pancreatitis. After excluding the diagnosis of a pseudocyst, the main goal is to differentiate a mucinous cyst from a serous cyst. If the diagnosis is a mucinous cyst, patients with MD-IPMN, combined-type IPMN, and MCN should be considered for surgical resection. Patients with BD-IPMN should be managed according to the guidelines. SCN should be followed, except for symptomatic ones or when they are larger than 4 cm.

EUS-FNA indications of PCL are not well defined in the guidelines. EUS-FNA is not generally recommended for all cystic lesions of pancreas when cross sectional imaging clearly diagnose it. In cases with an IPMN measuring more than 2 cm, and when the imaging shows benign features, the lesion should be aspirated. To make more certain, aspirated cystic fluid should be sent for CEA, *KRAS*, and GNAS evaluation. Evaluating the aspirated fluid for DNA mutations, especially when the aspirated cystic fluid is in a small amount, may enhance the results of cytology.

References

1. Yoon WJ, Brugge WR. Pancreatic cystic neoplasms: diagnosis and management. Gastroenterol Clin North Am. 2012;41:103–18.
2. Brugge WR. Diagnosis and management of cystic lesions of the pancreas. J Gastrointest Oncol. 2015;6:375–88.
3. Laffan TA, Horton KM, Klein AP, Berlanstein B, Siegelman SS, Kawamoto S, et al. Prevalence of unsuspected pancreatic cysts on MDCT. AJR Am J Roentgenol. 2008;191:802–7.

4. Moparty B, Brugge WR. Approach to pancreatic cystic lesions. Curr Gastroenterol Rep. 2007;9:130–5.

5. Spinelli KS, Fromwiller TE, Daniel RA, Kiely JM, Nakeeb A, Komorowski RA, et al. Cystic pancreatic neoplasms: observe or operate. Ann Surg. 2004;239:651–7. discussion 657–9.

6. Kimura W, Nagai H, Kuroda A, Muto T, Esaki Y. Analysis of small cystic lesions of the pancreas. Int J Pancreatol. 1995;18:197–206.

7. Kosmahl M, Pauser U, Peters K, Sipos B, Luttges J, Kremer B, et al. Cystic neoplasms of the pancreas and tumor-like lesions with cystic features: a review of 418 cases and a classification proposal. Virchows Arch. 2004;445:168–78.

8. Parra-Herran CE, Garcia MT, Herrera L, Bejarano PA. Cystic lesions of the pancreas: clinical and pathologic review of cases in a five year period. JOP. 2010;11:358–64.

9. Del Chiaro M, Verbeke C, Salvia R, Kloppel G, Werner J, McKay C, et al. European experts consensus statement on cystic tumours of the pancreas. Dig Liver Dis. 2013;45:703–11.

10. Goh BK, Tan YM, Chung YF, Chow PK, Ong HS, Lim DT, et al. Non-neoplastic cystic and cystic-like lesions of the pancreas: may mimic pancreatic cystic neoplasms. ANZ J Surg. 2006;76:325–31.

11. Silverman JF, Prichard J, Regueiro MD. Fine needle aspiration cytology of a pancreatic cyst in a patient with autosomal dominant polycystic kidney disease. A case report. Acta Cytol. 2001;45:415–9.

12. Valentini AL, Brizi MG, Mutignani M, Costamagna G, Destito C, Marano P. Adult medullary cystic disease of the kidney and pancreatic cystic disease: a new association. Scand J Urol Nephrol. 1999;33:423–5.

13. Monti L, Salerno T, Lucidi V, Fariello G, Orazi C, Manfredi R, et al. Pancreatic cystosis in cystic fibrosis: case report. Abdom Imaging. 2001;26:648–50.

14. Habashi S, Draganov PV. Pancreatic pseudocyst. World J Gastroenterol. 2009;15:38–47.

15. Banks PA, Bollen TL, Dervenis C, Gooszen HG, Johnson CD, Sarr MG, et al. Classification of acute pancreatitis 2012: revision of the Atlanta classification and definitions by international consensus. Gut. 2013;62:102–11.

16. Memis A, Parildar M. Interventional radiological treatment in complications of pancreatitis. Eur J Radiol. 2002;43:219–28.

17. Brun A, Agarwal N, Pitchumoni CS. Fluid collections in and around the pancreas in acute pancreatitis. J Clin Gastroenterol. 2011;45:614–25.
18. Aghdassi A, Mayerle J, Kraft M, Sielenkamper AW, Heidecke CD, Lerch MM. Diagnosis and treatment of pancreatic pseudocysts in chronic pancreatitis. Pancreas. 2008;36:105–12.
19. Pelaez-Luna M, Vege SS, Petersen BT, Chari ST, Clain JE, Levy MJ, et al. Disconnected pancreatic duct syndrome in severe acute pancreatitis: clinical and imaging characteristics and outcomes in a cohort of 31 cases. Gastrointest Endosc. 2008;68: 91–7.
20. Siegelman SS, Copeland BE, Saba GP, Cameron JL, Sanders RC, Zerhouni EA, et al. CT of fluid collections associated with pancreatitis. AJR Am J Roentgenol. 1980;134:1121–32.
21. Okuda K, Sugita S, Tsukada E, Sakuma Y, Ohkubo K. Pancreatic pseudocyst in the left hepatic lobe: a report of two cases. Hepatology. 1991;13:359–63.
22. Lankisch PG. The spleen in inflammatory pancreatic disease. Gastroenterology. 1990;98:509–16.
23. Fishman EK, Soyer P, Bliss DF, Bluemke DA, Devine N. Splenic involvement in pancreatitis: spectrum of CT findings. AJR Am J Roentgenol. 1995;164:631–5.
24. Lilienfeld RM, Lande A. Pancreatic pseudocysts presenting as thick-walled renal and perinephric cysts. J Urol. 1976;115:123–5.
25. Cannon JW, Callery MP, Vollmer Jr CM. Diagnosis and management of pancreatic pseudocysts: what is the evidence? J Am Coll Surg. 2009;209:385–93.
26. Brugge WR. Approaches to the drainage of pancreatic pseudocysts. Curr Opin Gastroenterol. 2004;20:488–92.
27. Desser TS, Sommer FG, Jeffrey Jr RB. Value of curved planar reformations in MDCT of abdominal pathology. AJR Am J Roentgenol. 2004;182:1477–84.
28. Sahani DV, Kadavigere R, Blake M, Fernandez-Del Castillo C, Lauwers GY, Hahn PF. Intraductal papillary mucinous neoplasm of pancreas: multi-detector row CT with 2D curved reformations correlation with MRCP. Radiology. 2006;238:560–9.
29. Garcea G, Ong SL, Rajesh A, Neal CP, Pollard CA, Berry DP, et al. Cystic lesions of the pancreas. A diagnostic and management dilemma. Pancreatology. 2008;8:236–51.
30. Balthazar EJ, Freeny PC, vanSonnenberg E. Imaging and intervention in acute pancreatitis. Radiology. 1994;193:297–306.

31. Brugge WR. The use of EUS to diagnose cystic neoplasms of the pancreas. Gastrointest Endosc. 2009;69:S203–9.
32. Pitman MB, Lewandrowski K, Shen J, Sahani D, Brugge W, Fernandez-del CC. Pancreatic cysts: preoperative diagnosis and clinical management. Cancer Cytopathol. 2010;118:1–13.
33. Johnson MD, Walsh RM, Henderson JM, Brown N, Ponsky J, Dumot J, et al. Surgical versus nonsurgical management of pancreatic pseudocysts. J Clin Gastroenterol. 2009;43:586–90.
34. Turner BG, Brugge WR. Pancreatic cystic lesions: when to watch, when to operate, and when to ignore. Curr Gastroenterol Rep. 2010;12:98–105.
35. Bennett S, Lorenz JM. The role of imaging-guided percutaneous procedures in the multidisciplinary approach to treatment of pancreatic fluid collections. Semin Intervent Radiol. 2012;29:314–8.
36. Neff R. Pancreatic pseudocysts and fluid collections: percutaneous approaches. Surg Clin North Am. 2001;81:399–403. xii.
37. Lerch MM, Stier A, Wahnschaffe U, Mayerle J. Pancreatic pseudocysts: observation, endoscopic drainage, or resection? Dtsch Arztebl Int. 2009;106:614–21.
38. Giovannini M. Endoscopic ultrasonography-guided pancreatic drainage. Gastrointest Endosc Clin N Am. 2012;22:221–30. viii.
39. Samuelson AL, Shah RJ. Endoscopic management of pancreatic pseudocysts. Gastroenterol Clin North Am. 2012;41:47–62.
40. Brugge WR, Lauwers GY, Sahani D, Fernandez-del Castillo C, Warshaw AL. Cystic neoplasms of the pancreas. N Engl J Med. 2004;351:1218–26.
41. Farrell JJ, Brugge WR. Intraductal papillary mucinous tumor of the pancreas. Gastrointest Endosc. 2002;55:701–14.
42. Sahani DV, Lin DJ, Venkatesan AM, Ainani N, Mino-Kenudson M, Brugge WR, et al. Multidisciplinary approach to diagnosis and management of intraductal papillary mucinous neoplasms of the pancreas. Clin Gastroenterol Hepatol. 2009;7:259–69.
43. Gaujoux S, Brennan MF, Gonen M, D'Angelica MI, DeMatteo R, Fong Y, et al. Cystic lesions of the pancreas: changes in the presentation and management of 1,424 patients at a single institution over a 15-year time period. J Am Coll Surg. 2011;212:590–600. discussion 600–3.
44. Salvia R, Fernandez-del Castillo C, Bassi C, Thayer SP, Falconi M, Mantovani W, et al. Main-duct intraductal papillary mucinous neoplasms of the pancreas: clinical predictors of malignancy and

long-term survival following resection. Ann Surg. 2004;239:678–85. discussion 685–7.

45. Crippa S, Fernandez-Del Castillo C, Salvia R, Finkelstein D, Bassi C, Dominguez I, et al. Mucin-producing neoplasms of the pancreas: an analysis of distinguishing clinical and epidemiologic characteristics. Clin Gastroenterol Hepatol. 2010;8:213–9.

46. Lafemina J, Katabi N, Klimstra D, Correa-Gallego C, Gaujoux S, Kingham TP, et al. Malignant progression in IPMN: a cohort analysis of patients initially selected for resection or observation. Ann Surg Oncol. 2013;20:440–7.

47. Schmidt CM, White PB, Waters JA, Yiannoutsos CT, Cummings OW, Baker M, et al. Intraductal papillary mucinous neoplasms: predictors of malignant and invasive pathology. Ann Surg. 2007;246:644–51. discussion 651–4.

48. Sohn TA, Yeo CJ, Cameron JL, Hruban RH, Fukushima N, Campbell KA, et al. Intraductal papillary mucinous neoplasms of the pancreas: an updated experience. Ann Surg. 2004;239:788–97. discussion 797–9.

49. Pelaez-Luna M, Chari ST, Smyrk TC, Takahashi N, Clain JE, Levy MJ, et al. Do consensus indications for resection in branch duct intraductal papillary mucinous neoplasm predict malignancy? A study of 147 patients. Am J Gastroenterol. 2007;102:1759–64.

50. Izawa T, Obara T, Tanno S, Mizukami Y, Yanagawa N, Kohgo Y, et al. Clonality and field cancerization in intraductal papillary-mucinous tumors of the pancreas. Cancer. 2001;92:1807–17.

51. Kang MJ, Lee KB, Jang JY, Kwon W, Park JW, Chang YR, et al. Disease spectrum of intraductal papillary mucinous neoplasm with an associated invasive carcinoma invasive IPMN versus pancreatic ductal adenocarcinoma-associated IPMN. Pancreas. 2013;42:1267–74.

52. Sakorafas GH, Smyrniotis V, Reid-Lombardo KM, Sarr MG. Primary pancreatic cystic neoplasms revisited. Part III. Intraductal papillary mucinous neoplasms. Surg Oncol. 2011;20:e109–18.

53. Andrejevic-Blant S, Kosmahl M, Sipos B, Kloppel G. Pancreatic intraductal papillary-mucinous neoplasms: a new and evolving entity. Virchows Arch. 2007;451:863–9.

54. Yopp AC, Katabi N, Janakos M, Klimstra DS, D'Angelica MI, DeMatteo RP, et al. Invasive carcinoma arising in intraductal papillary mucinous neoplasms of the pancreas: a matched

control study with conventional pancreatic ductal adenocarcinoma. Ann Surg. 2011;253:968–74.

55. Furukawa T, Hatori T, Fujita I, Yamamoto M, Kobayashi M, Ohike N, et al. Prognostic relevance of morphological types of intraductal papillary mucinous neoplasms of the pancreas. Gut. 2011;60:509–16.

56. Liszka L, Pajak J, Zielinska-Pajak E, Krzych L, Golka D, Mrowiec S, et al. Intraductal oncocytic papillary neoplasms of the pancreas and bile ducts: a description of five new cases and review based on a systematic survey of the literature. J Hepatobiliary Pancreat Sci. 2010;17:246–61.

57. Satoh K, Shimosegawa T, Moriizumi S, Koizumi M, Toyota T. K-ras mutation and p53 protein accumulation in intraductal mucinhypersecreting neoplasms of the pancreas. Pancreas. 1996;12:362–8.

58. Schonleben F, Qiu W, Bruckman KC, Ciau NT, Li X, Lauerman MH, et al. BRAF and KRAS gene mutations in intraductal papillary mucinous neoplasm/carcinoma (IPMN/IPMC) of the pancreas. Cancer Lett. 2007;249:242–8.

59. Shi C, Hruban RH. Intraductal papillary mucinous neoplasm. Hum Pathol. 2012;43:1–16.

60. Amato E, Molin MD, Mafficini A, Yu J, Malleo G, Rusev B, et al. Targeted next-generation sequencing of cancer genes dissects the molecular profiles of intraductal papillary neoplasms of the pancreas. J Pathol. 2014;233:217–27.

61. Schonleben F, Qiu W, Remotti HE, Hohenberger W, Su GH. PIK3CA, KRAS, and BRAF mutations in intraductal papillary mucinous neoplasm/carcinoma (IPMN/C) of the pancreas. Langenbecks Arch Surg. 2008;393:289–96.

62. Wu J, Matthaei H, Maitra A, Dal Molin M, Wood LD, Eshleman JR, et al. Recurrent GNAS mutations define an unexpected pathway for pancreatic cyst development. Sci Transl Med. 2011;3:92ra66.

63. Sato N, Rosty C, Jansen M, Fukushima N, Ueki T, Yeo CJ, et al. STK11/LKB1 Peutz-Jeghers gene inactivation in intraductal papillary-mucinous neoplasms of the pancreas. Am J Pathol. 2001;159:2017–22.

64. Konstantinou F, Syrigos KN, Saif MW. Intraductal papillary mucinous neoplasms of the pancreas (IPMNs): epidemiology, diagnosis and future aspects. JOP. 2013;14:141–4.

65. Clores MJ, Thosani A, Buscaglia JM. Multidisciplinary diagnostic and therapeutic approaches to pancreatic cystic lesions. J Multidiscip Health. 2014;7:81–91.

66. Jones MJ, Buchanan AS, Neal CP, Dennison AR, Metcalfe MS. Garcea G Imaging of indeterminate pancreatic cystic lesions: a systematic review. Pancreatology. 2013;13:436–42.
67. Sahani DV, Kambadakone A, Macari M, Takahashi N, Chari S, Fernandez-del CC. Diagnosis and management of cystic pancreatic lesions. AJR Am J Roentgenol. 2013;200:343–54.
68. Lee HJ, Kim MJ, Choi JY, Hong HS, Kim KA. Relative accuracy of CT and MRI in the differentiation of benign from malignant pancreatic cystic lesions. Clin Radiol. 2011;66:315–21.
69. Sainani NI, Saokar A, Deshpande V, Fernandez-del Castillo C, Hahn P, Sahani DV. Comparative performance of MDCT and MRI with MR cholangiopancreatography in characterizing small pancreatic cysts. AJR Am J Roentgenol. 2009;193:722–31.
70. Brugge WR. Endoscopic approach to the diagnosis and treatment of pancreatic disease. Curr Opin Gastroenterol. 2013;29:559–65.
71. Tanaka M, Fernandez-del Castillo C, Adsay V, Chari S, Falconi M, Jang JY, et al. International consensus guidelines 2012 for the management of IPMN and MCN of the pancreas. Pancreatology. 2012;12:183–97.
72. Grutzmann R, Niedergethmann M, Pilarsky C, Kloppel G, Saeger HD. Intraductal papillary mucinous tumors of the pancreas: biology, diagnosis, and treatment. Oncologist. 2010;15:1294–309.
73. Kadayifci A, Brugge WR. Endoscopic ultrasound-guided fine-needle aspiration for the differential diagnosis of intraductal papillary mucinous neoplasms and size stratification for surveillance. Endoscopy. 2014;46:357.
74. Lee LS, Saltzman JR, Bounds BC, Poneros JM, Brugge WR, Thompson CC. EUS-guided fine needle aspiration of pancreatic cysts: a retrospective analysis of complications and their predictors. Clin Gastroenterol Hepatol. 2005;3:231–6.
75. Brugge WR, Lewandrowski K, Lee-Lewandrowski E, Centeno BA, Szydlo T, Regan S, et al. Diagnosis of pancreatic cystic neoplasms: a report of the cooperative pancreatic cyst study. Gastroenterology. 2004;126:1330–6.
76. van der Waaij LA, van Dullemen HM, Porte RJ. Cyst fluid analysis in the differential diagnosis of pancreatic cystic lesions: a pooled analysis. Gastrointest Endosc. 2005;62:383–9.
77. Park WG, Wu M, Bowen R, Zheng M, Fitch WL, Pai RK, et al. Metabolomic-derived novel cyst fluid biomarkers for pancreatic cysts: glucose and kynurenine. Gastrointest Endosc. 2013;78: 295–302.e2.

78. Michaels PJ, Brachtel EF, Bounds BC, Brugge WR, Pitman MB. Intraductal papillary mucinous neoplasm of the pancreas: cytologic features predict histologic grade. Cancer. 2006;108: 163–73.
79. Pitman MB, Centeno BA, Daglilar ES, Brugge WR, Mino-Kenudson M. Cytological criteria of high-grade epithelial atypia in the cyst fluid of pancreatic intraductal papillary mucinous neoplasms. Cancer Cytopathol. 2014;122:40–7.
80. Sawhney MS, Devarajan S, O'Farrel P, Cury MS, Kundu R, Vollmer CM, et al. Comparison of carcinoembryonic antigen and molecular analysis in pancreatic cyst fluid. Gastrointest Endosc. 2009;69:1106–10.
81. Dal Molin M, Matthaei H, Wu J, Blackford A, Debeljak M, Rezaee N, et al. Clinicopathological correlates of activating GNAS mutations in intraductal papillary mucinous neoplasm (IPMN) of the pancreas. Ann Surg Oncol. 2013;20:3802–8.
82. Konda VJ, Meining A, Jamil LH, Giovannini M, Hwang JH, Wallace MB, et al. A pilot study of in vivo identification of pancreatic cystic neoplasms with needle-based confocal laser endomicroscopy under endosonographic guidance. Endoscopy. 2013;45:1006–13.
83. Rodriguez JR, Salvia R, Crippa S, Warshaw AL, Bassi C, Falconi M, et al. Branch-duct intraductal papillary mucinous neoplasms: observations in 145 patients who underwent resection. Gastroenterology. 2007;133:72–9. quiz 309–310.
84. Brugge WR. Management and outcomes of pancreatic cystic lesions. Dig Liver Dis. 2008;40:854–9.
85. Matthes K, Mino-Kenudson M, Sahani DV, Holalkere N, Fowers KD, Rathi R, et al. EUS-guided injection of paclitaxel (OncoGel) provides therapeutic drug concentrations in the porcine pancreas (with video). Gastrointest Endosc. 2007;65:448–53.
86. Pai M, Senturk H, Lakhtakia S, Reddy DN, Cicinnati V, Kabar I, et al. 351 endoscopic ultrasound guided radiofrequency ablation (EUS-RFA) for cystic neoplasms and neuroendocrine tumors of the pancreas. Gastrointest Endosc. 2013;77:AB143–4.
87. Kamata K, Kitano M, Kudo M, Sakamoto H, Kadosaka K, Miyata T, et al. Value of EUS in early detection of pancreatic ductal adenocarcinomas in patients with intraductal papillary mucinous neoplasms. Endoscopy. 2014;46:22–9.
88. Valsangkar NP, Morales-Oyarvide V, Thayer SP, Ferrone CR, Wargo JA, Warshaw AL, et al. 851 resected cystic tumors of the pancreas: a 33-year experience at the Massachusetts General Hospital. Surgery. 2012;152:S4–12.

89. Goh BK, Tan YM, Chung YF, Chow PK, Cheow PC, Wong WK, et al. A review of mucinous cystic neoplasms of the pancreas defined by ovarian-type stroma: clinicopathological features of 344 patients. World J Surg. 2006;30:2236–45.
90. Sakorafas GH, Smyrniotis V, Reid-Lombardo KM, Sarr MG. Primary pancreatic cystic neoplasms revisited: part II. Mucinous cystic neoplasms. Surg Oncol. 2011;20:e93–101.
91. Bai XL, Zhang Q, Masood N, Masood W, Zhang Y, Liang TB. Pancreatic cystic neoplasms: a review of preoperative diagnosis and management. J Zhejiang Univ Sci B. 2013;14:185–94.
92. Jimenez RE, Warshaw AL, Z'Graggen K, Hartwig W, Taylor DZ, Compton CC, et al. Sequential accumulation of K-ras mutations and p53 overexpression in the progression of pancreatic muci-nous cystic neoplasms to malignancy. Ann Surg. 1999;230:501–9. discussion 509–11.
93. Iacobuzio-Donahue CA, Wilentz RE, Argani P, Yeo CJ, Cameron JL, Kern SE, et al. Dpc4 protein in mucinous cystic neoplasms of the pancreas: frequent loss of expression in invasive carcinomas suggests a role in genetic progression. Am J Surg Pathol. 2000;24:1544–8.
94. Yamao K, Yanagisawa A, Takahashi K, Kimura W, Doi R, Fukushima N, et al. Clinicopathological features and prognosis of mucinous cystic neoplasm with ovarian-type stroma: a multi-institutional study of the Japan pancreas society. Pancreas. 2011;40:67–71.
95. Crippa S, Salvia R, Warshaw AL, Dominguez I, Bassi C, Falconi M, et al. Mucinous cystic neoplasm of the pancreas is not an aggressive entity: lessons from 163 resected patients. Ann Surg. 2008;247:571–9.
96. Procacci C, Carbognin G, Accordini S, Biasiutti C, Guarise A, Lombardo F, et al. CT features of malignant mucinous cystic tumors of the pancreas. Eur Radiol. 2001;11:1626–30.
97. Zamboni G, Scarpa A, Bogina G, Iacono C, Bassi C, Talamini G, et al. Mucinous cystic tumors of the pancreas: clinicopathological features, prognosis, and relationship to other mucinous cystic tumors. Am J Surg Pathol. 1999;23:410–22.
98. Sakorafas GH, Smyrniotis V, Reid-Lombardo KM, Sarr MG. Primary pancreatic cystic neoplasms revisited. Part I: serous cys-tic neoplasms. Surg Oncol. 2011;20:e84–92.
99. Moore PS, Zamboni G, Brighenti A, Lissandrini D, Antonello D, Capelli P, et al. Molecular characterization of pancreatic serous microcystic adenomas: evidence for a tumor suppressor gene on chromosome 10q. Am J Pathol. 2001;158:317–21.

100. Farrell JJ, Fernandez-del CC. Pancreatic cystic neoplasms: management and unanswered questions. Gastroenterology. 2013;144:1303–15.
101. Procacci C, Graziani R, Bicego E, Bergamo-Andreis IA, Guarise A, Valdo M, et al. Serous cystadenoma of the pancreas: report of 30 cases with emphasis on the imaging findings. J Comput Assist Tomogr. 1997;21:373–82.
102. Belsley NA, Pitman MB, Lauwers GY, Brugge WR, Deshpande V. Serous cystadenoma of the pancreas: limitations and pitfalls of endoscopic ultrasound-guided fine-needle aspiration biopsy. Cancer. 2008;114:102–10.
103. Papavramidis T, Papavramidis S. Solid pseudopapillary tumors of the pancreas: review of 718 patients reported in English literature. J Am Coll Surg. 2005;200:965–72.
104. Tipton SG, Smyrk TC, Sarr MG, Thompson GB. Malignant potential of solid pseudopapillary neoplasm of the pancreas. Br J Surg. 2006;93:733–7.
105. Choi JY, Kim MJ, Kim JH, Kim SH, Lim JS, Oh YT, et al. Solid pseudopapillary tumor of the pancreas: typical and atypical manifestations. AJR Am J Roentgenol. 2006;187:W178–86.
106. Jani N, Dewitt J, Eloubeidi M, Varadarajulu S, Appalaneni V, Hoffman B, et al. Endoscopic ultrasound-guided fine-needle aspiration for diagnosis of solid pseudopapillary tumors of the pancreas: a multicenter experience. Endoscopy. 2008;40:200–3.
107. Lee SE, Jang JY, Hwang DW, Park KW, Kim SW. Clinical features and outcome of solid pseudopapillary neoplasm: differences between adults and children. Arch Surg. 2008;143:1218–21.
108. Scheiman JM. Management of cystic lesions of the pancreas. J Gastrointest Surg. 2008;12:405–7.

Chapter 9
Bile Duct and Pancreas: Brief Anatomy, Investigations Used

Abdul H. Khan

Patient Information

Both the pancreas and liver are located in the upper abdomen and have many important functions, including the synthesis of digestive enzymes that are secreted through ducts into the duodenum, in a process largely controlled by hormones.

Pancreas

Anatomy

The pancreas is a yellowish, spongy-appearing gland situated across the upper abdomen in the retroperitoneal space. By convention, the pancreas is divided in thirds: the head/uncinate process towards the liver, the body in the middle, and the tail towards the spleen; however, there is no functional distinction between these regions, nor are there any visible landmarks to distinguish these regions. The main pancreatic

A.H. Khan, M.D. (✉)
Division of Gastroenterology and Hepatology—Froedtert Hospital, Medical College of Wisconsin, 9200 West Wisconsin Avenue, Milwaukee, WI 53226, USA
e-mail: ahkhan@mcw.edu

© Springer International Publishing Switzerland 2016   201
K. Dua, R. Shaker (eds.), *Pancreas and Biliary Disease*,
DOI 10.1007/978-3-319-28089-9_9

duct (duct of Wirsung) runs longitudinally in the center of the gland collecting digestive fluid from the peripheral ductules, and drains from the tail towards the head of the pancreas where it empties mainly through the major papilla (ampulla of Vater) into the 2nd portion of the duodenum. An accessory duct (duct of Santorini) branches off the main duct in the head of the pancreas and empties through the minor papilla a bit more proximally in the duodenum from the major papilla.

Anatomical variations can arise during the process of embryonic development. The most common is pancreas divisum where the ventral duct in the head of the pancreas fails to fuse with the dorsal duct in the body/tail resulting in the main pancreatic (dorsal) duct draining through the accessory duct via the minor papilla. A separate, small wispy ventral duct drains through the major papilla. The prevalence of pancreas divisum is approximately 5–10 % and it mostly has no clinical significance; however, these patients are at higher risk of developing acute pancreatitis [1]. Another anatomical variant is annular pancreas where the head of the pancreas completely encircles the 2nd portion of the duodenum resulting in gastric outlet obstruction often in early childhood but may also present in adulthood. These patients are best treated by surgical bypass of the obstructed duodenum [2, 3]. Ansa pancreas is an anatomic variant where the pancreatic duct forms an odd loop in the head of the pancreas as it drains towards the major papilla. This usually has no clinical significance but can make ERCP involving the pancreatic duct technically difficult in terms of passing a wire through the tortuous duct [4].

The arterial blood supply is through several separate arterial branches of the celiac artery and the superior mesenteric artery along with the splenic artery which takes an undulating course along the body/tail of the pancreas towards the spleen. The venous drainage mainly occurs through the splenic vein which runs along the inferior border of the pancreas along its entire length and drains into the portal vein at the portosplenic confluence located adjacent to the head of the pancreas. The pancreas is innervated by the splanchnic nerves and vagus nerve via the celiac and superior mesenteric plexi posterior to the pancreas.

Histologically, there are collections of neuroendocrine cells within the parenchyma that are not evident grossly, known as islets of Langerhans, which account for about 2 % of the pancreatic mass. These extremely important cells primarily regulate the body's glucose levels, and are composed of alpha, beta, and delta cells that secrete glucagon, insulin, and somatostatin, respectively. Large amounts of hormone can be produced from a small number of cells so pancreatic endocrine insufficiency requires loss of over 90 % of the pancreas gland's normal function, which can result from a number of scenarios including chronic pancreatitis, pancreatic atrophy, acute necrotizing pancreatitis, and surgical resection. The majority of the pancreas, roughly 85 % of its mass, is dedicated to its exocrine function and is composed of acinar and ductal cells. Acinar cells aggregate to form lobules which produce mostly zymogens, which are precursor digestive enzymes needed to breakdown fats, proteins, and carbohydrates. Acinar cells secrete their contents into a ductal system lined by a bicarbonate-secreting ductal epithelium which ultimately drains into the main pancreatic duct. The pancreatic exocrine function of providing digestive enzymes to the small bowel is much more susceptible to insufficiency than its endocrine function. Of all the pancreatic enzymes, lipase is the most sensitive to loss of function, and thus, steatorrhea, or fat malabsorption, is the first manifestation of pancreatic exocrine insufficiency.

Physiology

The two main hormones that regulate pancreatic exocrine function are secretin and cholecystokinin (CCK). Secretin is secreted by S cells of the gastric antrum and is released due to a drop in pH of the duodenum as acidic gastric contents are passed through the pylorus, and its main effect is to counter the acidity of the food bolus entering the small intestine from the stomach. Secretin stimulates pancreatic ductal cells to secrete bicarbonate which is released into the small bowel to raise duodenal pH. It also inhibits gastric G cells from secreting gastrin to reduce gastric secretion of acid. CCK is secreted from neuroendocrine I cells in the duodenal epithelium and acts mainly to provide digestive enzymes to the small bowel in response to a meal. CCK stimulates pancreatic acinar cells to secrete their zymogens into the ductal system which drains to the small bowel where enzymes along the duodenal brush border activate the zymogens to allow digestion to take place.

Biliary Tree

Anatomy

The biliary tree is a complex network of ducts in a tree like configuration with the common bile duct and common hepatic duct forming the extrahepatic trunk of the tree and the intrahepatic ductal system forming the branches. Bile from the liver parenchyma is delivered to the duodenum through the biliary tree for the purpose of digesting fats. The biliary system is lined by a cuboidal epithelium of cholangiocytes, which secrete bicarbonate in response to secretin, similar to pancreatic ductal cells. The intrahepatic ducts are part of the portal triad along with the portal venules and hepatic arterioles. The ductules drain the hepatocytes and join other ductules into larger ducts until uniting at a single duct inferior to the liver known as the common hepatic duct. The gallbladder is a distensible pouch that stores bile and is stimulated by CCK in response to a meal to contract and expel bile. The cystic duct is a spiral shaped duct due to the arrangement of its crescentic mucosal folds known as valves of Heister, and this can make it difficult to pass a wire through it during ERCP. The cystic duct drains the gallbladder and inserts into the common hepatic duct to form the common bile duct. Bile that crystallizes out of solution in the gallbladder can form sludge and stones which is generally has no clinical significance within the gallbladder, but can intermittently obstruct the cystic duct resulting in biliary colic or become impacted in the cystic duct leading to acute cholecystitis. If a stone passes into the bile duct causing obstruction, the patient will develop jaundice and possibly cholangitis. The common bile duct drains into the duodenum through the ampulla of Vater, which is a nipple like protrusion in the second portion of the duodenum. Surrounding the bile duct epithelium at the level of the ampulla is a round muscle known as the sphincter of Oddi. Normally it remains closed preventing passage of bile when there is no food present for digestion. CCK causes the sphincter of Oddi to relax allowing passage of bile from the gallbladder through the bile duct and into the duodenal lumen for digestion. In sphincter of Oddi dysfunction, this muscle inappropriately remains in a state of spasm preventing passage of bile resulting in elevated pressure within the biliary tree resulting in the sensation of biliary colic.

A small percentage of people have anatomic variants of the biliary tree that have no clinical significance but may result in complications during interventional procedures if not identified. The cystic duct may insert directly into the right hepatic duct rather than the common hepatic duct. There may be small ductules known as ducts of Luschka that connect the body of the gallbladder to the branches of the right hepatic duct at the inferior surface of the right lobe of the liver. Aberrant right hepatic ducts are ducts that drain a portion of the right lobe directly into the common bile duct rather than to the right main hepatic duct. These variants may result in bile leak and ductal injury after cholecystectomy.

Investigations Used

There are many diagnostic tools available to clinicians to investigate pancreaticobiliary disease.

Blood Tests

Amylase, Lipase

Two of the enzymes secreted by the pancreas, namely amylase and lipase, are also useful serum markers for acute pancreatitis and still widely used clinically. Amylase is a small enzyme that digests starch and is primarily produced by the pancreas and salivary glands. Serum amylase levels tend to rapidly rise with acute pancreatitis but normalize within 3–5 days due to rapid clearance through the kidneys and reticulo-endothelial system [5]. False positivity can occur when the amylase level is elevated from other causes such as mac-roamylasemia where an abnormal large protein binds amy-lase reducing its renal clearance [6]. Inflammation or trauma to the gastrointestinal tract can cause elevated amylase levels as well. In acute pancreatitis, gallstone pancreatitis tends to cause highly elevated amylase levels whereas pancreatitis due to hypertriglyceridemia or acute on chronic pancreatitis may result in normal amylase levels. Lipase is comparable in sensitivity but a more specific marker of pancreatitis than amylase at over 90 % [7]. Lipase levels rise with pancreatic inflammation but tend to remain elevated for many days due less rapid renal clearance than amylase. The degree of amylase and lipase elevation has not been shown to reliably predict severity of pancreatitis because necrosis of the pan-creas can result in a drop in enzyme levels. Therefore, the diagnosis of pancreatitis generally relies on meeting two of three criteria: pain typical of pancreatitis, elevation of amy-lase and/or lipase to 3 times the upper limit of normal, and imaging consistent with acute pancreatitis [8]. These markers are not useful in the diagnosis of chronic pancreatitis, how-ever, since the process involves the gradual replacement of normal parenchyma with scar tissue so there is no sudden release of amylase and lipase, but rather a diminishing of the total enzymatic content of the pancreas.

Hepatic Function Tests

A set of blood tests with high diagnostic utility are hepatic function tests: alkaline phosphatase, AST, ALT, and total/direct bilirubin. Any disease of the liver or biliary tree can cause a rise in all hepatic function tests but the proportion of elevation can suggest etiology. Biliary disease results in obstruction to flow through the biliary tree due to any number of conditions such as biliary stones, benign or malignant strictures, primary sclerosing cholangitis, sphincter of Oddi dysfunction, occluded biliary stents, or biliary atresia in early life. This tends to cause a rise in alkaline phosphatase and bilirubin more so than transaminases. Conversely, hepatocellular diseases cause a proportionally greater rise in transaminases. Bilirubin, a by-product of erythrocyte breakdown, is taken up by hepatocytes and conjugated enzymatically to make it soluble so that it can be excreted as a component of bile through the bile duct and into the GI tract where it can pass with stool. Failure in any step of bilirubin metabolism results in accumulation of bilirubin in the blood and failure to excrete bilirubin in the stool. In a patient with hyperbilirubinemia, if the conjugated (direct) fraction accounts for 50 % or more of the total bilirubin, the hyperbilirubinemia is most often due to downstream blockage of bile flow. It should be kept in mind that there are non-obstructive causes of elevated alkaline phosphatase such as intrahepatic cholestasis, which has numerous causes. Additional blood tests such as elevations in gamma glutamyl transpeptidase (GGT), 5-nucleotidase (5-NT), and fractionation of alkaline phosphatase can help confirm that the alkaline phosphatase elevation is hepatic in origin rather than from bone or elsewhere [9]. Also, there are non-obstructive causes of hyperbilirubinemia such as genetic conditions causing hepatocellular enzymatic insufficiency in processing bilirubin resulting in unconjugated hyperbilirubinemia (Gilbert's disease, Crigler–Najjar syndrome) or conjugated hyperbilirubinemia (Dubin–Johnson syndrome and Rotor syndrome) [10]. As with any test, hepatic function tests need to be correlated clinically in conjunction with imaging data to reach the correct diagnosis.

CA19-9 (Also Covered in the Chapter on Pancreas Cancer)

The tumor marker CA19-9 is often elevated in patients with adenocarcinoma of the pancreas or biliary tree including the gallbladder. It can be elevated in obstructive jaundice however, so it is important to recheck the level after a biliary stent is placed and the bilirubin has normalized. It has a sensitivity of 70 % and specificity of 80 % for pancreatic cancer which insufficiently accurate to replace the need for tissue diagnosis, but it can raise or lower suspicion in certain inconclusive cases [11]. Roughly 7–10 % of people lack the Lewis antigen glycosyltransferase enzyme and thus have no detectable serum CA19-9 at all [12]. In patients with elevated CA19-9 and proven pancreaticobiliary malignancy, the CA19-9 level can be useful as a marker of disease burden or recurrence, especially if it normalizes after treatment. An elevated CA19-9 may also trigger further evaluation in patients with PSC since it is difficult to distinguish benign from malignant biliary strictures [11].

Imaging Tests

Abdominal Ultrasound

Imaging tests have become increasingly more useful as the quality has improved through the years. Plain x-rays of the GI tract have little role in pancreaticobiliary disease. A "double bubble" sign reflecting air in the stomach and duodenal bulb consistent with duodenal obstruction is a nonspecific sign of annular pancreas. Calcified gallstones can be seen in the right upper quadrant. Dense opacities across the mid abdomen can be seen in severe calcific chronic pancreatitis, but X-ray is of low sensitivity for all of these conditions.

Abdominal ultrasound is still a useful test for the gallbladder and proximal biliary tree. It is relatively quick and does not expose the patient to radiation. It generally has a sensitivity as high as 98 % for evaluating the gallbladder in terms of stones, sludge, and polyps. In the diagnosis of acute cholecystitis, the finding of gallstones on ultrasound with a positive Murphy's sign in which pressing the ultrasound probe in the right upper quadrant causes tenderness, is associated with a positive predictive value of 92 %, whereas the absence of these two findings has a negative predictive value of 95 % [13]. It can show intrahepatic and proximal extrahepatic biliary ductal dilation suggesting obstruction with a sensitivity of 85–95 % in patients with jaundice [14]. However, it is poor in evaluating the distal bile duct and pancreas due to the frequent presence of small bowel anteriorly causing air artifact. Thus, its sensitivity for choledocholithiasis or pancreatic lesions in the setting of jaundice may only be 33 % [14]. Furthermore, the finding of bile duct dilation may not necessarily represent obstruction, especially in the setting of prior cholecystectomy after which the bile duct often develops mild dilatation.

Hepatobiliary Scintigraphy

Hepatobiliary scintigraphy, or hepatobiliary iminodiacetic acid (HIDA) scan, is a nuclear medicine test primarily used for the diagnosis of gallbladder disease. In patients with acute cholecystitis, the underlying pathology is usually an obstructed cystic duct from a gallstone. This test utilizes an intravenous injection of a technetium-labeled analogue of iminodiacetic acid, which is concentrated in the liver and expelled into the biliary tree. It is taken up by the gallbladder before being ejected through the common bile duct into the duodenum. The scan is performed in regular intervals allowing the radiologist to visualize the progress of the tracer through the biliary tree. If the cystic duct is obstructed, the gallbladder will not be visualized suggesting acute cholecystitis, and failure to see the gallbladder within 1 h has a sensitivity of 80–90 % for acute cholecystitis [15]. HIDA scan has been shown to be more accurate than abdominal ultrasound for acute cholecystitis but is usually reserved for cases in which there is clinical suspicion with an inconclusive ultrasound [15]. If the duodenum is not seen on a HIDA scan, it suggests obstruction of the bile duct. If the bile duct is never seen at all, either there is a very proximal biliary obstruction, such as a hilar cholangiocarcinoma, or there is hepatocellular dysfunction preventing uptake and secretion of the tracer at the hepatocyte level, such as in cirrhosis or acute hepatitis. In patients who have persistent abdominal pain after cholecystectomy, a HIDA scan may be used to detect a bile leak which would show as a blush of tracer at the cystic duct stump or elsewhere in the region. A CCK-HIDA scan is a modified version of the test in which an intravenous injection of CCK is given when the tracer has been taken up by the gallbladder, causing the gallbladder to contract and release the tracer into the bile duct. This allows calculation of the gallbladder ejection fraction which is normally 35 % or greater. The diagnosis of gallbladder dyskinesia can be considered in patients with biliary colic and abnormally low gallbladder ejection fractions, and the treatment is cholecystectomy, although due to variable outcomes in terms of symptom relief after cholecystectomy, this diagnosis is somewhat controversial.

CT Scan

CT is similar to abdominal ultrasound in being able to detect bile duct dilation and perhaps somewhat better than ultrasound for the distal bile duct, but it is similarly poor in visualizing stones within the bile duct and also less accurate in assessing the gallbladder. However, overall CT has greatly improved in resolution and is excellent in evaluating the pancreas and surrounding vessels for lesions, and is the best test for staging of pancreatic tumors. It can identify location and vascular involvement along with lymphadenopathy and distant metastases. To some degree it can differentiate pancreatic cysts from solid lesions but is still limited in characterizing cysts in terms of fluidity, septations, presence of mural nodules, and connection to the pancreatic duct. CT does cause radiation exposure and IV contrast is critical for evaluation of pancreaticobiliary disease so the patient must have suitable renal function and not be allergic to IV contrast.

MRCP (Magnetic Resonance Cholangiopancreatography)

Magnetic resonance cholangiopancreatography (MRCP) has gained usage through the years as well. It is a very slow test to perform and can be quite difficult on any patient that has trouble laying very still for a long period of time, and in such cases will likely result in a poor quality study. As with any MRI, any metal in the body or claustrophobia are contraindications. If done properly however, it gives an excellent detailed view of the biliary tree and the pancreatic ductal system in a non-invasive manner. For example, it is useful in determining if there are small biliary stones when there is conflicting clinical data such as improving hepatic function tests but persistent symptoms. It can show ductal changes of chronic pancreatitis better than abdominal ultrasound or CT scan. A secretin enhanced MRCP utilizes the increased volume of fluid within the pancreatic ductal system in response to secretin to further increase the sensitivity of MRCP in evaluating the pancreatic duct and its branches for subtle changes or to reveal a subtle ductal stricture. This test can be useful in evaluating recurrent acute pancreatitis or when suspecting early chronic pancreatitis [16, 17].

Secretin Stimulation Test

Secretin was also used in the pancreatic function test which was considered the best test for diagnosing early chronic pancreatitis because imaging may not be adequately sensitive. The test involved passing a collection tube to the second portion of the duodenum under fluoroscopy. After intravenous secretin injection, pancreatic fluid excreted from the major papilla is collected from the tube every 15 min for 1 h. Normally one would expect a predictable rise in the concentration of bicarbonate due to the effect of secretin on the pancreatic ductal cells. Patients with chronic pancreatitis, however, lose the ability to increase bicarbonate secretion in response to secretin rather early on in the disease and this difference can be detected by this test [18]. This test is rarely performed because it is rather invasive and time consuming, and there are alternative tests available.

Endoscopic Tests

Endoscopic Ultrasound

Endoscopic ultrasound has emerged as one of the most powerful diagnostic tools for pancreaticobiliary disease. Its complication risk is only slightly more than standard endoscopy which is quite low for most patients. It has the advantage over abdominal ultrasound in that the ultrasound probe is a very short distance from the pancreas and distal bile duct, without intervening small bowel, allowing a much more detailed view. Like MRCP, it is highly sensitive in evaluating the bile duct for stones/sludge in patients where other imaging tests are inconclusive, and has the advantage that an ERCP can be performed in the same setting [19]. It is the best test for evaluating pancreatic cysts, as it is more sensitive than CT in detecting septations and differentiating cystic from solid lesions. Furthermore, it allows sampling by FNA for tissue diagnosis and fluid analysis which is important in distinguishing benign cysts from pre-malignant pancreatic cystic neoplasms. EUS is the most sensitive test for detecting pancreatic lesions less than 2 cm in size [20]. FNA is highly effective in determining cell type for solid pancreatic lesions and can differentiate adenocarcinoma, neuroendocrine tumor, autoimmune pancreatitis, lymphoma, metastatic lesions, and other more rare tumors. More recently, cytology from FNA is being used in molecular profiling of tumors to optimize chemotherapy [21]. EUS-FNA has replaced CT-guided sampling of the pancreas due to being at least as accurate as CT and its lower risk of tumor seeding along the needle tract as a result of the proximity of the echoendoscope to the lesion [22, 23]. EUS can closely evaluate the pancreas parenchyma and duct for changes of early chronic pancreatitis such as cysts, calcifications, ductal stones/strictures, and dilated side branches, although this is operator dependent and there can be considerable interobserver disagreement [24]. EUS is very effective in draining large pseudocysts that are in physical proximity with the GI tract, even with necrotic debris since a cystgastrostomy can be created endoscopically allowing passage of an endoscope directly into the cyst cavity for necrosectomy and then placement of stents and, if necessary, a nasocystic drain for continued flushing of the cyst. In cases of biliary ductal obstruction where ERCP fails or is not possible, EUS can be used to access the dilated left intrahepatic ductal branches transgastrically or the dilated common bile duct transduodenally to place a stent between the duct and GI tract or to pass a wire down across the papilla to facilitate ERCP. The advantage of this technique to percutaneous transhepatic cholangiostomy (PTC) is that it allows internal drainage without the presence of an external drain. It is especially advantageous in cases with complete biliary obstruction in which PTC would require external drainage of bile which may lead to dehydration.

ERCP (Endoscopic Retrograde Cholangiopancreatography)

ERCP is a test combining endoscopy and radiology to evaluate the biliary tree and pancreatic duct where the duodenoscope is advanced into the duodenum and contrast is injected, usually through the major papilla, into the bile duct and/or pancreatic duct to obtain a cholangiogram and/or pancreatogram, along with ductal access using a guidewire. Due to a relatively high complication rate of pancreatitis and the emergence of other effective diagnostic tests such as MRCP and EUS, ERCP should no longer be performed solely as a diagnostic test, but instead be performed with the intention of providing a specific therapeutic benefit [25]. Virtually all ERCP requires a sphincterotomy in which cautery is applied through a metal wire to the papilla to cut through the sphincter muscle to allow passage of instruments over the guide wire and allow better drainage. ERCP is highly effective with over 90 % success rate in the removal of biliary stones [26] but considerably less effective for pancreatic duct stones [27]. Biliary and pancreatic duct strictures can be sampled by biopsy and cytology brushing, stretched with dilation balloons, and drained with temporary plastic or permanent metal stents. Bile leaks and pancreatic ductal leaks can be identified and treated with temporary stenting. Cholangiograms can define hilar strictures by Bismuth classification and pancreatograms can define the pancreatic duct for changes of chronic pancreatitis based on the Cambridge classification, but EUS and MRCP have generally replaced the purely diagnostic ERCP.

In select patients with symptoms of biliary colic without obvious cause, sphincter of Oddi manometry can be performed. A manometry probe is passed through the ERCP duodenoscope into the bile duct and/or pancreatic duct to obtain pressure readings across the ductal openings with a baseline reading in the duodenal lumen. Pressures that are elevated compared with an accepted standard pressure are suggestive of sphincter of Oddi dysfunction, for which the treatment is biliary sphincterotomy. This diagnosis is controversial due to the difficulty in diagnosis and inconsistent response to endoscopic sphincterotomy. Furthermore, ERCP in such patients is associated with a very elevated risk of post-ERCP pancreatitis. As a result, it is being recommended not to offer ERCP to patients with unexplained biliary colic without any objective finding of elevated LFTs or biliary dilation [28].

Cholangioscopy and pancreatoscopy, in which a small endoscope is passed through the duodenoscope and into the ducts, allow direct visualization of the ducts for better analysis and more directed tissue sampling. In addition, electrohydraulic lithotripsy, in which a thin fiber that passes through the cholangioscope, can be used to apply high current to large bile duct stones under direct visualization to break stones that are too large for standard removal techniques. Recent technological advancement is greatly improving the image quality of cholangioscopy. ERCP does have considerably more risk than standard endoscopy, specifically pancreatitis, bleeding, and perforation, and it has been shown that both technical success and complication rates correlate with operator experience and case volume [29].

References

1. Feldman M, Friedman, LS, Brandt LJ, editors. Sleisenger and Fordtran's Gastrointestinal and Liver Disease, 10th ed. Vol 1. Chapter 55, p. 931.
2. Wani AA, Maqsood S, Lala P, Wani S. Annular pancreas in adults: a report of two cases and review of literature. JOP. 2013;14(3):277–9.
3. Jimenez JC, Emil S, Podnos Y, Nguyen N. Annular pancreas in children: a recent decade's experience. J Pediatr Surg. 2004;39(11):1654–7.
4. Bhasin DK, Rana SS, Nanda M, Gupta R, Nagi B, Wig JD. Ansa pancreatica type of ductal anatomy in a patient with idiopathic acute pancreatitis. JOP. 2006;7(3):315–20.
5. Pieper-Bigelow C, Strocchi A, Levitt MD. Where does serum amylase come from and where does it go? Gastroenterol Clin North Am. 1990;19(4):793.
6. Sachdeva CK, Bank S, Greenberg R, Blumstein M, Weissman S. Fluctuations in serum amylase in patients with macroamylasemia. Am J Gastroenterol. 1995;90(5):800.
7. Steinberg WM, Goldstein SS, Davis ND, Shamma'a J, Anderson K. Diagnostic assays in acute pancreatitis. A study of sensitivity and specificity. Ann Intern Med. 1985;102(5):576.
8. Banks PA, Freeman ML, Practice Parameters Committee of the American College of Gastroenterology. Practice guidelines in acute pancreatitis. Am J Gastroenterol. 2006;101(10):2379–400.
9. Pratt DS, Kaplan MM. Chapter 302. Evaluation of liver function. In: Longo DL, Fauci AS, Kasper DL, Hauser SL, Jameson J, Loscalzo J, editors. Harrison's principles of internal medicine. New York, NY: McGraw-Hill; 2012. p. 18e.
10. Dennery PA, Seidman DS, Stevenson DK. Neonatal hyperbilirubinemia. N Engl J Med. 2001;344:581–90.
11. Ong SL, Sachdeva A, Garcea G, Gravante G, Metcalfe MS, Lloyd DM, et al. Elevation of carbohydrate antigen 19.9 in benign hepatobiliary conditions and its correlation with serum bilirubin concentration. Dig Dis Sci. 2008;53(12):3213–7.
12. Lamerz R. Role of tumour markers, cytogenetics. Ann Oncol. 1999;10 Suppl 4:145.
13. Ralls PW, Colletti PM, Lapin SA, et al. Real-time sonography in suspected acute cholecystitis: prospective evaluation of primary and secondary signs. Radiology. 1985;155:767–71.

14. Scharschmidt BF, Goldberg HI, Schmid R. Current concepts in diagnosis. Approach to the patient with cholestatic jaundice. N Engl J Med. 1983;308(25):1515–9.
15. Strasberg SM. Clinical practice. Acute calculous cholecystitis. N Engl J Med. 2008;358(26):2804–11.
16. Sherman S, Freeman ML, Tarnasky PR, Wilcox CM, Kulkarni A, Aisen AM, et al. Administration of secretin (RG1068) increases the sensitivity of detection of duct abnormalities by magnetic resonance cholangiopancreatography in patients with pancreatitis. Gastroenterology. 2014;147(3):646–54.
17. Czakó L, Endes J, Takács T, Boda K, Lonovics J. Evaluation of pancreatic exocrine function by secretin-enhanced magnetic resonance cholangiopancreatography. Pancreas. 2001;23(3):323–8.
18. Ochi K, Mizushima T, Harada H, Matsumoto S, Matsumura N, Seno T. Chronic pancreatitis: functional testing. Pancreas. 1998;16(3):343–8.
19. de Lédinghen V, Lecesne R, Raymond JM, Gense V, Amouretti M, Drouillard J, et al. Diagnosis of choledocholithiasis: EUS or magnetic resonance cholangiography? A prospective controlled study. Gastrointest Endosc. 1999;49(1):26–31.
20. Wang W, Shpaner A, Krishna SG, Ross WA, Bhutani MS, Tamm EP, et al. Use of EUS-FNA in diagnosing pancreatic neoplasm without a definitive mass on CT. Gastrointest Endosc. 2013;78(1):73–80.
21. Bournet B, Pointreau A, Souque A, Oumouhou N, Muscari F, Lepage B, et al. Gene expression signature of advanced pancreatic ductal adenocarcinoma using low density array on endoscopic ultrasound-guided fine needle aspiration samples. Pancreatology. 2012;12(1):27–34.
22. Horwhat JD, Paulson EK, McGrath K, Branch MS, Baillie J, Tyler D, et al. A randomized comparison of EUS-guided FNA versus CT or US-guided FNA for the evaluation of pancreatic mass lesions. Gastrointest Endosc. 2006;63(7):966–75.
23. Micames C, Jowell PS, White R, Paulson E, Nelson R, Morse M, et al. Lower frequency of peritoneal carcinomatosis in patients with pancreatic cancer diagnosed by EUS-guided FNA vs. percutaneous FNA. Gastrointest Endosc. 2003;58(5):690–5.
24. Catalano MF, Sahai A, Levy M, Romagnuolo J, Wiersema M, Brugge W, et al. EUS-based criteria for the diagnosis of chronic pancreatitis: the Rosemont classification. Gastrointest Endosc. 2009;69(7):1251–61.

25. Adler DG, Baron TH, Davila RE, Egan J, Hirota WK, Leighton JA, et al. ASGE guideline: the role of ERCP in diseases of the biliary tract and the pancreas. Gastrointest Endosc. 2005;62:1–8.
26. Costi R, Gnocchi A, Di Mario F, Sarli L. Diagnosis and management of choledocholithiasis in the golden age of imaging, endoscopy and laparoscopy. World J Gastroenterol. 2014;20(37): 13382–401.
27. Talukdar R, Nageshwar Reddy D. Endoscopic therapy for chronic pancreatitis. Curr Opin Gastroenterol. 2014;30(5):484–9.
28. Cotton PB, Durkalski V, Romagnuolo J, Pauls Q, Fogel E, Tarnasky P, et al. Effect of endoscopic sphincterotomy for suspected sphincter of Oddi dysfunction on pain-related disability following cholecystectomy: the EPISOD randomized clinical trial. JAMA. 2014;311(20):2101–9.
29. Freeman ML, Nelson DB, Sherman S, Haber GB, Herman ME, Dorsher PJ, et al. Complications of endoscopic biliary sphincterotomy. N Engl J Med. 1996;335(13):909–18.

Part 5
Clinical Scenario: Pain/Fever/Jaundice

Chapter 10
Gallstone Disease

Travis P. Webb

How Did I Get Gallstones?

Gallstones form in the gallbladder due to many factors and are very common in the USA. Women are most commonly affected, and by 50 years of age, nearly 20 % of women and 5 % of men have gallstones. Most of the stones are made of cholesterol and are formed due to cholesterol settling out of the bile as bile is being stored in the gallbladder between meals. The biggest risk factors for developing gallstones include family history of gallstones, ethnicity, being female, pregnancy, taking oral contraceptives, obesity, diabetes, and age over 40. Other diseases such as Crohn's disease, sickle cell disease, and thalassemia are commonly associated with gallstones as well. Correlation between specific dietary intake and gallstone formation is not as clear but there may be an increased risk of gallstones for those eating diets high in simple sugars and saturated fat and low in fiber.

T.P. Webb (✉)
Department of Surgery, Medical College of Wisconsin,
9200 W. Wisconsin Avenue, Milwaukee, WI 53226, USA
e-mail: trwebb@mcw.edu

© Springer International Publishing Switzerland 2016
K. Dua, R. Shaker (eds.), *Pancreas and Biliary Disease*,
DOI 10.1007/978-3-319-28089-9_10

Do I Have to Have My Gallbladder Removed or Are There Other Options?

Most people remain asymptomatic from their gallstones, but once you have developed symptoms, it is likely that you will have recurrent episodes of symptoms and these episodes may progress to complications. So in general if you have incidentally found asymptomatic gallstones, you do not need to have surgery. When symptoms develop, surgery is recommended to remove the gallbladder. There are no good alternatives to surgery such as medications or lithotripsy to break up stones such as is done for kidney stones. While awaiting surgery, refraining from large meals and fatty foods may be helpful to decrease the risk of developing worsening symptoms or complications. The good news is that about 90 % of patients with typical biliary symptoms and gallstones are rendered symptom free after cholecystectomy.

How Will the Surgery Affect Me?

Surgical removal of the gallbladder can be performed using a laparoscopic or open technique. Laparoscopic cholecystectomy is the preferred approach and is a safe and highly effective treatment for the majority of patients. Most people can have the surgery and go home the same day with some pain medication and stool softeners as the only needed post operative medications. There are typically four small incisions made on the abdomen, but this may vary depending upon the difficulty of the case. Patients are generally advised to eat like they are getting over the flu (plenty of liquids and small meals consisting of bland food) for a couple days after the operation. Once feeling a bit better, a normal diet may be resumed. Some people experience looser than normal stools when eating diets high in fatty foods. This is usually self-limited and can be fairly easily managed with simple dietary modification. Most surgeons recommend taking a week or two off work to recover and discourage lifting heavy objects over 10 pounds for 2–6 weeks after the operation to allow the abdominal wall to fully heal.

Brief Review of Gallstone Disease

Gallstone disease is a common problem affecting the digestive tract of more than 30 million people in the USA. The incidence rises with age, leading to 20 % of women and 5 % of men being affected by 65 years of age. However, less than 20 % of people with gallstones actually develop symptoms such as biliary colic or chronic cholecystitis during their lifetime. Even fewer people develop acute cholecystitis, gallstone pancreatitis, or other complications related to their gallstones. Therefore, most people with gallstones never know that they have them and do not require any particular intervention or counseling.

Population-based risk factors for gallstone formation and gallstone disease have been widely studied and are well established. Ethnicity including the Native American populations in both North and South Americas has been linked to a high prevalence of cholelithiasis. Caucasians are the next most commonly affected, while the incidence of gallstone disease is lowest in the African American population. Other well-described risk factors for development of cholesterol stones include: family history of gallstones, female gender, pregnancy, oral contraceptive use, obesity, diabetes, and metabolic syndrome. In addition, rapid weight loss, particularly after operations for morbid obesity, is strongly related to cholesterol gallstone formation.

Seventy-five percent of gallstones are composed primarily of cholesterol and the remaining 25 % are pigmented stones. Cholesterol gallstones result from secretion by the liver of bile supersaturated with cholesterol that then precipitates from solution. Cholesterol is insoluble and must be transported in the bile within salt micelles and phospholipid vesicles. When the amount of cholesterol exceeds the holding capacity of the bile, cholesterol crystals precipitate. These cholesterol crystals then form into macroscopic stones within the gallbladder. Most stones remain in the gallbladder but some pass into the common bile duct leading to choledocholithiasis and possibly cholangitis or gallstone pancreatitis.

Pigment stones account for 25 % of gallstones in the USA and 60 % of those in Japan. Pigment stones are black or dark brown, 2–5 mm in diameter, and amorphous. They are composed primarily of a mixture of calcium bilirubinate, complex bilirubin polymers, and bile acids. Predisposing factors include cirrhosis, bile stasis (due to bile duct strictures or markedly dilated common duct), and chronic hemolysis. Some patients have high concentrations of unconjugated bilirubin in their bile and bacteria within the stones. This high bacterial presence suggests that bacteria may have a primary role in stone development and may explain why patients with pigment stone have a higher rate of sepsis than those with cholesterol stones. Unlike cholesterol stones, the incidence of pigment stones is low in Native Americans, and similar in blacks and whites, men and women.

Several studies have attempted to evaluate the impact of dietary intake on the formation of cholesterol stones. Some studies have demonstrated a correlation of gallstone formation and the intake of diets high in simple sugars and saturated fats as well as low in fiber. Though a western diet appears to correlate with gallstone incidence, the impact of diet remains controversial and has not been definitively tied to the incidence of gallstone formation.

Regardless of the composition, the natural history and clinical sequelae of gallstones are the same. The majority of patients found to have incidental asymptomatic cholelithiasis can be managed nonoperatively without complication. Patients with symptoms generally should have their gallbladder removed to manage symptoms and prevent worsening complications.

The majority of patients who become symptomatic will first note symptoms of biliary colic prior to the onset of acute cholecystitis, choledocholithiasis, cholangitis, or gallstone pancreatitis. Once patients develop symptomatic cholelithiasis, they are most likely to develop recurrent bouts of biliary colic or less frequently progress to more severe complications. Thus, patients with symptomatic cholelithiasis should be considered for laparoscopic cholecystectomy in a timely manner.

In studies of patients presenting to the emergency room with biliary colic or acute cholecystitis, nearly 40 % will return to the hospital within 2 years with recurrent symptoms if cholecystectomy is not performed at the time of the index event.

Prophylactic cholecystectomy in the setting of asymptomatic cholelithiasis is generally not warranted except in special situations such as in patients who are candidates for organ transplantation or in the presence of hemolytic anemias such as sickle cell or thalassemia. Asymptomatic patients with large stones (>2 cm diameter) or a calcified gallbladder may have an increased risk for gallbladder cancer. Studies supporting expectant management of large gallstones recommend ultrasound surveillance and ultimately cholecystectomy if symptoms develop or imaging demonstrates changes in gallbladder characteristics. Studies have been inconclusive in demonstrating an increased risk of cancer thus definitive recommendations are not available. Of particular note and contrary to previous beliefs, diabetic patients with asymptomatic stones do not benefit from cholecystectomy over watchful waiting.

The diagnosis of gallstone disease is typically based on clinical signs and symptoms, laboratory studies, and imaging of the gallbladder with ultrasound. The typical presentation of biliary colic includes episodes of right upper quadrant or epigastric pain that lasts for several minutes to a few hours after meals. The pain may radiate to the right flank or across the abdomen to the left substernal area thus prompting a cardiac evaluation to rule out myocardial infarction. The episodes tend to follow large fatty meals and thus frequently occur in the evening when people eat their largest meal of the day. Other symptoms such as fatty food intolerance, nausea, vomiting, flatulence, and dyspepsia are common as well and should prompt the clinician to consider the diagnosis.

The constellation of symptoms associated with gallstones in the gallbladder is due to the blockage of the cystic duct as the gallbladder contracts to expel bile into the common bile duct as an aid to digestion. When gallstones fail to move and the cystic duct remains obstructed, acute cholecystitis may develop. Acute cholecystitis can be distinguished from biliary colic by the persistent nature of the pain or less frequently signs of systemic inflammation or infection. Patients with pain that fails to subside several hours after onset are much more likely to have acute cholecystitis and benefit from urgent cholecystectomy. Laboratory tests should include white blood cell count, liver function tests, and serum lipase. These laboratory tests may alert the provider to the complications of gallstones such as acute cholecystitis, choledocholithiasis, cholangitis, or gallstone pancreatitis and the need for further interventions or treatment.

Ultrasound is the preferred imaging modality for the diagnosis of gallstones and gallstone related complications (Fig. 10.1). It is both highly sensitive and specific (>95 %) for cholelithiasis but has a lower sensitivity (60 %) for acute cholecystitis. Based on this lower sensitivity for acute cholecystitis, patients with symptoms consistent with acute cholecystitis but evidence only of cholelithiasis on ultrasound should be presumed to have acute cholecystitis based on the clinical diagnosis rather than imaging alone. The presence of a "large" gallbladder seen on imaging is not an indication for cholecystectomy and does not independently correlate with clinical symptoms. CT scanning is more sensitive for acute cholecystitis but less sensitive for cholelithiasis and should not be used as a first line imaging modality.

Medical management of gallstones has been marginally effective and is not recommended as a first line therapy. Most patients are counseled to avoid offending foods, but this strategy is not a consistent or durable solution for most patients. Dissolution of gallstones has been attempted with variable and poor overall results. Chronic treatment with ursodiol reduces the cholesterol saturation of bile by inhibiting cholesterol secretion and may result in slow dissolution of solid cholesterol stones over time. However, few patients are candidates for this type of treatment. The gallstones must be small (<5 mm) and devoid of calcium, and the cystic duct must not be obstructed in order for the bile in the gallbladder to be exposed to the medication. Only about 15 % of patients with gallstones are candidates for this treatment. Dissolution occurs in only 50 % of these highly selected

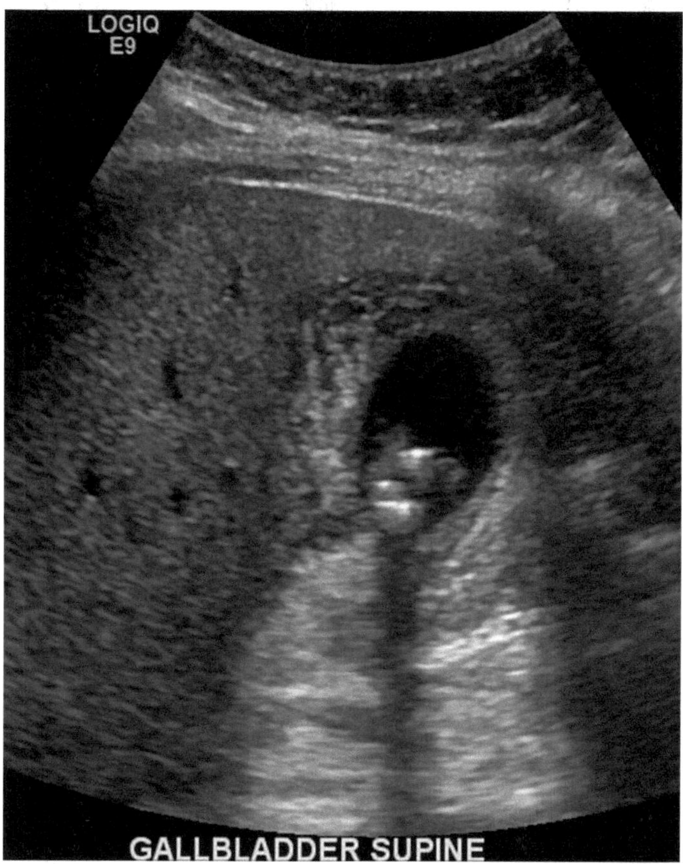

Fig. 10.1 Gallbladder ultrasound. Gallbladder with gallstones and posterior shadowing

patients and takes 2 years of constant therapy. Finally, stones recur in 50 % of cases within 5 years. Given these poor outcomes, dissolution therapy, alone or in conjunction with lithotripsy, is used very rarely for gallstones.

Cholecystectomy is one of the most common procedures performed by the general surgeon with over 700,000 operations performed annually in the USA. Currently approximately 90 % of all cholecystectomies are performed laparoscopically.

Benefits of laparoscopic cholecystectomy over open cholecystectomy include the shorter length of hospital stay, shorter recovery time, fewer surgical site complications (infections, seromas, hematomas, dehiscence), fewer hernias, and better cosmesis. The rate of common bile duct injury remains higher for laparoscopic cholecystectomy but is overall quite low with a rate of 0.4 %. The need to convert to an open procedure varies based on surgeon expertise and the presence of complicated gallbladder disease. Other complications can certainly occur and include bile leaks (cystic duct leaks or liver bed leak), hematomas, infections, and intestinal injury.

Recovery after cholecystectomy is similar to many other abdominal surgeries and is dependent upon many factors including surgeon and patient expectations. Patients can frequently undergo laparoscopic cholecystectomy and go home the same day without complication. Even patients undergoing laparoscopic cholecystectomy for acute cholecystitis are now being sent home the same day at some institutions. When patients require open cholecystectomy due to technical reasons or contraindications, their recovery is slower and they frequently stay in the hospital for 3–4 days post operatively.

After cholecystectomy, patients are allowed to eat a general diet and are not restricted from fatty foods. However, some patients experience a change in their bowel habits for a limited period of time that may concern them. Due to the increased presence of bile salts within the small bowel and colon, looser stools are frequently noted. This change is self-limited as the bowel is able to compensate over time by increasing the absorption of bile salts into the enterohepatic circulation. There does not appear to be any negative long-term sequelae of this increased volume of bile within the digestive system.

In conclusion, gallstone disease is one of the most common problems associated with the digestive system and knowledge of the basics for diagnosis and treatment are important for the healthcare provider. Future studies will continue to elucidate risk factors and optimal treatment strategies including medical and surgical techniques to manage the disease.

References

1. Cuevas A, Miguel JF, Reyes MS, Zanlungo S, Nervi F. Diet as a risk factor for cholesterol gallstone disease. J Am Coll Nutr. 2004;23(3):187–96.
2. Duncan CB, Riall TS. Evidence-based current surgical practice: calculous gallbladder disease. J Gastrointest Surg. 2012;16: 2011–25.
3. Gracie WA, Ransohoff DF. The natural history of silent gallstones: the innocent gallstone is not a myth. N Engl J Med. 1982;307:798–800.
4. Gurusamy KS, Davidson BR. Surgical treatment of gallstones. Gastroenterol Clin North Am. 2010;39:229–44.
5. Internal Clinical Guidelines Team (UK). Gallstone disease: diagnosis and management of cholelithiasis, cholecystitis and choledocholithiasis. London, UK: National Institute for Health and Care Excellence; 2014.
6. Mendez-Sanchez N, Zamora-Valdes D, Chavez-Tapia NC, Uribe M. Role of diet in cholesterol gallstone formation. Clinica Chimica Acta. 2007;376:1–8.
7. Peitzman AB, Watson GA, Marsh JW. Acute cholecystitis: when to operate and how to do it safely. J Trauma Acute Care Surg. 2014;78(1):1–12.
8. Portincasa P, Moschetta A, Palasciano G. Cholesterol gallstone disease. Lancet. 2006;368:230–9.
9. Psaila J, Agrawal S, Fountain U, Whitfield T, Murgatroyd B, Dunsire MF, et al. Day-surgery laparoscopic cholecystectomy: factors influencing same-day discharge. World J Surg. 2008;32: 76–81.
10. Stinton LM, Myers RP, Shaffer EA. Epidemiology of gallstones. Gastroenterol Clin North Am. 2010;39:157–69.

Chapter 11
Choledocholithiasis Including Acute Cholangitis

Srinivas Gaddam and Simon Lo

Abbreviations

CT	Computed tomography
ERCP	Endoscopic retrograde cholangiopancreatography
EUS	Endoscopic ultrasound
MRCP	Magnetic resonance cholangiopancreatography

Patient Questions and Answers

What Are Gallstones and What Is the Difference Between Gallbladder Stones and Common Bile Duct Stones?

The liver produces bile which then flows into the small intestine through drainage channels called bile ducts. The gallbladder acts as a temporary storage sac for bile which is released into the small intestine after a meal. Stones can precipitate from bile fluid within the gallbladder and they are

S. Gaddam, M.D., M.P.H. (✉) • S. Lo, M.D., F.A.C.P.
Digestive Diseases Center, Cedars-Sinai Medical Center,
8700 Beverly Boulevard, ST, Suite 7751, Los Angeles, CA
90048, USA
e-mail: srinivas.gaddam@cshs.org

© Springer International Publishing Switzerland 2016
K. Dua, R. Shaker (eds.), *Pancreas and Biliary Disease*,
DOI 10.1007/978-3-319-28089-9_11

known as gallbladder stones or simply gallstones. Gallstones generally do not cause any symptoms, as they usually stay within the gallbladder without causing irritation. They may rarely cause gallbladder inflammation or chronic cholecystitis, block the gallbladder outlet to cause acute cholecystitis, or migrate into the common bile duct. The presence of gallstones in the bile duct is called choledocholithiasis. These stones can cause symptoms like episodic pain in the right upper abdomen with abnormal liver function tests. The exact reasons that increase the risk for migration of gallstones into the common bile duct are not well-understood, although it is generally believed that a large number and small size of stones are contributing factors. Unfortunately, there is no effective way to prevent migration of stones or dissolve stones once they have migrated into the common bile duct. When choledocholithiasis occurs, patients are at risk for serious abdominal pain or other complications. Therefore, these common bile duct stones must be removed to prevent complications from occurring.

What Are the Complications of Common Bile Duct Stones?

A gallstone that has entered the large bile duct may flow downstream and quietly escape from a bile duct valve, known as sphincter of Oddi, into the duodenum without causing any problem. During this downward passage, it may lodge temporarily at the sphincter and bring about abdominal symptoms, abnormal blood tests and possibly blockage of the pancreatic duct (pancreatic duct joins the bile duct at the sphincter of Oddi). Whether it is stone wedging at the sphincter or within the common bile duct, the blockage leads to a sudden increase in bile duct pressure that in turn brings about intense pain and nausea that lasts for hours. The pressure buildup may be transmitted back up to affect the liver, leading to abnormal liver blood tests. When the bile duct impaction is let up, these stones then become free floating again and the symptoms and abnormal blood test may temporarily resolve without any medical interventions. However, it may be a matter of time when symptoms recur or serious complications take place.

In the event that stone impaction persists and causes complete blockage of bile flow, jaundice and itching can occur because of failure of the body to clear the yellow bile pigment from the liver. Eventually, the obstructed biliary fluid can be infected and lead to the condition known as ascending cholangitis. The reason for the propensity of choledocholithiasis to cholangitis is not fully established. It is probable that a bile duct stone, in the process of passage into the duodenum, stretches and partially open up the biliary sphincter. This provides the opportunity of duodenal bacteria to enter the normally clean bile duct. If the stone is not able to get through, it would invariably retreat into the bile duct and recreate a closed system wherein the bacteria can multiply and ultimately lead to infection.

As mentioned, a passing gallstone can obstruct the pancreatic duct, impede the flow of pancreatic juice and cause inflammation of the pancreas. Pancreatic inflammation, referred to as acute pancreatitis, occurs because the sphincter of Oddi is shared by both the bile duct and pancreatic duct. In a vast majority of the time, this pancreatic duct blockage is a transient process and the stone would eventually pass through and enter the duodenum. However, the damage on the pancreas set forth by the sphincter obstruction can be severe and lasting. Acute pancreatitis manifests as severe upper abdominal pain and vomiting, and is associated with elevation of blood levels of enzymes released from the pancreas called amylase and lipase.

There are other less common complications of bile duct stones. Long-standing presence of untreated stones can induce irritation and inflammation of the bile duct lining, leading to its narrowing. An indolent progression of untreated bile duct strictures can cause long-term liver damage. Although strictures may be caused by gallstone induced chronic inflammation, the opposite may also be true. In some situations, the existence of a stricture may cause disturbance to bile flow and result in formation of stones within the partially blocked bile duct. These so-called de novo bile duct stones may occur in patients with a slow growing bile duct cancer, bile duct parasites, or a surgically induced bile duct injury. Once formed within the bile duct, these stones can result in cholangitis, jaundice, and pain just like those stones that have migrated from the gallbladder.

How Is the Diagnosis Made?

Common bile duct stones may present in an unpredictable or subtle manner. The diagnosis of stones in the common bile duct can be difficult and easily missed. Therefore, a clinician should exercise a high level of suspicion in the setting of abnormal liver function tests and right upper abdominal pain so as to accurately make an early diagnosis. Bedside, examination typically produces tenderness on palpation of the right upper abdomen, which may indicate liver, gallbladder, or bile duct problem. Tenderness of the liver is usually mild and it may involve a wide area of the right upper abdomen. Gallbladder tenderness is commonly sharply focused, very intense and may lead to extreme pain when the patient is asked to take a deep breath. Finally, pushing on the deep seated bile duct produces localized but not very pronounced tenderness. Another important distinction between a gallbladder and a bile duct issue is minimally abnormal for the former vs. significantly elevated liver blood tests in the latter condition. Unfortunately, these bedside clinical findings are insufficient to make a definitively diagnosis of bile duct stones and imaging tests are needed for confirmation. There are several radiographic imaging studies available to evaluate the common bile duct and each has its strengths and weaknesses.

Transabdominal ultrasound is the cheapest, most easily available and least invasive test to evaluate for choledocholithiasis. While the liver and gallbladder are located close to the body surface and easily examined with ultrasound, the common bile duct tends to run deeper towards the duodenum and can be difficult to study from across the abdominal wall. This is especially true of the distal bile duct. The ability of the ultrasound to evaluate for stones also depends on the medium surrounding the site of interest. For example, in the case of the distal bile duct which is closer to the duodenum, bowel gas can interfere with the transmission of sound waves and thus obscure visualization of a potential stone in the region. While a CT scan is more expensive and subjects patients to ionization radiation, the visualization of common bile duct is better as X-rays have higher penetration than ultrasound waves through the various nearby structures. However, most gallstones contain cholesterol and tend to be radiolucent on CT images. When stones have high calcium content, CT scan can readily make a diagnosis of choledocholithiasis. Neither a normal transabdominal ultrasound nor a normal CT scan provide conclusive evidence to exclude common bile duct stones in patients with suspicion for common bile duct stones. Therefore, when CBD stones are still suspected, further testing with either an endoscopic ultrasound (EUS) or magnetic resonance cholangiopancreatography (MRCP) is recommended. In rare occasions, bile duct stones can be detected only by directly injecting radiologic contrast solution into the bile duct at endoscopic retrograde cholangiopancreatography (ERCP).

What Is an ERCP? Why Is It Necessary to Perform This Procedure When Patients Have Common Bile Duct Stones?

Historically, common bile duct stones were removed at the time of surgery. Over the last few decades, endoscopic removal of stones has become the standard of care sparing patients an extensive operation. This involves the use of a special kind of a flexible endoscope that is passed through the mouth to the duodenum, where the opening of the bile duct is identified. The bile duct opening, or sphincter of Oddi, may be accessed with a narrow plastic tube or a slippery wire. Once the bile duct is entered, contrast material is injected to identify the bile duct abnormalities. If a gallstone is confirmed on X-ray, miniature tools can be passed through the endoscope into the common bile duct to extract the stone. A plastic drainage tube may be placed during the ERCP to facilitate bile flow.

ERCP may be performed either electively within a few days or urgently to remove the stones from the common bile duct. A nonemergent procedure is done for patients with confirmed or high likelihood of bile duct stones without ongoing signs of infection, pancreatitis or severe abdominal pain. Cholangitis typically manifests with right upper quadrant pain, fever, and jaundice and is treated with ERCP urgently or emergently. If it is not treated promptly with antibiotics and stone removal, it can result in dissemination of infection into the blood stream, leading to unstable blood pressure, poor mentation, and even death. Since infection can only occur within a clogged bile duct, placement of a hollow tube or a stent without stone removal would reestablish bile flow and temporarily resolve the cholangitis. Placement of a stent is usually done during a serious bile duct infection, when thoroughly cleaning out the bile duct may not be technically feasible or safe to carry out.

The other feared complication of retained common bile duct stones is acute pancreatitis, which is an inflammation of pancreas that is believed to be caused by gallstone blockage of the pancreatic duct. While majority of gallstone pancreatitis are mild and complete recovery is expected within a few days, severe pancreatitis may lead to irreparable damage to the pancreas and other organs and even death. ERCP may be performed to remove common bile duct stones to prevent pancreatitis. It may also be done if a stone is believed to remain within the bile duct after a bout of pancreatitis has occurred.

The many risks of choledocholithiasis, including the development of cholangitis and acute pancreatitis, are too great to ignore. Therefore, it is imperative that all common bile duct stones be treated immediately without undue delay.

The current standard of care is to perform an ERCP for removal of these stones. Another important reason to perform an ERCP is to evaluate the common bile duct for other conditions that may mimic choledocholithiasis and predisposing diseases such as benign or malignant strictures.

My Elderly Mother Has No More Pain or Fever Since the Bile Duct Infection 2 Days Ago. Also, She Is Very Tired and Needs to Get More Sleep. Should We Hold Off on the ERCP for Now?

In the elderly, fever and pain may be less pronounced and such patients may have nonspecific symptoms including fatigue and somnolence. In fact, an elderly person suffering from worsening cholangitis may appear sleepy and seemingly be improving without further fever or pain. This change in mental alertness is a bad prognostic sign and should be treated immediately with unclogging of the bile duct through ERCP. The window of time to performing a safe and effective ERCP may be as short as a few minutes, beyond which point the body shuts down and death may ensue. Holding off on performing ERCP may not be a good idea in this setting. Likewise, elderly patients who suffer from acute gallstone pancreatitis may rarely have only mild abdominal pain and even no symptoms at all. The diagnosis may only be established by imaging studies alone. Therefore, a high degree of suspicion is needed to make a diagnosis of cholangitis and acute pancreatitis due to common bile duct stones in the elderly.

Brief Review of Literature

Epidemiology

Cholelithiasis is a very common condition. Six percent of men and 9 % of women have gallbladder stones in the USA [1]. Based on a gallbladder ultrasonography on a sample survey of subjects enrolled in the National Health and Nutrition Examination Survey III, it is estimated that 20 million Americans have cholelithiasis [1]. Majority of these patients do not develop symptoms in their lifetime and therefore are said to have incidental gallbladder stones. In patients undergoing cholecystectomy for symptomatic cholelithiasis, about 5–10 % of patients are found to have common bile duct stones [2–5]. This may be significantly higher (18–33 %) in patients with acute biliary pancreatitis [6–9].

Risk Factors

Most stones that are detected in the common bile duct originate from the gallbladder. This is known as secondary choledocholithiasis. However, rarely, stones can form de novo in the bile duct and are known as primary choledocholithiasis. Bile stasis secondary to benign or malignant stricture, large bile ducts, recurrent pyogenic cholangitis, and periampullary diverticula is the key factor for primary choledocholithiasis [10].

Risk factors for formation of gallbladder stones have been widely reported. Older age [11], female sex [12], pregnancy [13], use of oral contraceptive therapy [14], family history [15], obesity [16], rapid weight loss [17], and diabetes mellitus [18] are some of the known causes. The risk factors for migration of gallstones from the gallbladder to the common bile duct have not been well-studied. Prior studies have suggested that the size and number of stones within the gallbladder may predict the possibility of concurrent choledocholithiasis [19, 20]. In a study of 511 patients undergoing intraoperative cholangiography, small size of gall bladder stones (<1 cm) was an independent risk factor for migration into the common bile duct [19]. In a study involving 300 consecutive patients undergoing laparoscopic cholecystectomy, the presence of multiple small (<5 mm) or multiple variable stones sizes (small and large) was a significant independent risk factor for choledocholithiasis [20]. These studies suggest that the presence of numerous small stones in the gall bladder may be suggestive of higher risk of choledocholithiasis.

Clinical Presentation

Patients with uncomplicated choledocholithiasis may complain of episodes of biliary colic, indistinguishable from symptoms of acute cholecystitis. Often, this is accompanied by nausea and vomiting. The term colic is a misnomer, as it implies phasic, minute to minute pain. Rather, biliary pain is a rapid rise of pain to a severe plateau that lasts for hours. Besides the common right upper quadrant location, biliary pain may present as a belt like pain that spread across the entire upper abdomen and even around the back. On physical examination, the patients typically have localized right upper quadrant or epigastric tenderness, though the intensity is not dramatic and the Murphy sign is usually lacking. These classic signs and symptoms are not pathognomonic of cholelithiasis or choledocholithiasis. A prospective evaluation of 37 signs and symptoms for gall stones in 192 patients showed that these symptoms are poor in establishing the diagnosis but their absence was a good indicator in excluding the diagnosis of gall stone disease [21].

In patients with complicated choledocholithiasis, the clinical presentation may be more pronounced and manifest with symptoms and signs of either acute cholangitis or acute pancreatitis. Acute cholangitis should be suspected when patients have fevers or shaking chills, jaundice, and abdominal pain (Charcot's triad) [22]. Rarely, patients can present with suppurative cholangitis that is associated with confusion and hypotension (Reynolds pentad) [23]. When a patient with choledocholithiasis presents with acute pancreatitis, severe abdominal pain that radiates to the back, elevated lipase levels, and imaging evidence of pancreatic inflammation should dominate the clinical picture.

Diagnosis

Laboratory

Choledocholithiasis should always be suspected in patients presenting with right upper quadrant pain and abnormal liver function tests (LFT). LFT abnormalities are almost an obligatory finding; their absence has an excellent utility in excluding common bile duct stones [24]. In a study of 1002 patients who underwent laparoscopic cholecystectomy, completely normal LFTs had a negative predictive value for common bile duct stones of 97 % [25]. Conversely, the positive predictive value of abnormal LFTs in findings choledocholithiasis was only 15 % [25]. Other case series evaluating a combination of abnormal bilirubin, alkaline phosphatase or gamma glutamyl transpeptidase (GGT) have only reported modest improvement in positive predictive value to 25–50 % [26–28]. Elevation of aminotransferases is seen during the initial phases when the patient is acutely symptomatic. The condition is commonly misdiagnosed as acute hepatitis, although it typically has much less pronounced pain than in choledocholithiasis. Cholestatic enzyme pattern is usually evident in the latter phase of choledocholithiasis. Higher levels of LFT abnormalities are generally indicative of increased likelihood of choledocholithiasis [27, 28]. Studies evaluating patients with established common bile ducts stones have shown mean bilirubin levels to be around 1.5–1.9 mg/dL [26, 27] and rarely above 4 mg/dL [27, 28]. The data suggests that liver function tests may vary widely, from normal results to extreme abnormalities, and that a high degree of suspicion is needed to detect choledocholithiasis.

Imaging

Transabdominal ultrasound is an inexpensive, noninvasive, and readily available first line diagnostic test in the management of patients with suspected choledocholithiasis. Although transabdominal or external ultrasound has poor sensitivity (22–55 %) in the detection of bile duct stones, it is quite sensitive (sensitivity range 77–87 %) in detecting dilation of the common bile duct [24] (Fig. 11.1). Ultrasound is also highly valuable in evaluating for acute cholecystitis, which can present with similar symptoms. Although ultrasound is the first imaging study of choice, the technical difficulties in its ability to detect stones within the distal bile duct limit its role in completely ruling out choledocholithiasis.

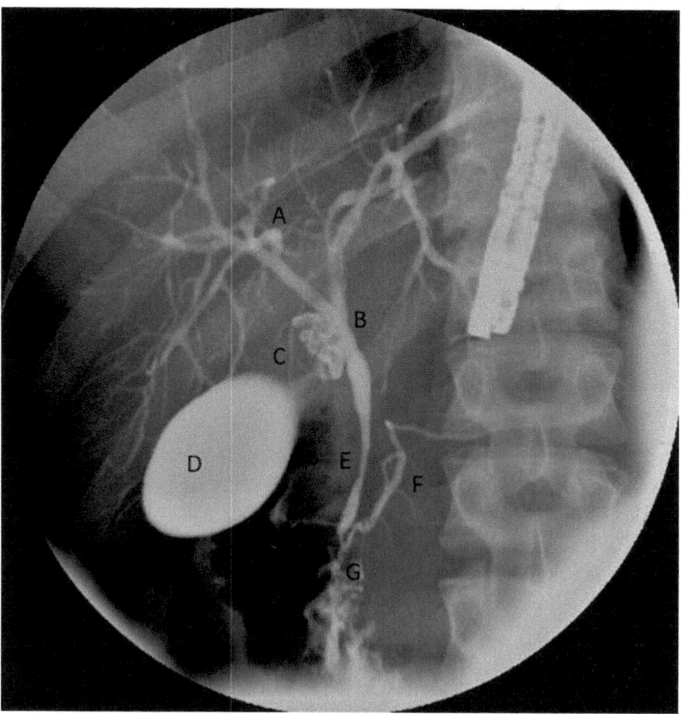

FIG. 11.1 A cholangiogram obtained at ERCP illustrating different parts of the biliary tree and the pancreatic duct. They include (**a**) intrahepatic bile ducts, (**b**) common hepatic duct, (**c**) cystic duct, (**d**) gall bladder, (**e**) common bile duct, (**f**) pancreatic duct, and (**g**) common pancreatobiliary channel

While conventional CT scan of the abdomen has low sensitivity and specificity for the detection of CBD stones, newer multidetector CT scans have much improved sensitivity and specificity [29, 30]. Studies evaluating conventional CT scans in detection of direct and indirect evidence of choledocholithiasis have shown widely varying sensitivities (25–90 %) [31]. Direct visualization of choledocholithiasis on CT occurs in less than 75 % [32]. Although helical CT cholangiography has comparable diagnostic characteristic to MRCP [33] (Fig. 11.3), concerns regarding toxicity of the chole-

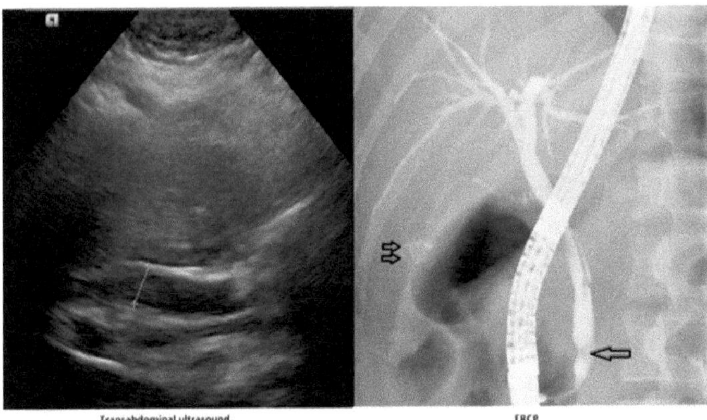

Fig. 11.2 Patient with suspected choledocholithiasis on ultrasound which showed dilation of the common bile duct to 1 cm. Patient was deemed to be high risk for choledocholithiasis and underwent ERCP. Findings of common bile duct stone (*arrow*) and cholelithiasis (*two arrows*) as shown on this cholangiogram taken at ERCP

graphic agents and significant dosage of radiation have limited its widespread use [24]. Of all imaging modalities used in the detection of biliary stones, EUS and MRCP have the highest sensitivity and specificity for the detection of choledocholithiasis. Based on a Cochrane meta-analysis of 18 studies evaluating both modalities of diagnosis, the overall sensitivities of EUS and MRCP were equal and more than 95 % [34] (Fig. 11.2). However, MRCP has a lower sensitivity in the setting of small stones (<6 mm) in the range of 33–71 % [35, 36]. EUS continues to be highly sensitive in detecting small stones less than 5 mm [37, 38]. Despite EUS being somewhat invasive, the risks from a diagnostic EUS are rare (0.1–0.3 %) [39, 40]. Given its high accuracy in the detection of small common bile duct stones, EUS may be preferred over MRCP in some circumstances such as in patients with claustrophobia or morbid obesity. Finally, ERCP is considered the gold standard when it comes to diagnosis of choledocholithiasis. Rarely, some stones can only be detected on ERCP [37].

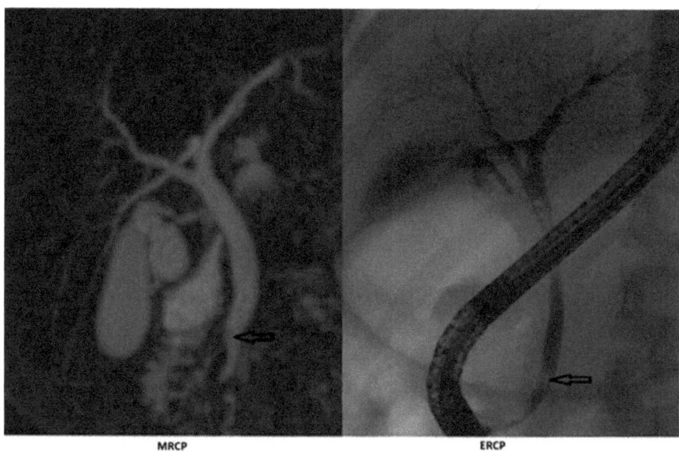

FIG. 11.3 Patient with choledocholithiasis established on MRCP. On the right are cholangiographic images from ERCP which demonstrate the common bile duct stone (*arrow*)

Management

In patients with suspected choledocholithiasis, the 2010 ASGE guidelines recommend a risk stratification process to evaluate the probability of choledocholithiasis [24]. This process involves the use of predictors to help assess for risk. Patients are classified into low, intermediate and high risk for common bile duct stone. High risk patients have more than 50 % risk of choledocholithiasis and hence are recommended for ERCP. Patients who are considered low risk have less than 10 % risk of choledocholithiasis and are recommended to pursue laparoscopic cholecystectomy. Patients who are deemed to be intermediate risk can either be evaluated preoperatively with EUS or MRCP or undergo laparoscopic cholecystectomy with an intraoperative cholangiogram. The confirmation of stones with either of these two methods would require an ERCP for endoscopic therapy (Fig. 11.4).

ERCP has become the main stay of common bile duct stone extraction in the last 20 years. If a definitive diagnosis

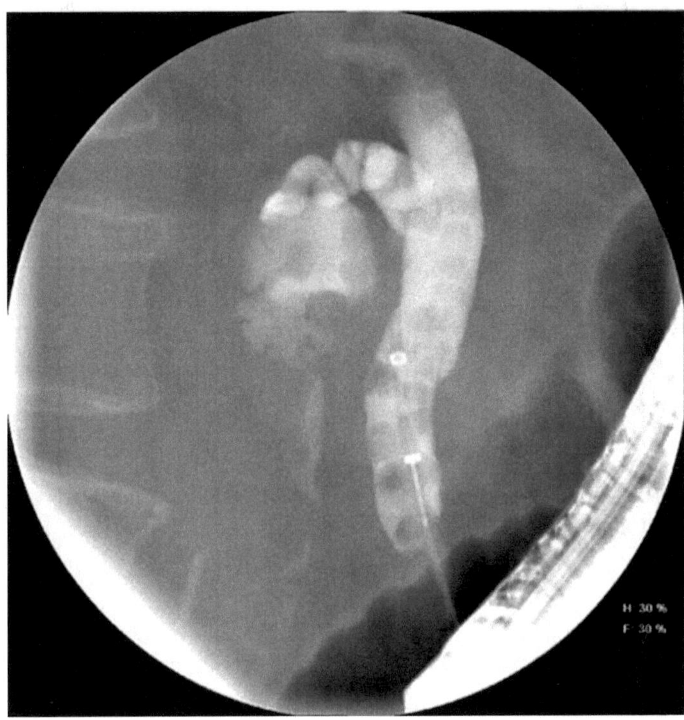

F𝖨𝖦. 11.4 Cholangiogram showing multiple gallstones within the gallbladder, cystic duct, hepatic duct, and common bile duct

of choledocholithiasis has been obtained by imaging studies, ERCP is the first line of therapy [41]. In the setting of acute cholangitis, an urgent ERCP is indicated. In cholangitis patients who do not respond to empiric antibiotics or who present with unstable blood pressure or altered mentation, immediate ERCP is mandatory. The timing of ERCP in the setting of acute pancreatitis is not entirely clear. A meta-analysis of randomized trials comparing early ERCP vs. conservative management without ERCP in patients with acute biliary pancreatitis showed no morbidity or mortality benefit in patients with early ERCP [42]. The American Society of Gastrointestinal Endoscopy (ASGE) currently recommends against emergent ERCP in patients with mild acute pancreatitis without definitive evidence of persistent acute pancreatitis [24]. When patients have concomitant cholangitis, an emergent ERCP is recommended. Future studies are needed to help determine the timing of ERCP in patients with severe acute pancreatitis [41].

Diagnosis and Management of Choledocholithiasis in the Elderly

While about 5 % of all patients with acute cholecystitis have choledocholithiasis; this number is dramatically higher in the elderly [43]. About 10–20 % of the elderly with acute cholecystitis present with choledocholithiasis [44]. In the older patients who undergo emergent cholecystectomy, the rate of choledocholithiasis can be as high as 50 % [43]. In a study on 191 patients, Sugiyama et al. show that when elderly patients develop cholangitis, they have a much higher incidence of septic shock or altered mentation (43 % vs. 25 %) when compared to the young [45]. In addition, they have significantly higher morbidity (38 % vs. 17 %) and mortality (11 % vs. 3 %).

In elderly patients with acute pancreatitis, gallstones were responsible for nearly 55 % of the cases [46]. This incidence is much higher than those reported in younger individuals with acute pancreatitis. Acute pancreatitis in this cohort of patients does not manifest with typical symptoms of abdominal pain but rather with nonspecific symptoms [47]. A high degree of clinical suspicion is needed to make a correct diagnosis. In one study the primary manifestation of acute pancreatitis was shock, organ failure, hyperglycemia and hypothermia [48]. Older studies even showed acute pancreatitis being discovered during postmortem studies in 30–42 % of older patients [48, 49]. Failing to diagnose acute pancreatitis is not likely today because of a high utilization of computed tomography and lab investigations. Nonetheless, reliance on bedside investigations alone may be insufficient to make a diagnosis of acute pancreatitis in the sick elderly.

Given the high morbidity and mortality associated with complications from choledocholithiasis in the elderly, it is important to promptly diagnose and treat prior to development of complications. The preferred modality of treatment is ERCP. Several studies have demonstrated the safety and efficacy of ERCP in the elderly. In a large study of approximately 2600 patients, the efficacy rate of ERCP in clearing out common bile duct stones was 97 %, with the overall complication rate actually significantly lower than that in the younger age group (1.6 % vs. 3.5 %) [50]. Another large study of approximately 750 patients showed that the feared post-ERCP pancreatitis is lower in the elderly (0.9 % vs. 5 %) [51].

Future Trends

While there have been tremendous developments and advancements in detection and management of choledocholithiasis over the last few decades, there remain several unknowns in the natural history, diagnosis, and prevention of choledocholithiasis. Future large studies should address prevention and predictors of gallbladder stones and stone migration into the common bile duct. Newer, noninvasive, safe imaging modalities are needed to detect small bile duct stones with high sensitivity and specificity.

Conflicts of interest: No conflicts of interest relevant to this chapter.

References

1. Everhart JE, Khare M, Hill M, Maurer KR. Prevalence and ethnic differences in gallbladder disease in the United States. Gastroenterology. 1999;117:632–9.
2. Hunter JG. Laparoscopic transcystic common bile duct exploration. Am J Surg. 1992;163:53–6. discussion 57–8.
3. O'Neill CJ, Gillies DM, Gani JS. Choledocholithiasis: overdiagnosed endoscopically and undertreated laparoscopically. ANZ J Surg. 2008;78:487–91.

4. Petelin JB. Laparoscopic common bile duct exploration. Surg Endosc. 2003;17:1705–15.
5. Robinson BL, Donohue JH, Gunes S, et al. Selective operative cholangiography. Appropriate management for laparoscopic cholecystectomy. Arch Surg. 1995;130:625–30. discussion 630–1.
6. Chang L, Lo SK, Stabile BE, Lewis RJ, de Virgilio C. Gallstone pancreatitis: a prospective study on the incidence of cholangitis and clinical predictors of retained common bile duct stones. Am J Gastroenterol. 1998;93:527–31.
7. Chak A, Hawes RH, Cooper GS, Hoffman B, Catalano M, Wong R et al. Prospective assessment of the utility of EUS in the evaluation of gallstone pancreatitis. Gastrointest Endosc. 1999;49:599–604.
8. Liu CL, Lo CM, Chan JK, Poon R, Lam C, Fan S et al. Detection of choledocholithiasis by EUS in acute pancreatitis: a prospective evaluation in 100 consecutive patients. Gastrointest Endosc. 2001;54:325–30.
9. Cohen ME, Slezak L, Wells CK, Andersen DK, Topazian M. Prediction of bile duct stones and complications in gallstone pancreatitis using early laboratory trends. Am J Gastroenterol. 2001;96:3305–11.
10. Kim MH, Myung SJ, Seo DW, Lee S, Kim Y, Lee M et al. Association of periampullary diverticula with primary choledocholithiasis but not with secondary choledocholithiasis. Endoscopy. 1998;30:601–4.
11. Barbara L, Sama C, Morselli-Labate A, Taroni F, Rusticali A, Festi D. A ten year incidence of gallstone disease: the Sirmione study. J Hepatol. 1993;18:S43.
12. Attili AF, Carulli N, Roda E, Barbara B, Capocaccia L, Menotti A et al. Epidemiology of gallstone disease in Italy: prevalence data of the Multicenter Italian Study on Cholelithiasis (M.I.COL.). Am J Epidemiol. 1995;141:158–65.
13. Valdivieso V, Covarrubias C, Siegel F, Cruz F. Pregnancy and cholelithiasis: pathogenesis and natural course of gallstones diagnosed in early puerperium. Hepatology. 1993;17:1–4.
14. Racine A, Bijon A, Fournier A, Hampe J, Doren M. Menopausal hormone therapy and risk of cholecystectomy: a prospective study based on the French E3N cohort. CMAJ. 2013;185:555–61.
15. Gilat T, Feldman C, Halpern Z, Dan M, Bar-Meir S. An increased familial frequency of gallstones. Gastroenterology. 1983;84:242–6.
16. Stampfer MJ, Maclure KM, Colditz GA, Manson JE, Willett WC. Risk of symptomatic gallstones in women with severe obesity. Am J Clin Nutr. 1992;55:652–8.

17. Liddle RA, Goldstein RB, Saxton J. Gallstone formation during weight-reduction dieting. Arch Intern Med. 1989;149:1750–3.
18. De Santis A, Attili AF, Ginanni Corradini S, Scafato E, Cantagalli A, De Luca C, et al. Gallstones and diabetes: a case-control study in a free-living population sample. Hepatology. 1997;25:787–90.
19. Huguier M, Bornet P, Charpak Y, Houry S, Chastang C. Selective contraindications based on multivariate analysis for operative cholangiography in biliary lithiasis. Surg Gynecol Obstet. 1991;172:470–4.
20. Costi R, Sarli L, Caruso G, Iusco D, Gobbi S, Violi V, et al. Preoperative ultrasonographic assessment of the number and size of gallbladder stones: is it a useful predictor of asymptomatic choledochal lithiasis? J Ultrasound Med. 2002;21:971–6.
21. Wegge C, Kjaergaard J. Evaluation of symptoms and signs of gallstone disease in patients admitted with upper abdominal pain. Scand J Gastroenterol. 1985;20:933–6.
22. Kiriyama S, Takada T, Strasberg SM, Solomkin J, Mayumi T, Pitt H et al. TG13 guidelines for diagnosis and severity grading of acute cholangitis (with videos). J Hepatobiliary Pancreat Sci. 2013;20:24–34.
23. Takada T, Kawarada Y, Nimura Y, Yoshida M, Mayumi T, Sekimoto M, et al. Background: Tokyo guidelines for the management of acute cholangitis and cholecystitis. J Hepatobiliary Pancreat Surg. 2007;14:1–10.
24. Committee ASoP, Maple JT, Ben-Menachem T, Appalaneni V, Banerjee S, Cash B, et al. The role of endoscopy in the evaluation of suspected choledocholithiasis. Gastrointest Endosc. 2010;71:1–9.
25. Yang MH, Chen TH, Wang SE, Tsai Y, Su C, Wu C, et al. Biochemical predictors for absence of common bile duct stones in patients undergoing laparoscopic cholecystectomy. Surg Endosc. 2008;22:1620–4.
26. Peng WK, Sheikh Z, Paterson-Brown S, Nixon SJ. Role of liver function tests in predicting common bile duct stones in acute calculous cholecystitis. Br J Surg. 2005;92:1241–7.
27. Onken JE, Brazer SR, Eisen GM, Williams D, Bouras E, DeLong E, et al. Predicting the presence of choledocholithiasis in patients with symptomatic cholelithiasis. Am J Gastroenterol. 1996;91:762–7.
28. Barkun AN, Barkun JS, Fried GM, Ghitulescu G, Steinmetz O, Pham C et al. Useful predictors of bile duct stones in patients

undergoing laparoscopic cholecystectomy. McGill Gallstone Treatment Group. Ann Surg. 1994;220:32–9.

29. Anderson SW, Lucey BC, Varghese JC, Soto JA. Accuracy of MDCT in the diagnosis of choledocholithiasis. Am J Roentgenol. 2006;187:174–80.

30. Anderson SW, Rho E, Soto JA. Detection of biliary duct narrowing and choledocholithiasis: accuracy of portal venous phase multidetector CT. Radiology. 2008;247:418–27.

31. Miller FH, Hwang CM, Gabriel H, Goodhartz LA, Omar AJ, Parsons 3rd WG. Contrast-enhanced helical CT of choledocholithiasis. Am J Roentgenol. 2003;181:125–30.

32. Neitlich JD, Topazian M, Smith RC, Gupta A, Burrell MI, Rosenfield AT. Detection of choledocholithiasis: comparison of unenhanced helical CT and endoscopic retrograde cholangiopancreatography. Radiology. 1997;203:753–7.

33. Soto JA, Alvarez O, Munera F, Velez SM, Valencia J, Ramirez N. Diagnosing bile duct stones: comparison of unenhanced helical CT, oral contrast-enhanced CT cholangiography, and MR cholangiography. Am J Roentgenol. 2000;175:1127–34.

34. Giljaca V, Gurusamy KS, Takwoingi Y, Higgie D, Poropat G, Stimac D, et al. Endoscopic ultrasound versus magnetic resonance cholangiopancreatography for common bile duct stones. Cochrane Database Syst Rev. 2015;2:CD011549.

35. Boraschi P, Neri E, Braccini G, Gigoni R, Caramella D, Perri G, et al. Choledocolithiasis: diagnostic accuracy of MR cholangiopancreatography. Three-year experience. Magn Reson Imaging. 1999;17:1245–53.

36. Zidi SH, Prat F, Le Guen O, Rondeau Y, Rocher L, Fritsch J, Rondeau Y, Rocher L, Fritsch J, et al. Use of magnetic resonance cholangiography in the diagnosis of choledocholithiasis: prospective comparison with a reference imaging method. Gut. 1999;44:118–22.

37. Kondo S, Isayama H, Akahane M, Toda N, Sasahira N, Nakai Y, et al. Detection of common bile duct stones: comparison between endoscopic ultrasonography, magnetic resonance cholangiography, and helical-computed-tomographic cholangiography. Eur J Radiol. 2005;54:271–5.

38. Sugiyama M, Atomi Y. Endoscopic ultrasonography for diagnosing choledocholithiasis: a prospective comparative study with ultrasonography and computed tomography. Gastrointest Endosc. 1997;45:143–6.

39. Mortensen MB, Fristrup C, Holm FS, Pless T, Durup J, Ainsworth A, et al. Prospective evaluation of patient tolerability, satisfaction with patient information, and complications in endoscopic ultrasonography. Endoscopy. 2005;37:146–53.
40. Bournet B, Migueres I, Delacroix M, Vigouroux D, Bornet J, Escourrou J, et al. Early morbidity of endoscopic ultrasound: 13 years' experience at a referral center. Endoscopy. 2006;38: 349–54.
41. Committee ASoP, Maple JT, Ikenberry SO, Appalaneni V, Decker G, Early D, et al. The role of endoscopy in the management of choledocholithiasis. Gastrointest Endosc. 2011;74: 731–44.
42. Petrov MS, van Santvoort HC, Besselink MG, van der Heijden GJ, van Erpecum KJ, Gooszen HG. Early endoscopic retrograde cholangiopancreatography versus conservative management in acute biliary pancreatitis without cholangitis: a meta-analysis of randomized trials. Ann Surg. 2008;247:250–7.
43. Siegel JH, Kasmin FE. Biliary tract diseases in the elderly: management and outcomes. Gut. 1997;41:433–5.
44. Beaton HL. Surgical considerations. In: Gelb A ed. Clinical Gastroenterology in the Elderly. New York: Marcel Dekker, 1996, pp. 271–82.
45. Sugiyama M, Atomi Y. Treatment of acute cholangitis due to choledocholithiasis in elderly and younger patients. Arch Surg. 1997;132:1129–33.
46. Park J, Fromkes J, Cooperman M. Acute pancreatitis in elderly patients. Pathogenesis and outcome. Am J Surg. 1986;152: 638–42.
47. Gloor B, Ahmed Z, Uhl W, Buchler MW. Pancreatic disease in the elderly. Best Pract Res Clin Gastroenterol. 2002;16:159–70.
48. Wilson C, Imrie CW. Deaths from acute pancreatitis: why do we miss the diagnosis so frequently? Int J Pancreatol. 1988;3: 273–81.
49. Lankisch PG, Schirren CA, Kunze E. Undetected fatal acute pancreatitis: why is the disease so frequently overlooked? Am J Gastroenterol. 1991;86:322–6.
50. Lukens FJ, Howell DA, Upender S, Sheth SG, Jafri SM. ERCP in the very elderly: outcomes among patients older than eighty. Dig Dis Sci. 2010;55:847–51.
51. Finkelmeier F, Tal A, Ajouaou M, Filmann N, Zeuzem S, Waidmann O, et al. ERCP in elderly patients: increased risk of sedation adverse events but low frequency of post-ERCP pancreatitis. Gastrointest Endosc. 2015;82:1051–9.

Chapter 12
Benign Biliary Strictures

Sheeva K. Parbhu and Douglas G. Adler

What Is a Biliary Stricture and Why Do I Have One?

Suggested Response to the Patient

Bile is a substance made by the liver and gallbladder that aids in digestion, primarily of fats. The function of the biliary tree is to facilitate the drainage of bile from the liver and the gallbladder into the small intestine via multiple ducts. Benign (noncancerous) disease of the biliary tree includes strictures, leaks, or stones, which occur alone or in combination. Benign biliary strictures (BBS) account for about 15 % of strictures seen in the Western world.

S.K. Parbhu, M.D.
Gastroenterology and Hepatology, University of Utah School of Medicine, Salt Lake City, UT, USA

D.G. Adler, M.D., F.A.C.G., A.G.A.F. (✉)
Gastroenterology and Hepatology, Huntsman Cancer Center, University of Utah School of Medicine,
30N 1900E 4R118, Salt Lake City, UT 84132, USA
e-mail: douglas.adler@hsc.utah.edu

© Springer International Publishing Switzerland 2016
K. Dua, R. Shaker (eds.), *Pancreas and Biliary Disease*,
DOI 10.1007/978-3-319-28089-9_12

Etiology and Classification

The most common cause of BBS is a postoperative stricture, occurring most commonly after laparoscopic cholecystectomy. BBS can develop after other surgeries that affect the bile duct, such as liver transplantation or liver resection. Another common etiology is chronic pancreatitis.

BBS are classified based on location in the bile ducts themselves. This system is known as the Bismuth classification, and ranges from distal (Bismuth I) to proximal (Bismuth V). A majority of the BBS seen after surgery or in chronic pancreatitis are distal (Bismuth I or II) strictures.

Signs and Symptoms

The presentation and diagnosis of BBS can vary from mild subclinical disease to severe disease resulting in a high degree of morbidity and mortality. Common findings include an elevation in transaminases ("liver function tests") and high levels of bilirubin buildup leading to jaundice (yellow eyes and yellow skin). Chronic low-grade biliary obstruction by stricture formation can lead to the development of chronic bile duct injury, which is often referred to as secondary sclerosing cholangitis (SSC), or less frequently, as biliary cirrhosis. This can lead to jaundice, recurrent or persistent infection within the bile ducts (cholangitis), and even end-stage liver disease if left untreated.

Postoperative Biliary Strictures

Cholecystectomy

The most common cause of benign biliary strictures is associated with laparoscopic cholecystectomy. This has become the most commonly performed operation in the digestive tract, and it is first-line surgical treatment for symptomatic gallbladder disease. Although, when compared to the open approach, the use of laparoscopy results in less pain, shorter hospital stay, and expedited return to normal activity, there is a two to four times increase in the incidence of bile duct strictures, likely due to limited visualization of the biliary anatomy.

Today, there remains an incidence of biliary tract injury (including BBS) of about 0.2–1.4 %. This is caused by direct surgical injury of the ducts with scalpels, clips, trocars, cautery, or misidentification of biliary structures. There is good evidence to show that using an intraoperative cholangiogram improves detection rate of biliary tract injuries and is predictive of decreased future complications.

Liver Transplant

Surgeries that require end-to-end connection (anastomosis) of the biliary tree include liver transplantation and liver resection, and have a much higher incidence of biliary strictures. Biliary injury is the most frequently noted complication after transplantation and this includes BBS. The most common type of BBS after transplant is called an anastomotic stricture (AS) and accounts for 87 % of lesions. It is commonly due to lack of blood flow (ischemia) or surgical injury. Nonanastomotic strictures (NAS) can also be seen, most commonly as a result of organ rejection or ischemic injury. A majority of patients who develop BBS will have symptoms within 1 year of transplantation. Risk factors include hepatic artery thrombosis, chronic ductopenic rejection, ABO incompatibility, and the characteristics of the liver donor. BBS can lead to infection, graft failure requiring repeat transplant, and carry an associated mortality rate of 5 %.

Biliary Strictures Secondary to Pancreatitis

Chronic pancreatitis (CP) is most commonly caused by alcohol abuse and is a progressive disease characterized by pancreatic functional decline and ultimately failure. Approximately one-third of patients with CP will develop

BBS, accounting for about 10 % of all benign strictures. The common bile duct runs through the pancreas, and in the setting of inflammation and fibrosis in CP, strictures can form due to repeated compression and damage of the duct. Imaging studies such as Computed Tomography (CT), Magnetic Resonance Imaging (MRI), and Endoscopic Ultrasound (EUS) are commonly used to diagnose CP.

Infectious, Inflammatory, and Rare Causes of Biliary Strictures

Other causes of BBS include conditions that are seen in the setting of inflammation, infection, or direct mechanical injury. Blunt or penetrating abdominal trauma can sometimes lead to the development of biliary strictures, typically with a delayed presentation.

Sequelae of cancer treatment such as abdominal radiation and chemotherapeutic agents such as bevacizumab, adriamycin, 5-fluorodeoxyuridine, and mitomycin C are associated with the formation of BBS. A rare condition known as Mirizzi syndrome may present as a BBS, but is actually an acute obstruction in which the hepatic duct is compressed due to impacted gallstones.

HIV cholangiopathy was once common, but now is a relatively rare cause of biliary strictures in the era of highly active antiretroviral therapy. It is seen in patients with CD4 T-cell counts less than $100/mm^3$, and is associated with Cryptosporidium or Cytomegalovirus in more than 90 % of cases. Tuberculosis and histoplasmosis are other rare infectious causes of BBS seen independently of HIV infection.

An immune-mediated condition called immunoglobulin G subclass 4-related disease (IgG4-RD) is a relatively recently described etiology of BBS. This disease is twice as likely to occur in males as in females and primarily affects middle-aged to elderly (50–70 year-old) patients. Other autoimmune conditions such as polyarteritis nodosa and systemic lupus erythematosus may result in development of BBS.

Brief Review of the Literature

The function of the biliary tree is to facilitate the drainage of bile from the liver and the gallbladder to the small intestine via multiple ducts. Benign disease of the biliary tree includes biliary strictures, leaks, and stones [1]. These can occur alone or in combination. Benign biliary strictures themselves account for about 15 % of strictures in the Western world, and the etiologies are diverse, ranging from postoperative injury, anastomotic strictures, acute and chronic pancreatitis, gallstone disease, and other less common inflammatory and infectious conditions [2, 3]. Primary sclerosing cholangitis (PSC) is another well-described cause of benign biliary strictures and will be covered in a separate chapter.

The most common cause of a benign biliary stricture is a postoperative stricture, occurring most commonly after laparoscopic cholecystectomy as well as after other surgeries that involve the bile duct, such as orthotopic liver transplantation or liver resection. Benign strictures can also develop in the setting of chronic pancreatitis [4].

When evaluating and treating biliary strictures, it is helpful to classify them based on their location in the bile ducts themselves. A classification system, known as the Bismuth classification system, exists for just this purpose. Bismuth I strictures are located >2 cm distal to the hepatic bifurcation, while Bismuth II strictures are < 2 cm distal to the hepatic bifurcation. Bismuth III strictures occur at the level of the hepatic bifurcation, Bismuth IV strictures involve the right or left hepatic ducts, and Bismuth V strictures extend into the right or left hepatic branch ducts [5]. Once the benign nature of the stricture has been confirmed, endoscopy has surpassed surgery as the first-line approach for therapy of Bismuth I and II (distal) postoperative strictures as well as many proximal strictures [4].

The presentation and diagnosis of benign biliary strictures can vary from mild subclinical disease to severe disease resulting in a high degree of morbidity and mortality. Chronic low-grade biliary obstruction by stricture formation can lead to the development of chronic bile duct injury, often referred to as secondary sclerosing cholangitis (SSC) or, less frequently, as biliary cirrhosis. SSC can lead to jaundice, recurrent cholangitis, and even end-stage liver disease if left untreated. Other conditions associated with biliary strictures include recurrent cholangitis, as well as biliary stone formation and persistent or recurrent biliary infections [6]. Other common findings include mild transaminitis and hepatic obstruction with hyperbilirubinemia. One case series of 300 patients evaluated over 15 years described the most common presentation of clinically significant strictures to be jaundice, seen in approximately 77 % of patients. Other common presenting features were cholangitis, seen in 70 % of patients, pruritis in 49.6 %, and portal hypertension with evidence of esophageal varices in 3.7 % [7].

Postoperative Biliary Strictures

Cholecystectomy

The most common cause of benign bile duct strictures, laparoscopic cholecystectomy, has become the most commonly performed operation in the digestive tract and the first-line surgical treatment for symptomatic gallbladder disease over the past 30 years [8]. While the laparoscopic approach has been shown to result in less postoperative pain, a shorter hospital stay, and expedited return to normal activity when compared to the open approach, it is also associated with a two to four times increase in the incidence of bile duct strictures [9]. This is likely due to limited visualization as compared to the open approach.

In the early 1990s, there was a peak of iatrogenic biliary tract injuries that was thought to be a result of the surgeon learning curve with a novel surgical procedure [7]. Even today, there still exists an incidence of biliary tract injury associated with laparoscopic cholecystectomy that ranges from 0.2 to 1.4 % and can result in increased number of hospitalizations, decreased quality of life, and high rates of malpractice litigation [10] (Fig. 12.1).

The cause of these strictures is thought to be most likely due to direct surgical injury with scalpels, clips, trocars, cautery, or misidentification of biliary structures. While majority of 114 surgeons in one published survey indicated that these injuries were unavoidable [11], there is significant evidence that bile duct injury should be regarded as preventable. Approximately 70–80 % of injuries are due to misidentification of biliary anatomy, and multiple techniques have been described to facilitate anatomical orientation before dissection with the goal of reducing risk of injury [12].

Although often these strictures are discovered after patients develop clinical sequela as previously described (infection, hyperbilirubinemia, cirrhosis, and portal hypertension), there is evidence that intraoperative cholangiograms do help to increase the likelihood of earlier detection of bile duct injury. In a study involving 565 surgeons, the likelihood of identifying a bile duct injury when using intraoperative cholangiography was greatly improved (80.9 %) when compared to no intraoperative evaluation (45.1 %) [8]. A smaller series of 65 patients also described a significantly improved operative detection rate of injury (68 % vs. 32 %) with the use of intraoperative cholangiogram that was importantly found to be a predictive factor for decreased future complications [13]. A large population-based retrospective study of over 4000 laparoscopic cholecystectomies similarly reported an eightfold reduction in biliary tract injury with the use of concurrent cholangiograms. While bile duct injury cannot be prevented by cholangiography, it is a cost-effective means of early detection that allows for more thorough assessment as well as a decreased risk of future morbidity [14].

Liver Transplant

Surgeries that require biliary anastomosis such as orthotopic liver transplantation or liver resection have a much higher incidence of biliary strictures. Biliary complications are the most frequently noted complication after liver transplantation, and include a wide variety of injuries, including strictures,

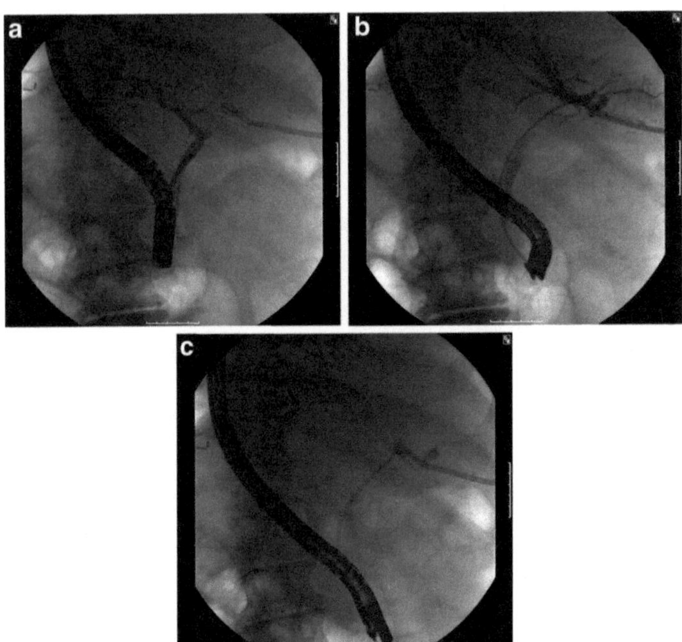

Fig. 12.1 Biliary stricture following laparoscopic cholecystectomy. (a) ERCP cholangiogram showing contrast injection without opacification of the right hepatic duct. Note a percutaneous drain has been placed in the abdomen. (b) A guidewire is advanced across the stricture, and contrast injection reveals the completely obstructed, dilated right hepatic ductal system. (c) A plastic biliary stent is placed across the stricture to provide dilation and drainage

biliary leaks, biliary casts, stones, or debris [15]. Of those, biliary strictures are the most common, occurring in 5.8–39 % of cases. The causes of these biliary strictures are multifactorial and are usually produced by the combination of local ischemia, fibrosis, immunosuppression and infectious issues, and primary surgical injury [16].

There are two separate classifications of post-transplant biliary strictures: anastomotic strictures (AS) and nonanastomotic strictures (NAS) (Fig. 12.2). AS are commonly due to ischemia or surgical injury, while NAS are seen as a result of rejection or ischemic injury [17]. AS account for the majority of lesions (87 %), and involve the choledochojejunostomy or choledochocholedochostomy, while NAS involve the donor hepatic ducts [18]. Most liver transplants involve the creation of a choledochocholedochostomy, and this is overwhelmingly the most common site of injury.

Although strictures can present at any time, the mean time to presentation is 5–8 months, and a majority present within one year of transplantation. Early postoperative bile strictures usually occur at the anastomotic site and are caused by problems related to surgical technique in combination with fibrotic healing. Strictures that present late are often due to ischemia or rejection, and can often be associated with multiple strictures involving the intrahepatic ducts [19]. Risk factors include hepatic artery thrombosis, chronic ductopenic rejection, ABO incompatibility, and characteristics of the liver donor including use of vasopressors, older age, and presence of cardiac death [20].

The complication rate has been noted to be higher in living-related liver transplantation versus orthotopic liver transplantation, a complication that is attributed to increased difficulty in defining the dissection plane around the right hepatic duct [15, 19]. Although classified as a "benign" complication, post-transplantation strictures have been shown to be responsible for mortality in 5 % of patients, usually as they can lead to infection and graft failure, which can sometimes require repeat transplant [17].

Biliary Strictures Secondary to Pancreatitis

While acute pancreatitis (often in the setting of pancreatic necrosis) can present with common bile duct obstruction as a result of direct compression due to periductal swelling, chronic pancreatitis is a more common etiology of benign biliary strictures [21]. Chronic pancreatitis (CP), most commonly due to alcohol abuse, is a progressive disease characterized by pancreatic exocrine and endocrine decline and ultimately failure, associated with a mortality rate of 50 %

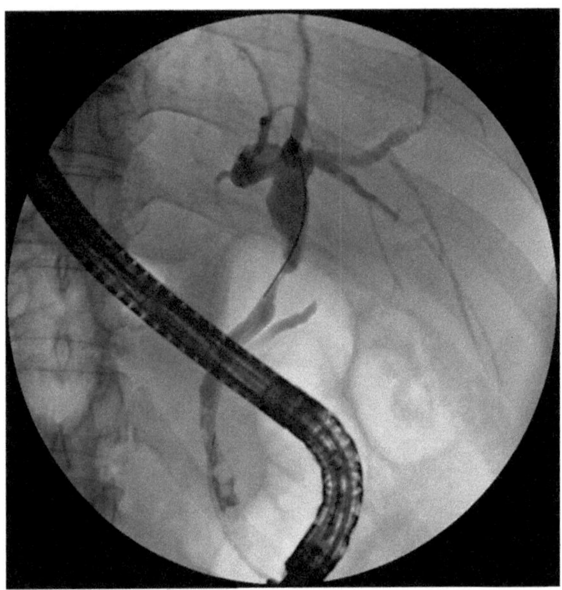

Fig. 12.2 Cholangiogram showing an anastomotic stricture following liver transplantation. Note the proximal ductal dilation above the stricture

over 20–25 years. Patients with CP tend to present with significant pain and have many complications including malabsorption, pseudocyst formation, pleural fistulas, and duodenal or biliary obstruction [22].

Approximately one-third of patients with chronic pancreatitis will develop biliary strictures, accounting for about 10 % of benign strictures of the biliary system. These strictures arise in the setting of inflammation and fibrosis in the pancreatic head. As the distal common bile duct (CBD) runs "through" the pancreatic head, the duct at this location is subject to extrinsic compression by the surrounding diseased pancreas. Fibrosis of the pancreatic head from chronic inflammation and fibrosis often results in biliary strictures that can be very difficult to treat [23]. One study saw an incidence of biliary strictures of 46 % in patients with moderate to severe CP [24].

The diagnosis of pancreatitis is typically made with a detailed history, physical examination, laboratory data, and findings on imaging. Imaging modalities such as CT, MRI, and EUS are most commonly used in the diagnosis and evaluation of chronic pancreatitis, while ERCP remains useful for further ductal characterization and therapeutics [23, 24].

Infectious, Inflammatory, and Rare Causes of Biliary Strictures

Other causes of benign biliary strictures (excluding PSC) include conditions that are seen in the setting of inflammation, infection, as well as direct mechanical injury to the biliary system [2].

Mirizzi syndrome may present similarly to a biliary stricture, but is actually a condition in which the common hepatic duct is compressed. In this syndrome, gallstones are impacted in the cystic duct or an out-pouching of the gallbladder at the junction of the gallbladder and cystic duct (referred to as Hartmann's pouch) and can cause repeated episodes of injury leading to obstruction and occasionally fistulas [25]. Blunt or penetrating abdominal trauma can sometimes lead to the development of biliary strictures, typically with a delayed presentation [26].

Sequelae of cancer treatment can cause long-term effects including biliary injuries. Strictures have been seen to arise in the setting of abdominal radiation for treatment of lymphoma and other intra-abdominal malignancies and may present many years after the original exposure [27]. Chemotherapy, including hepatic artery infusion of 5-fluorodeoxyuridine, as well as other systemic agents such as bevacizumab, adriamycin, and mitomycin C have also been associated with a form of secondary sclerosing cholangitis and the formation of biliary strictures [28].

HIV cholangiopathy, once common, is now a relatively rare cause of biliary strictures in the era of highly active antiretroviral therapy (HAART). HIV cholangiopathy is typically seen in advanced disease, in patients with CD4 T-cell counts less than $100/mm^3$. It is associated with Cryptosporidium and Cytomegalovirus in more than 90 % of cases, but other implicated pathogens include Mycobacterium Avium-Intracellulare, Cyclospora, Isospora, Cryptococcus, and Giardia [29, 30]. Tuberculosis and Histoplasmosis are other rare infectious causes of biliary strictures seen independently of HIV infection [31].

An immune-mediated condition called immunoglobulin G subclass 4–related disease (IgG4-RD) is a relatively recently described etiology of biliary strictures [28]. IgG4-RD was first described in younger Asian males, although it is thought that this disease has probably been underdiagnosed in the past due to poor awareness among physicians [32]. Further studies suggest that men are twice as likely to develop IgG4-RD, and it mainly affects middle-aged to elderly (50–70 year-old) patients with mass-forming or nodular lesions in various organs. A subset of IgG4-RD is IgG4-related sclerosing cholangitis (IgG4-SC) and presents with circular thickening and extensive fibrosis of the bile duct wall, progressing to stenotic lesions and strictures [33]. This can mimic PSC, but in contrast to PSC often responds to immunosuppressive therapy [32].

Other immune-mediated conditions such as polyarteritis nodosa and systemic lupus erythematosus result in multisystem disease states involving inflammation of small to medium-sized arteries, occasionally presenting with biliary obstruction due to biliary strictures. Unfortunately, a small percentage of biliary strictures are idiopathic, and no clear etiology is ever elucidated [2, 26].

Can You Fix My Benign Biliary Stricture?

Suggested Response to the Patient

BBS represent a significant clinical problem of diverse etiology, with three general management options available: surgery, interventional radiology approaches, or endoscopy.

Surgery

Standard surgical technique offers a good chance at cure for the majority of BBS. Surgical management of BBS involves drainage via the creation of an anastomosis between uninjured bile duct and the proximal intestine, with an end-to-side ("roux-en Y") reconstruction. For many years, this was the only option and was considered first-line treatment for this condition. While this approach is still considered the most definitive treatment, operative repair is very invasive and has been shown to have a high stricture recurrence rate.

Interventional Radiology

The main indication for interventional radiology (IR) intervention in BBS is the presence of anatomy that does not permit easy endoscopic access or critical illness requiring immediate biliary decompression in patients not suitable for sedation and/or endoscopy. In IR procedures, the biliary system is accessed percutaneously, or through the skin. Once a catheter has been placed into the biliary tree, the bile duct may be drained by an "external" biliary catheter, which drains the obstructed bile into a drainage bag attached to the patient. Another type of drain is the "internal-external" biliary catheter, which drains both externally into a drainage bag as well as internally into the small bowel. These drain catheters are left in place and replaced with increasingly larger drains to dilate the stricture. A recurrence rate of up to 58 % is seen in these patients, and downsides include an increased rate of infection with an external catheter as well as discomfort due to the necessity of an external drainage bag.

Endoscopy

Endoscopic retrograde cholangiopancreatography (ERCP) is now first-line therapy in the therapeutic treatment of benign strictures. It provides the advantage of successfully establishing internal drainage without the need for an external catheter, and has been shown to have long-term success rates equal to that of surgical treatment while being markedly less invasive. Benefits of endoscopy include its minimally invasive nature, safety, repeatability, and utility in chronically and critically ill patients. Drawbacks include a less than 100 % success rate, technically demanding procedures, and the need for multiple (average number of 5) ERCPs, which can be burdensome for the patient.

When endoscopic treatment was first introduced, balloon dilation alone was the primary treatment modality. This offered good short-term resolution, but it was often followed by both symptom and stricture recurrence. Standard endoscopic therapy now involves initial balloon dilation followed by placement of an internal biliary stent. A stent is a plastic or metal tube which is inserted into a bile duct to mechanically relieve a stenosis or obstruction. The use of stents almost tripled the success rate of the procedure and offered long-term stricture resolution.

A standard protocol of placing multiple plastic stents at one time was developed and showed an even greater success rate than placement of a single stent. Plastic stents will "clog" and require replacement on average every 3–4 months, and so protocol includes scheduled stent removal every 3 months, or earlier when clinically necessary. The placement of multiple, simultaneous plastic stents over multiple endoscopic procedures until stricture resolution has been shown in multiple studies to be successful in post-laparoscopic cholecystectomy strictures, post-transplant strictures, and in strictures related to chronic pancreatitis (Fig. 12.3).

Although placement of multiple plastic stents has been shown to be effective, due to their short duration of patency and technical difficulty of placement of multiple stents at one time, they are not able to effectively treat all strictures. Many, newer studies have emerged to evaluate alternative types of stents to manage BBS. Fully covered self-expandable metal stents (FCSEMS) specifically have been studied in randomized controlled fashion compared to multiple plastic stents.

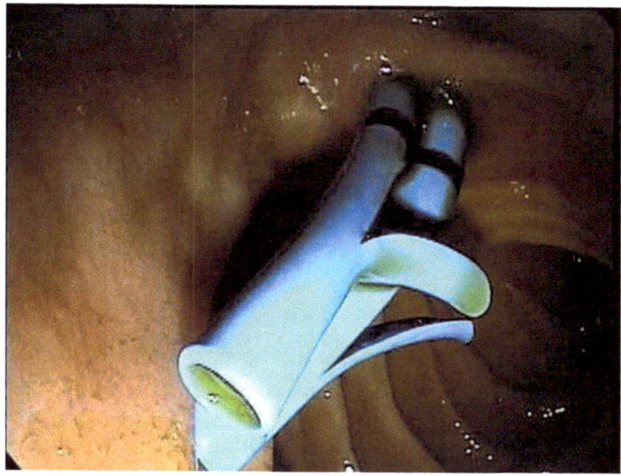

FIG. 12.3 Endoscopic image of side-by-side plastic biliary stents being used to treat a benign biliary stricture

These FCSEMS have an expansile force, and because they are covered, they have less complications with mucosal ingrowth, stent retrieval, and stricture recurrence. Because a single FCSEMS can expand to a diameter approximately equivalent to three plastic stents, these devices are able to stay patent for longer than plastic stents. While FCSEMS are more expensive than plastic stents, studies have been able to show a reduced number of ERCPs, similar rates of stricture resolution, fewer complications, and greater cost-effectiveness. For these reasons, FCSEMS are now in widespread use for the treatment of BBS and are often used as the initial treatment modality (Fig. 12.4).

Brief Review of the Literature

Surgical, Interventional Radiology, or Endoscopic Approaches to the Treatment of Biliary Strictures

Benign biliary strictures (BBS) represent a significant clinical problem of diverse etiologies, with three general management options available: surgery, interventional radiology approaches, or endoscopy [34]. Surgery involves drainage via

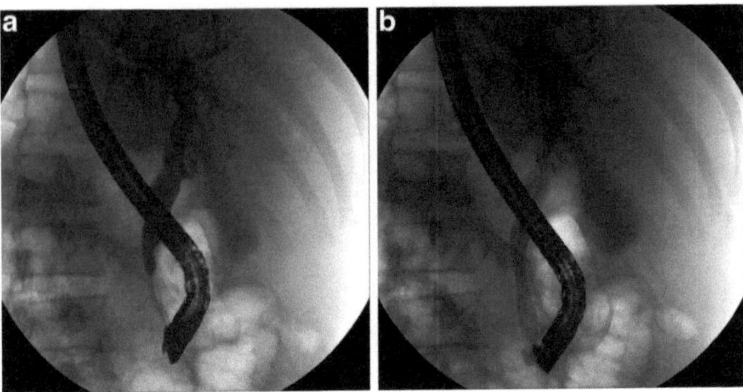

Fig. 12.4 FCSEMS to treat a benign biliary stricture in a patient with chronic pancreatitis. (**a**) Cholangiogram shows a distal common bile duct stricture due to surrounding pancreatic inflammation and fibrosis. (**b**) A FCSEMS is placed across the stricture in a transampullary manner. The stent was left in place for 3 months, after which the stricture resolved

the creation of an anastomosis between uninjured bile duct and the proximal small bowel (usually by hepaticojejunostomy). Interventional radiologists insert percutaneous catheters across duct strictures and can perform dilations. Endoscopic management involves stricture dilation with or without stent insertion [35, 36].

Surgery

Standard surgical technique offers a good chance at cure for the majority of benign biliary strictures and was the only option for these complications for many years [35]. In patients treated with surgery, continuity between the biliary and enteric system is achieved with a Roux-enY reconstruction via the creation of either a hepaticojejunostomy, choledochojejunostomy, or an intrahepatic cholangiojejunostomy [37]. Surgery was formerly considered first-line treatment for this condition, and while this approach is still considered the most definitive treatment, operative repair is very invasive and has been shown to have a stricture recurrence rate of 10–30 %.

Interventional Radiology

Interventional radiology (IR) also has an established role in the management of patients with BBS by percutaneous access to the biliary system. The main indication for IR intervention in patients with biliary strictures is the presence of anatomy that does not permit easy endoscopic access to the stricture or critical illness that requires an immediate decompression of the biliary obstruction in patients who are not suitable for sedation and/or endoscopy [38]. In patients with BBS in the setting of surgically altered anatomy (most commonly the presence of a Roux-en Y reconstruction), a percutaneous approach is able to access the stricture successfully over 90 % of the time [39]. Once the biliary tree has been accessed percutaneously, the bile duct may be drained by a so-called "external" biliary catheter, which is placed above the blockage and drains externally into a drainage bag attached to the patient. The most common type of drainage catheter is a so-called "internal-external" biliary drain. To place this type of drain, a guidewire is inserted and crosses the stenotic lesion, and is advanced down through the bile duct, through the ampulla, and into the duodenum. The drainage catheter that is placed over the wire also follows this path and terminates in the duodenum; hence it is both "internal" and "external." The internal-external catheter facilitates drainage externally into a drainage bag, but also anterograde into the small intestine [40]. The drain catheter is left in place and replaced with drains of increasingly large diameter often in conjunction with balloon dilation of the stenosis with gradually increasing sizes of balloons. Although highly effective, downsides of this approach include a decreased quality of life and increased rate of infections with the presence of an external catheter (which most patients find very unpleasant), as well as a prolonged follow-up period requiring multiple procedures [38]. While IR drainage has a high success rate at temporary decompression and drainage of the biliary system, recurrent stenosis after dilation is seen in up to 58 % of cases, highlighting the recalcitrant nature of many biliary strictures [41]. A newer technique involves placement via percutaneous catheter of a covered stent across the stricture, with subsequent removal and replacement of the stent. Although this can lead to shorter indwelling catheter periods, this approach is not commonly performed and is generally reserved for patients who are not suitable for endoscopy [42].

Endoscopy

ERCP is now first-line therapy in the therapeutic treatment of benign strictures, as it provides the advantage of successfully establishing internal drainage without the need for an external catheter, and has been shown to have long-term success rates equal to that of surgical treatment [24, 35, 43, 44]. In a retrospective study of 101 patients treated for BBS, surgery and endoscopy were shown to have similar long-term success rates in regard to mortality, morbidity, and recurrence rate, with endoscopy being markedly less invasive [35]. A larger study followed over 5000 patients undergoing surgery over the span of 11 years, 77 of which developed postoperative strictures. The success rate of nonsurgical treatment in this group was over 70 %, and the study concluded that endoscopic management should be the initial treatment for this disorder [9]. The benefits of endoscopy include its minimally invasive nature, safety, repeatability, and utility in chronically and critically ill patients when compared to surgery. Drawbacks include a less than 100 % success rate, technically demanding procedures, and when accounting for an average number of 5 ERCPs to stricture resolution, can be burdensome for the patient [45].

When endoscopic treatment was first introduced, balloon dilation alone was the primary treatment modality.

This offered good short-term resolution, but was often followed by stricture (and symptom) recurrence, with a success rate of less than 50 % [17, 24, 45]. Standard endoscopic therapy now involves initial balloon dilation followed by placement of an internal biliary stent, a plastic or metal tube inserted into a bile duct to mechanically relieve a stenosis or obstruction. Once endoscopists progressed to placements of stents, operators saw improved results when compared to balloon dilation alone and almost tripled the success rate of the procedure [17]. Plastic stents are available in a variety of lengths and diameters, can be easily tailored for a particular stricture, and remain patent for an average of 3 months [46].

An early study described 74 patients with postoperative BBS who received placement of 1–2 plastic stents at least every 3 months, more frequently if clinically indicated, with stent removal at 1 year. Although technically successful with immediate biliary drainage in all patients, there was a higher than expected recurrence rate, with the majority of the 20 % of patients who experienced recurrent stricture presenting within 6 months of stent removal [47]. This progressed to placement of multiple, simultaneous plastic stents over multiple endoscopic procedures until resolution of a given stricture was seen, often around 12 months. In this approach, the diameter and number of inserted stents varies, with up to five stents placed at once, limited only by the ability of the stricture to accommodate the stents and the technical challenges of placing so many stents at one time [16]. Placement of multiple simultaneous plastic stents was shown to have a success rate in treatment of BBS of 92 % compared with 24 % for single stent placement in short-term follow-up studies [23].

As discussed earlier, AS and NAS represent different etiologies of strictures after liver transplantation. AS, the more common stricture type seen, respond more readily to endoscopic stents and balloon dilation, while NAS are more difficult to treat [48]. Success rates of endoscopic therapy in post-transplant anastomotic strictures can vary widely, from 27 % to 91 %, with lower success rates associated with more conservative forms of endoscopic therapy such as balloon dilation alone or single plastic stent placement [49, 50]. More aggressive endoscopic approaches have been studied in this population, during which multiple plastic stents are placed simultaneously after maximal balloon dilation of the stricture. In a series of 25 patients treated with balloon dilation and "maximal stent placement," 22 (88 %) experienced immediate success, and 20/22 (91 %) of patients who successfully completed endoscopic therapy were able to avoid surgical intervention [18]. One study described an "accelerated" protocol, during which maximal stent exchange occurred every 2 weeks over an average of 3.6 months instead of 12 months, and showed a comparable 87 % success rate of stricture resolution [51].

NAS are less amenable to endoscopic stent placement, mostly due to the complex etiology of autoimmune rejection and ischemia. They are also found to be associated with increased amounts of biliary sludge, debris, and casts, which may contribute to recurrent stent occlusion and cholangitis [52]. Stent placement is often performed, but can be less successful overall due to multiple strictures of variable lengths and location [48]. Typically, smaller balloons and stents are used in these strictures [52].

As living-donor liver transplantation has become more common in recent years, there has been a rise in the incidence of complications, including BBS. These strictures are similar to NAS in that they have proven to be more difficult to treat, although NAS are less frequently seen in this population due to short ischemia times and relatively healthy donors. While there have been fewer studies directly comparing different interventions in this specific population, a combination of balloon dilation and multiple stent placement is first-line therapy, successful in about 60–75 % of these living-donor post-transplant patients [53, 54].

Similar results are seen in patients with post-laparoscopic cholecystectomy BBS. In a study of 45 patients enrolled to have the maximum number of plastic stents inserted every 3 months until disappearance of stricture on cholangiography, 89 % of strictures morphologically resolved after a mean treatment duration of 12.1 months [55]. A different study of 43 patients prospectively followed BBS which developed after laparoscopic cholecystectomy and placed between 3 and 5 stents per ERCP at intervals over a period of 1 year. These patients were followed for an average of 16 months after conclusion of therapy, and a 100 % success rate was reported [56]. A retrospective study of 110 patients treated for BBS with multiple plastic stents cited a greater than 80 % success rate with a mean follow-up time of over 7 years. The remaining patients were eventually referred for surgical management of the stricture, most commonly due to "stent-dependence" (the need for persistent stent placement and removal past 1 year). Other factors cited in the decision to refer to surgery included restenosis, patient preference, and stricture of segmental bile duct [10]. More recent data and long-term follow-up over 10 years have identified increasing success, possibly due to better technical proficiency with the procedure. This study, following postcholecystectomy BBS, found a 95 % success rate over 10 years in patients who were able to complete the course of multiple plastic stents placed over the span of one year [57].

Endoscopic therapy with stent placement is also the first-line therapy for BBS due to chronic pancreatitis (CP), despite the fact that these strictures have been found to be more difficult to treat than postoperative lesions. These patients often have comorbidities and are at a greater risk of developing pancreatic cancer, which must be evaluated before treatment decisions are made [24, 62]. Similarly to postoperative BBS, results of balloon dilation and/or single plastic stent placement were disappointing, due to increased occlusion and migration of the stents. These early studies cited success rates ranging from 12 to 30 % [23, 45, 58]. With the utilization of dilation and multiple stent placements as described above, the success rate increased when compared to single stent placement alone, with a long-term success rate of around 60–70 %, with one study reporting a success rate as high as 92 %. While the protocol of stent exchange every 3 months or when clinically necessary is similar to that described in postoperative BBS, CP patients will often require 1–2 years of treatment before stricture resolution is achieved [23, 36, 59]. The decreased responsiveness to stent placement in CP is likely due to the fact that BBS develop in patients with advanced disease and diffuse fibrosis, and especially occurs in the setting of chronic calcific pancreatitis. Around 30 % of patients will not respond to endoscopic therapy, and these patients may need to be referred for surgical management [59, 60].

Although placement of multiple plastic stents has been shown to be effective therapy, due to their short duration of patency and technical difficulty of placement of multiple plastic stents, they are not able to effectively treat all strictures. Many studies have emerged to evaluate alternative types of stents to manage BBS. Uncovered self-expandable metal stents (SEMS) are primarily used in malignant biliary strictures, mainly due to their longer patency when compared to plastic stents. However, in BBS, uncovered SEMS are associated with long-term failure due to mucosal hyperplasia leading to premature stent obstruction [45, 61]. Fully covered self-expandable metal stents (FCSEMS) are being increasingly used and have been studied in randomized controlled fashion compared to multiple plastic stents. These fully covered stents have the same expansile force as uncovered SEMS, but because they are covered, have less complications with mucosal in-growth, stent retrieval, and stricture recurrence. A downside of FCSEMS is a higher risk of migration [16, 62, 63]. FCSEMS are now in widespread use for the treatment of benign biliary strictures.

One prospective study of 79 patients with BBS involved monitoring of LFTs every 3 months until stent dysfunction or death, with the primary endpoint being stricture resolution after the FCSEMS was removed. The majority of patients in this study had BBS due to chronic pancreatitis or postsurgical injury. The median time before stent removal in this protocol was 4 months, and successful treatment was confirmed by symptom resolution, LFT normalization, and repeat imaging. While the intention-to-treat group achieved a success rate of

75 %, of the patients who tolerated the treatment, a 90 % success rate was seen at 1 year [62]. Another study with 23 patients studied patients prospectively after placement of FCSEMS. While one patient had short-term failure due to persistent stricture, 96 % (22/23) of patients had stricture resolution after the stenting period. These patients continued to be followed over a median of 19 months, with an 82 % long-term success rate. Failures in this study were all seen in patients with chronic pancreatitis with calcifications, suggesting intractable fibrosis around the duct [63]. Similarly, several other studies in patients with BBS of diverse etiologies have also been able to show a clinical success rate of stricture resolution to be greater than 80 % [64, 65].

Because a single FCSEMS can expand to a diameter approximately equivalent to three 10 Fr plastic stents and these devices are able to remain patent for longer than plastic stents, it is thought that the use of these stents may increase the tolerance of the multiple-procedure protocol and lead to better long-term outcomes [65]. For this reason, there are also a fewer number of procedures required until stricture resolution, which decreases risk, time, and cost of treatment. While FCSEMS are more expensive than plastic stents, these studies have been able to show a reduced number of ERCPs, similar rates of stricture resolution, fewer complications, and more cost-effectiveness [16, 62, 63]. Although more randomized trials comparing efficacy are needed, especially in subgroups of patients with different etiologies of BBS, FCSEMS represent an important endoscopic therapy and are often now used as the initial treatment modality.

Will My Benign Biliary Stricture Return and What Are the Complications of Treatment?

Suggested Response to the Patient

While there are multiple different modalities used in the treatment of BBS, none have been shown to have a 100 %

success rate. The first-line treatment is now endoscopy, as it is less invasive, with multiple sequential plastic stents or FCSEMS, but the incidence of recurrence is significant. Recurrence is important not just because it requires further medical or surgical management, but has an important impact on quality of life for many patients. Frequent follow-up is necessary in almost all BBS patients, with close clinical monitoring and treatment plan which includes stent removal and exchanging every 3 months. While surgical management is reserved for BBS refractory to endoscopic management, surgical repair carries a mortality risk approaching 2 % and morbidity as high as 35 %.

Benign Biliary Stricture Recurrence

In liver transplant patients, endoscopy with balloon dilation alone in treatment of BBS has a recurrence rate of greater than 60 %. Any modest benefit is seen in patients who have an immediate, transient narrowing of a duct-to-duct anastomosis. Most strictures are representative of underlying injury that requires stent placement and frequent follow-up. Anastomotic strictures are less likely to recur when compared to nonanastomotic strictures, likely due to the different location and cause of the strictures. In AS, the mean number of ERCPs required for successful treatment is between 3 and 5, with a recurrence rate between 0 and 20 %. In NAS, due to technically difficult endoscopy and difficult to treat strictures, the recurrence rate is 25–30 %.

In patients with post-laparoscopic cholecystectomy BBS, early identification is a good prognostic indicator for successful treatment. Early studies reported recurrence rates as high as 30 %, but with newer endoscopic therapies, the recurrence rate has decreased to 0–12 %. The longest study followed patients for almost 14 years, and noted an 11.4 % recurrence rate.

The highest rates of recurrence can be seen in BBS in the setting of CP, which are more resistant to endoscopic treatment. Although some of these strictures resolve with time as the chronic inflammation and underlying cause are treated, the vast majority are permanent. While the placement of multiple plastic stents was able to decrease treatment failure, it remained as high as 40–56 %. This disappointing result is thought to be due to tissue in-growth and more frequent stent replacement than in BBS of other etiologies. More recent studies with FCSEMS in CP patients have been promising, with recurrence rate of around 23–30 % of patients. In addition to increased stricture resolution, these patients undergo fewer procedures and associated complications. Pancreatic head calcifications or presence of pancreatic duct strictures requiring stenting is a poor prognostic factor for successful BBS resolution.

Complications Related to Endoscopy

As with any procedure, there is an inherent risk of complication. Specific complications of ERCP have been well described and include pancreatitis, bleeding, sepsis, and perforation. These occur in around 6–7 % of patients, with a majority of complications being mild to moderate in severity, with post-ERCP pancreatitis being the most common complication.

Complications can either be immediate (related to the procedure itself), early (within 30 days), or late (after 30 days). Some patients experience complications due to endoscopically placed biliary stents, including cholangitis, cholecystitis, bleeding, pancreatitis, stent occlusion, and migration. The use of FCSEMS is associated with an increased rate of stent migration, but also a longer patency when compared to plastic stents, decreasing the overall risk by decreasing the number of procedures needed for stricture resolution.

Brief Review of the Literature

While there are multiple different modalities used in the treatment of benign biliary strictures, none have been shown to have a 100 % success rate. The first-line treatment is now endoscopy with multiple sequential plastic stents or FCSEMS, but the incidence of recurrence is significant. Recurrence is important not just because it requires further medical or surgical management, but has important impact on quality of life for many patients. The etiology of BBS plays the biggest role in treatment as well as complications and recurrence. Other factors such as location of stricture and time to diagnosis also are prognostic indicators of successful treatment and possibility of stricture recurrence [9].

Benign Biliary Stricture Recurrence

Recurrence Rate in Liver Transplant Patients

As previously discussed, endoscopy with balloon dilation alone in both AS and NAS has a recurrence rate of greater than 60 %. Any modest benefit is likely seen in patients who have an immediate, often transient narrowing of a duct-to-duct anastomosis within the first 1–2 months after transplantation [17]. Most strictures, however, are representative of underlying injury that requires stent placement with longer-term treatment and follow-up.

AS develop recurrence less commonly when compared to NAS. This is thought to be due to the fact that stent placement is easier in these strictures because biliary anastomosis is usually located at the level of the middle common bile duct, far from the main biliary confluence [48]. The mean number of ERCPs required for successful treatment is between 3 and 5, with a recurrence rate between 0 and 20 % [17, 46, 51]. In NAS, the strictures can be multiple and variably extend to the biliary confluence and sometimes into intrahepatic branches. This leads to technically difficult endoscopy, and stricture recurrence in greater than 25–30 % of patients in various studies [66, 67].

When BBS are diagnosed within 3–6 months after OLT, patients trended towards a statistically significant better prognosis and response to endoscopic therapy [36, 66]. Unfortunately, in patients who do not have morphologic disappearance of the stricture, persistent cholestasis and recurrent cholangitis can be seen [67]. Regardless of the etiology, these patients often require long-term follow-up.

Recurrence Rate in Postcholecystectomy BBS

The most common postoperative BBS occur after cholecystectomy, and are due to direct surgical trauma, dissection, or thermal injury causing ischemia. These BBS are usually diagnosed within 6 to 12 months, and in all patients without complete transection and/or complete closure (usually from clipping) of the duct, endoscopic treatment is first-line therapy [7]. Therapy has transitioned from placing 1–2 stents at a time to a more aggressive approach with maximal stent placement at more frequent intervals or FCSEMS placement, with a concurrent decreased recurrence rate. These earlier studies of more conservative therapy reported a recurrence rate of 20–30 %, while more recent, aggressive approaches have shown the recurrence rate to be 0–12 % [47, 55, 56]. The study with the longest follow-up period evaluated patients over a mean of almost 14 years, with an 11.4 % stricture recurrence rate. Of those patients who experienced stricture recurrence, all were able to be successfully retreated endoscopically [55].

Frequent follow-up is necessary in almost all BBS patients, with close clinical monitoring and treatment plan which includes stent removal and exchanging every 3 months. While surgical management is reserved for BBS refractory to endoscopic management, surgical repair carries a mortality risk approaching 2 % and morbidity as high as 35 % [2, 7].

BBS Recurrence in CP

In contrast to postoperative strictures, BBS in CP are more resistant to endoscopic treatment. Although some of these strictures resolve with time as the chronic inflammation and underlying cause are treated, the vast majority are permanent [24]. The stricture recurrence rate was shown in one study to decrease from 76 % to 8 % with the introduction of maximal stent placement and frequent stent replacement [23]. This low recurrence rate, however, has not been seen in similar studies involving plastic stents, with the recurrence rate ranging from 40 to 56 % [36, 59]. Long-term results of plastic stents have been disappointing due to tissue in-growth and more frequent stent replacement than in postoperative strictures [68]. More recent studies with FCSEMS in CP patients have been promising, with recurrence rates seen in 23–30 % of strictures. In addition to the decreased recurrence rate, these patients undergo fewer procedures and complications related to the technical difficulty of placing multiple plastic stents [62, 68].

Poor outcomes and a trend to failure in stricture resolution have been seen in patients with pancreatic head calcifications. If calcifications are present, there is an associated 17-fold increased risk of treatment failure. The need for concurrent stenting of the pancreatic duct (PD) is another factor associated with poor outcomes in these patients [60]. As evidenced by higher recurrence rates, BBS in chronic pancreatitis are difficult to treat and are associated with a lower odds ratio of treatment success compared with other biliary disease [69].

Complications Related to Endoscopy

As with any procedure, there is an inherent risk of complication. Specific complications of ERCP have been well described and include pancreatitis, bleeding, sepsis, and perforation. These occur in around 6–7 % of patients, with a majority of complications being mild to moderate in severity, with post-ERCP pancreatitis being the most common complication [70].

Complications can either be immediate (related to the procedure itself), early (within 30 days), or late (after 30 days). Around 8–10 % of patients experience complications due to endoscopically placed biliary stents, including cholangitis, cholecystitis, bleeding, pancreatitis, stent occlusion, and proximal or distal stent migration [45, 71]. The use of FCSEMS is associated with an increased rate of stent migration, but also a longer patency when compared to plastic stents, decreasing the overall risk by decreasing the number of procedures needed for stricture resolution [69].

Conclusion

Biliary strictures remain commonly encountered clinical entities. These strictures can be postoperative, inflammatory, infectious, or from other etiologies. Surgical, radiologic, and endoscopic approaches are available, and currently endoscopic therapy is the first-line treatment for most biliary injuries. Surgery and interventional radiology are generally reserved for patients with endoscopically inaccessible strictures or in those whom endoscopic approaches have failed.

References

1. Lillemore KD, Melton GB, Cameron JL, Pitt HA, Campbell KA, Talamini MA, et al. Postoperative bile duct strictures: management and outcome in the 1990s. Ann Surg. 2000;232(3):430–41.
2. Byrne MF. Management of benign biliary strictures. Gastroenterol Hepatol (NY). 2008;4(10):694–7. PubMed PMID: 21960889, PubMed Central PMCID: PMC3104180.
3. Bakhru MR, Kahaleh M. Expandable metal stents for benign biliary disease. Gastrointest Endosc Clin N Am. 2011;21(3):447–62. doi:10.1016/j.giec.2011.04.007. PubMed PMID: 21684464, viii. Review.
4. Judah JR, Draganov PV. Endoscopic therapy of benign biliary strictures. World J Gastroenterol. 2007;13(26):3531–9. PubMed PMID: 17659703, PubMed Central PMCID: PMC4146792, Review.
5. Bismuth H. Postoperative strictures of the bile duct. In: Blumgart LH, editor. The biliary tract. Edinburgh: Churchill Livingstone; 1982. p. 209–18.

6. Warshaw AL, Schapiro RH, Ferrucci JT, Galdabini JJ. Persistent obstructive jaundice, cholangitis, and biliary cirrhosis due to common bile duct stenosis in chronic pancreatitis. Gastroenterology. 1976;70:562–7.

7. Sikora SS, Pottakkat B, Srikanth G, Kumar A, Saxena R, Kapoor VK. Postcholecystectomy benign biliary strictures—long-term results. Dig Surg. 2006;23(5-6):304–12. PubMed PMID: 17164542, Epub 2006 Dec 11.

8. Archer SB, Brown DW, Smith CD, Branum GD, Hunter JG. Bile duct injury during laparoscopic cholecystectomy: results of a national survey. Ann Surg. 2001;234(4):549–58. PubMed PMID: 11573048, discussion 558–9.

9. Eum YO, Park JK, Chun J, Lee SH, Ryu JK, Kim YT, et al. Non-surgical treatment of post-surgical bile duct injury: clinical implications and outcomes. World J Gastroenterol. 2014;20(22):6924–31. doi:10.3748/wjg.v20.i22.6924. PubMed PMID: 24944484.

10. de Reuver PR, Rauws EA, Vermeulen M, Dijkgraaf MG, Gouma DJ, Bruno MJ. Endoscopic treatment of post-surgical bile duct injuries: long term outcome and predictors of success. Gut. 2007;56(11):1599–605. PubMed PMID: 17595232, Epub 2007 Jun 26.

11. Francoeur JR, Wiseman K, Buczkowski AK, Chung SW, Scudamore CH. Surgeons' anonymous response after bile duct injury during cholecystectomy. Am J Surg. 2003;185(5):468–75.

12. Connor S, Garden OJ. Bile duct injury in the era of laparoscopic cholecystectomy. Br J Surg. 2006;93(2):158–68. Review.

13. Gigot J, Etienne J, Aerts R, Wibin E, Dallemagne B, Deweer F, et al. The dramatic reality of biliary tract injury during laparoscopic cholecystectomy. An anonymous multicenter Belgian survey of 65 patients. Surg Endosc. 1997;11(12):1171–8.

14. Fletcher DR, Hobbs MS, Tan P, Valinsky LJ, Hockey RL, Pikora TJ, et al. Complications of cholecystectomy: risks of the laparoscopic approach and protective effects of operative cholangiography: a population-based study. Ann Surg. 1999;229(4):449–57. PubMed PMID: 10203075, PubMed Central PMCID: PMC1191728.

15. Traina M, Tarantino I, Barresi L, Volpes R, Gruttadauria S, Petridis I, et al. Efficacy and safety of fully covered self-expandable metallic stents in biliary complications after liver transplantation: a preliminary study. Liver Transpl. 2009;15(11):1493–8. doi:10.1002/lt.21886. PubMed PMID: 19877248.

16. Kaffes A, Griffin S, Vaughan R, James M, Chua T, Tee H, et al. A randomized trial of a fully covered self-expandable metallic stent versus plastic stents in anastomotic biliary strictures after liver transplantation. Therap Adv Gastroenterol. 2014;7(2):64–71. doi:10.1177/1756283X13503614. PubMed PMID: 24587819.

17. Zoepf T, Maldonado-Lopez EJ, Hilgard P, Malago M, Broelsch CE, Treichel U, et al. Balloon dilatation vs. balloon dilatation plus bile duct endoprostheses for treatment of anastomotic biliary strictures after liver transplantation. Liver Transpl. 2006;12(1):88–94.

18. Pasha SF, Harrison ME, Das A, Nguyen CC, Vargas HE, Balan V, et al. Endoscopic treatment of anastomotic biliary strictures after deceased donor liver transplantation: outcomes after maximal stent therapy. Gastrointest Endosc. 2007;66(1):44–51.

19. Thuluvath PJ, Pfau PR, Kimmey MB, Ginsberg GG. Biliary complications after liver transplantation: the role of endoscopy. Endoscopy. 2005;37(9):857–63.

20. Sharma S, Gurakar A, Jabbour N. Biliary strictures following liver transplantation: past, present and preventive strategies. Liver Transpl. 2008;14(6):759–69. doi:10.1002/lt.21509.

21. Cahen DL, van Berkel AM, Oskam D, Rauws EA, Weverling GJ, Huibregtse K, et al. Long-term results of endoscopic drainage of common bile duct strictures in chronic pancreatitis. Eur J Gastroenterol Hepatol. 2005;17(1):103–8. PubMed PMID: 15647649.

22. Steer ML, Waxman I, Freedman S. Chronic pancreatitis. N Engl J Med. 1995;332(22):1482–90. Review.

23. Catalano MF, Linder JD, George S, Alcocer E, Geenen JE. Treatment of symptomatic distal common bile duct stenosis secondary to chronic pancreatitis: comparison of single vs. multiple simultaneous stents. Gastrointest Endosc. 2004;60(6):945–52.

24. Adler DG, Lichtenstein D, Baron TH, Davila R, Egan JV, Gan SL, et al. The role of endoscopy in patients with chronic pancreatitis. Gastrointest Endosc. 2006;63(7):933–7.

25. Elhanafy E, Atef E, El Nakeeb A, Hamdy E, Elhemaly M, Sultan AM. Mirizzi Syndrome: How it could be a challenge. Hepatogastroenterology. 2014;61(133):1182–6. PubMed PMID: 25513064.

26. Dadhwal US, Kumar V. Benign bile duct strictures. Med J Armed Forces India. 2012;68(3):299–303. doi:10.1016/j.mjafi.2012.04.014.

PubMed PMID: 24532893, PubMed Central PMCID: PMC3862965.

27. Cherqui D, Palazzo L, Piedbois P, Charlotte F, Duvoux C, Duron JJ, et al. Common bile duct stricture as a late complication of upper abdominal radiotherapy. J Hepatol. 1994;20(6):693–7.

28. Shanbhogue AK, Tirumani SH, Prasad SR, Fasih N, McInnes M. Benign biliary strictures: a current comprehensive clinical and imaging review. AJR Am J Roentgenol. 2011;197(2):W295–306. doi:10.2214/AJR.10.6002. Review.

29. Nash JA, Cohen SA. Gallbladder and biliary tract disease in AIDS. Gastroenterol Clin North Am. 1997;26(2):323–35.

30. Zuckerman MJ, Peters J, Fleming RV, Boman D, Calleros JE, Adler DG. Cholangiopathy associated with giardiasis in a patient with human immunodeficiency virus infection. J Clin Gastroenterol. 2008;42(3):328–9.

31. Fan ST, Ng IO, Choi TK, Lai EC. Tuberculosis of the bile duct: a rare cause of biliary stricture. Am J Gastroenterol. 1989;84(4):413–4.

32. Beyer G, Schwaiger T, Lerch MM, Mayerle J. IgG4-related disease: a new kid on the block or an old acquaintance? United European Gastroenterol J. 2014;2(3):165–72. doi:10.1177/2050640614532457. PubMed PMID: 25360299, PubMed Central PMCID: PMC4212459, Review.

33. Okazaki K, Uchida K, Ikeura T, Takaoka M. Current concept and diagnosis of IgG4-related disease in the hepato-bilio-pancreatic system. J Gastroenterol. 2013;48(3):303–14. doi:10.1007/s00535-012-0744-3. PubMed PMID: 23417598, PubMed Central PMCID: PMC3698437, Epub 2013, Review.

34. Roslyn JJ, Ferdinand FD. Biliary strictures and neoplasms. In: Bayless TM, editor. Current therapy in Gastroenterology and liver disease. 4th ed. St. Louis: Mosby Yearbook; 1994. p. 613–8.

35. Davids PH, Tanka AK, Rauws EA, van Gulik TM, van Leeuwen DJ, de Wit LT, et al. Benign biliary strictures. Surgery or endoscopy? Ann Surg. 1993;217(3):237–43. PubMed PMID: 8452402, PubMed Central PMCID: PMC1242775.

36. Draganov P, Hoffman B, Marsh W, Cotton P, Cunningham J. Long-term outcome in patients with benign biliary strictures treated endoscopically with multiple stents. Gastrointest Endosc. 2002;55(6):680–6.

37. Tocchi A, Mazzoni G, Liotta G, Costa G, Lepre L, Miccini M, et al. Management of benign biliary strictures: biliary enteric

anastomosis vs endoscopic stenting. Arch Surg. 2000;135(2):153–7.
38. Krokidis M, Orgera G, Rossi M, Matteoli M, Hatzidakis A. Interventional radiology in the management of benign biliary stenoses, biliary leaks and fistulas: a pictorial review. Insights Imaging. 2013;4(1):77–84. doi:10.1007/s13244-012-0200-1. PubMed PMID: 23180415, PubMed Central PMCID: PMC3579997, Epub 2012 Nov 24.
39. Fontein DBY, Gibson RN, Collier NA, Tse G, Wang L, Speer TG, et al. Two decades of percutaneous transjejunal biliary intervention for benign biliary disease; a review of the intervention nature and complication. Insights Imaging. 2011;2(5):557–65.
40. Westwood DA, Fernando C, Connor SJ. Internal-external percutaneous transhepatic biliary drainage for malignant biliary obstruction: a retrospective analysis. J Med Imaging Radiat Oncol. 2010;54(2):108–10. doi:10.1111/j.1754-9485.2010.02147.x.
41. Kuo MD, Lopresti DC, Gover DD, Hall LD, Ferrara SL. Intentional retrieval of viabil stent-grafts from the biliary system. J Vasc Interv Radiol. 2006;17(2 Pt 1):389–97.
42. Kim JH, Gwon DI, Ko GY, Sung KB, Lee SK, Yoon HK, et al. Temporary placement of retrievable fully covered metallic stents versus percutaneous balloon dilation in the treatment of benign biliary strictures. J Vasc Interv Radiol. 2011;22(6):893–9.
43. Costamagna G, Boškoski I. Current treatment of benign biliary strictures. Ann Gastroenterol. 2013;26(1):37–40. PubMed PMID: 24714594, PubMed Central PMCID: PMC3959511, Review.
44. Adler DG, Baron TH, Davila RE, Egan J, Hirota WK, Leighton JA, et al. Standards of Practice Committee of American Society for Gastrointestinal Endoscopy. ASGE guideline: the role of ERCP in diseases of the biliary tract and the pancreas. Gastrointest Endosc. 2005;62:1–8.
45. Devière J, Nageshwar Reddy D, Püspök A, Ponchon T, Bruno MJ, Bourke MJ, et al. Successful management of benign biliary strictures with fully covered self-expanding metal stents. Gastroenterology. 2014;147(2):385–95; quiz e15. doi:10.1053/j.gastro.2014.04.043. Epub 2014 May 4.
46. Elmi F, Silverman WB. Outcome of ERCP in the management of duct-to-duct anastomotic strictures in orthotopic liver transplant. Dig Dis Sci. 2007;52(2346):2350.
47. Bergman JJ, Burgemeister L, Bruno MJ, Rauws EA, Gouma DJ, Tytgat GN, et al. Long-term follow-up after biliary stent placement

for postoperative bile duct stenosis. Gastrointest Endosc. 2001;54(2):154–61.
48. Perri V, Familiari P, Tringali A, Boskoski I, Costamagna G. Plastic biliary stents for benign biliary diseases. Gastrointest Endosc Clin N Am. 2011;21(3):405–33. doi:10.1016/j.giec.2011.04.012. viii. Review.
49. Rossi AF, Grosso C, Zanasi G, Gambitta P, Bini M, De Carlis L, et al. Long-term efficacy of endoscopic stenting in patients with stricture of the biliary anastomosis after orthotopic liver transplantation. Endoscopy. 1998;30(4):360–6.
50. Theilmann L, Küppers B, Kadmon M, Roeren T, Notheisen H, Stiehl A, et al. Biliary tract strictures after orthotopic liver transplantation: diagnosis and management. Endoscopy. 1994; 26(6):517–22.
51. Morelli G, Fazel A, Judah J, et al. Rapid-sequence endoscopic management of posttransplant anastomotic biliary strictures. Gastrointest Endosc. 2008;67:879–85.
52. Londono MC, Balderramo D, Cardenas A. Management of biliary complications after orthotopic liver transplantation: the role of endoscopy. World J Gastroenterol. 2008;14:493–7.
53. Gomez CM, Dumonceau JM, Marcolongo M, de Santibañes E, Ciardullo M, Pekolj J, et al. Endoscopic management of biliary complications after adult living-donor versus deceased-donor liver transplantation. Transplantation. 2009;88(11):1280–5. doi:10.1097/TP.0b013e3181bb48c2.
54. Kato H, Kawamoto H, Tsutsumi K, Harada R, Fujii M, Hirao K, et al. Long-term outcomes of endoscopic management for biliary strictures after living donor liver transplantation with duct-to-duct reconstruction. Transpl Int. 2009;22(9):914–21. doi:10.1111/j.1432-2277.2009.00895.x. Epub 2009 May 20.
55. Costamagna G, Pandolfi M, Mutignani M, Spada C, Perri V. Long-term results of endoscopic management of postoperative bile duct strictures with increasing numbers of stents. Gastrointest Endosc. 2001;54(2):162–8.
56. Kuzela L, Oltman M, Sutka J, Hrcka R, Novotna T, Vavrecka A. Prospective follow-up of patients with bile duct strictures secondary to laparoscopic cholecystectomy, treated endoscopically with multiple stents. Hepatogastroenterology. 2005;52(65):1357–61.
57. Kuroda Y, Tsuyuguchi T, Sakai Y, K C S, Ishihara T, Yamaguchi T, Saisho H, Yokosuka O.. Long-term follow-up evaluation for more than 10 years after endoscopic treatment for postoperative

bile duct strictures. Surg Endosc. 2010;24(4):834–40. doi: 10.1007/s00464-009-0673-2.
58. Smits ME, Rauws EA, van Gulik TM, Gouma DJ, Tytgat GN, Huibregtse K. Long-term results of endoscopic stenting and surgical drainage for biliary stricture due to chronic pancreatitis. Br J Surg. 1996;83(6):764–8.
59. Pozsár J, Sahin P, László F, Forró G, Topa L. Medium-term results of endoscopic treatment of common bile duct strictures in chronic calcifying pancreatitis with increasing numbers of stents. J Clin Gastroenterol. 2004;38(2):118–23.
60. Kahl S, Zimmermann S, Genz I, Glasbrenner B, Pross M, Schulz HU, et al. Risk factors for failure of endoscopic stenting of biliary strictures in chronic pancreatitis: a prospective follow-up study. Am J Gastroenterol. 2003;98(11):2448–53.
61. Irani S, Baron TH, Akbar A, Lin OS, Gluck M, Gan I, et al. Endoscopic treatment of benign biliary strictures using covered self-expandable metal stents (CSEMS). Dig Dis Sci. 2014;59(1):152–60. doi:10.1007/s10620-013-2859-7. Epub 2013 Sep 24.
62. Kahaleh M, Behm B, Clarke BW, Brock A, Shami VM, De La Rue SA, et al. Temporary placement of covered self-expandable metal stents in benign biliary strictures: a new paradigm? (with video). Gastrointest Endosc. 2008;67(3):446–54. doi:10.1016/j.gie.2007.06.057.
63. Wagh MS, Chavalitdhamrong D, Moezardalan K, Chauhan SS, Gupte AR, Nosler MJ, et al. Effectiveness and safety of endoscopic treatment of benign biliary strictures using a new fully covered self expandable metal stent. Diagn Ther Endosc. 2013;2013:183513. doi:10.1155/2013/183513. PubMed PMID: 23956613, Epub 2013 May 11.
64. Mahajan A, Ho H, Sauer B, Phillips MS, Shami VM, Ellen K, et al. Temporary placement of fully covered self-expandable metal stents in benign biliary strictures: midterm evaluation (with video). Gastrointest Endosc. 2009;70(2):303–9. doi:10.1016/j.gie.2008.11.029. PubMed PMID: 19523620, Epub 2009 Jun 11.
65. Park do H, Lee SS, Lee TH, Ryu CH, Kim HJ, Seo DW, et al. Anchoring flap versus flared end, fully covered self-expandable metal stents to prevent migration in patients with benign biliary strictures: a multicenter, prospective, comparative pilot study (with videos). Gastrointest Endosc. 2011;73(1):64–70. doi:10.1016/j.gie.2010.09.039. PubMed PMID: 21184871.

66. Rizk RS, McVicar JP, Emond MJ, et al. Endoscopic management of biliary strictures in liver transplant recipients: effect on patient and graft survival. Gastrointest Endosc. 1998;47:128–35.
67. Verdonk RC, Buis CI, van der Jagt EJ, Gouw AS, Limburg AJ, Slooff MJ, et al. Nonanastomotic biliary strictures after liver transplantation, part 2: management, outcome, and risk factors for disease progression. Liver Transpl. 2007;13(5):725–32.
68. Perri V, Boškoski I, Tringali A, Familiari P, Mutignani M, Marmo R, et al. Fully covered self-expandable metal stents in biliary strictures caused by chronic pancreatitis not responding to plastic stenting: a prospective study with 2 years of follow-up. Gastrointest Endosc. 2012;75(6):1271–7. doi:10.1016/j.gie.2012.02.002. Epub 2012 Mar 29.
69. Tringali A, Blero D, Boškoski I, Familiari P, Perri V, Devière J, et al. Difficult removal of fully covered self expandable metal stents (SEMS) for benign biliary strictures: the "SEMS in SEMS" technique. Dig Liver Dis. 2014;46(6):568–71. doi:10.1016/j.dld.2014.02.018. PubMed PMID: 24661988, Epub 2014 Mar 22.
70. Andriulli A, Loperfido S, Napolitano G, Niro G, Valvano MR, Spirito F, et al. Incidence rates of post-ERCP complications: a systematic survey of prospective studies. Am J Gastroenterol. 2007;102(8):1781–8. PubMed PMID: 17509029, Epub 2007 May 17. Review.
71. Johanson JF, Schmalz MJ, Geenen JE. Incidence and risk factors for biliary and pancreatic stent migration. Gastrointest Endosc. 1992;38:341–6.

Chapter 13
Point-of-Care Clinical Guide: Cholangiocarcinoma

Abdulrahman Y. Hammad, Nicholas G. Berger, and T. Clark Gamblin

Patient's Perspective: Questions on Cholangiocarcinoma

Question: I have been recently diagnosed with cholangiocarcinoma, which my primary care physician told me is lethal. What is my prognosis, and what can I expect for my treatment?

Answer: Unfortunately, only about 5–10 % of all patients with cholangiocarcinoma will live 5 years after their initial diagnosis, and cure requires that the cancer be surgically removed. There are three types of cholangiocarcinoma: intrahepatic (in the liver), extrahepatic (outside the liver), and hilar (next to the liver by the bile duct). Extrahepatic cholangiocarcinoma is most likely to be amenable to removal. Surgery consists of removing the tumor, and depending on the location, part of

A.Y. Hammad, M.D. • N.G. Berger, M.D. • T.C. Gamblin, M.D., M.S., M.B.A. (✉)
Department of Surgery, The Medical College of Wisconsin, 9200 West Wisconsin Ave., Milwaukee, WI, USA
e-mail: ahammad@mcw.edu; nberger@mcw.edu; tcgamblin@mcw.edu

© Springer International Publishing Switzerland 2016
K. Dua, R. Shaker (eds.), *Pancreas and Biliary Disease*,
DOI 10.1007/978-3-319-28089-9_13

287

your liver, intestine, and/or bile ducts. If your cancer cannot be surgically removed, your oncologist will give you chemotherapy and possibly radiation to slow the progression of your cancer. The amount of time patients survive depends on all of these factors, as well as other medical conditions and the stage of the disease. You and your cancer doctors, and primary doctor will develop a treatment plan tailored to you.

Question: I have been recently diagnosed with cholangiocarcinoma, and I have heard that some cancers are inheritable, and can run in families. Should I have my children tested for cholangiocarcinoma?

Answer: Cholangiocarcinoma itself does not have a strong genetic association. However, there are some heritable conditions which are risk factors for developing cholangiocarcinoma. Primary Sclerosing Cholangitis (PSC) or multiple biliary papillomatosis can be inherited in families, and are associated with a higher risk for the development of cholangiocarcinoma. Testing for these syndromes is disease-specific, but there is no known hereditary association of cholangiocarcinoma, even in first-degree relatives.

Cholangiocarcinoma

Overview

Cholangiocarcinoma is a neoplasm arising from the epithelial lining of the biliary tree; the cholangiocytes. Cholangiocarcinoma encompasses three types based on anatomical location: intrahepatic (IHCC), extrahepatic (EHCC), and hilar (HiCC) type; with the hilar type being the most common. Although cholangiocarcinoma is a rare tumor, its incidence is rising worldwide. Late presentation of the disease contributes to the poor prognosis and occurs due to subtle symptoms that often initially go unrecognized. Although surgical resection remains the best available option for cholangiocarcinoma, late presentation can limit surgical resection as an option, stressing the need for alternative interventions. Current therapeutic options beside surgical resection include liver transplantation, systematic chemotherapy, radiotherapy, and liver directed therapies. Palliative care is a valuable tool for those entering a non-curative paradigm in order to potentially minimize symptoms and improve the patient's quality of life. In this chapter, we discuss factors most commonly associated with disease development, available treatments, and anticipated outcomes for cholangiocarcinoma.

Epidemiology

Cholangiocarcinoma accounts for approximately 3 % of all gastrointestinal cancers worldwide [1]. The majority of patients are Caucasian males with a peak incidence in the seventh decade [2–4]. Incidence varies according to geographical distribution. For example, intrahepatic cholangiocarcinoma (IHCC) is the highest in Thailand (96/100,000 in males), followed by China, Mali and Japan; whereas the lowest incidence is reported in Australia (0.1–0.2/100,000) (Fig. 1) [2]. The incidence of IHCC has been rising over the last 20 years in North America, Europe, Asia, and Japan, with subsequent increase in mortality rates in the USA, Japan, Australia, England, and Wales [5]. Studies suggest that the increase in incidence and mortality may be the result of changes in risk factors, such as choledocholithiasis, cirrhosis, and hepatitis C infection [3].

Conversely, the incidence and mortality of extrahepatic cholangiocarcinoma (EHCC) is decreasing worldwide [6–10]. Data from the Surveillance, Epidemiology, and End Results (SEER) database suggest a decrease in EHCC age adjusted mortality from 0.6/100,000 in 1979 to 0.3/100,000 in 1998 [2, 9]. The reason for the decrease in disease incidence was not related to the decrease in risk factors of the disease [7].

Currently, hilar cholangiocarcinoma is the most common type of cholangiocarcinoma, followed by extrahepatic and intrahepatic cholangiocarcinoma [4, 11]. In the USA, 1–2 cases

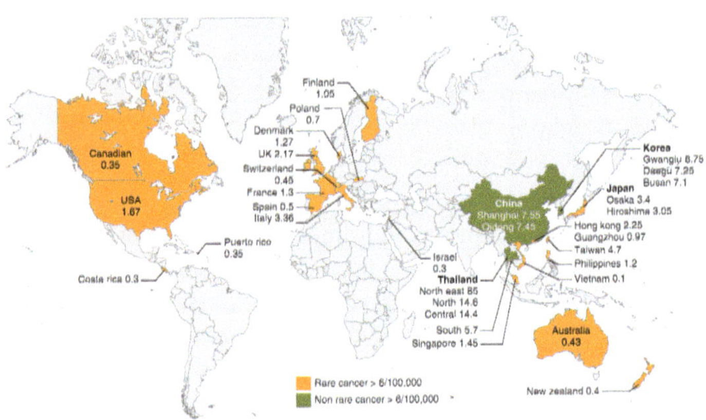

FIG. 1 Worldwide incidence of cholangiocarcinoma 1997–2007 (Cases/100,000)

per 100,000 occur annually. According to the last report from the American Cancer Society, an estimate of 35,660 new liver cancer cases (including intrahepatic and hilar cholangiocarcinoma) are reported annually, compared to 10,910 gallbladder and other biliary cancers (extrahepatic cholangiocarcinoma included) [12]. Identification of different risk factors and disease etiologies followed by careful monitoring may impact the survival rates of this challenging disease.

Etiology

Primary Sclerosing Cholangitis (PSC) (Also Refer to the Separate Chapter on PSC)

PSC is an autoimmune disease affecting the biliary tree, and results in fibrosis and stricture formation of the intrahepatic and/or extrahepatic bile ducts. Patients with this disease have a higher incidence of developing cholangiocarcinoma, ranging from 9 % to 15 % lifetime risk, with a yearly incidence of 0.6 %–1.5 % [13–16]. A recent study suggests that a lower percentage of cholangiocarcinoma cases are discovered in the first year following the PSC diagnosis than previously thought (15 % vs. 30 %) [15, 17]. However, it remains that many PSC patients are often diagnosed late at the time of liver transplant or at autopsy [14]. Due to the established risk of cholangiocarcinoma in PSC patients, surveillance through annual imaging and CA19-9 levels has been proposed [18].

Parasitic Liver Infection

Infection with the liver flukes *Opisthorchis viverrini* or *Clonorchis sinensis* is a risk factor of cholangiocarcinoma. Reports from Asia, especially from Thailand and Korea, have shown an increased risk in patients harboring flukes [19–22]. The exact mechanism behind cancer development is not fully understood, although the state of chronic inflammation is thought to be responsible. Sripa et al. suggested that mechanical irritation by the fluke or its metabolic products may result in chronic inflammation and biliary epithelial desquamation. The subsequent release of nitric oxide and other reactive oxygen intermediates, combined with the nitrosamine and its precursors found in some sea foods may collectively result in the development of cholangiocarcinoma [22].

Hepatolithiasis

Hepatolithiasis (intrahepatic biliary stones) is more prevalent in eastern Asia and is considered a risk factor for cholangiocarcinoma [23, 24]. A case–control study including 370 hepatolithiasis patients reported a higher odds of developing cholangiocarcinoma in this population (odds ratio: 6.7 [95 % CI: 1.3–33.4]) [25]. Furthermore, recurrent pyogenic cholangitis, a common disease in Eastern Asia characterized by hepatolithiasis, stricture formation and recurrent attacks of cholangitis, is also associated with a 2.8 % incidence of cholangiocarcinoma in a 10-year follow-up period [26]. Although duct stricture alone is a risk factor of cancer, its association with hepatolithiasis and infection carries a higher risk towards cholangiocarcinoma development.

Congenital Biliary Malformation

Choledochal cysts, a congenital bile duct abnormality presenting with cystic dilatation of extrahepatic ducts, intrahepatic radicles, or both carry 10–28 % incidence of developing cholangiocarcinoma if untreated [27–29]. Although the excision of the choledochal cyst is thought to decrease the risk of cholangiocarcinoma, cancer may still develop [30]. Similarly, Caroli disease—a rare disorder characterized by multifocal dilatation of intrahepatic bile ducts—is linked to the development of cholangiocarcinoma, necessitating close surveillance [31]. The mechanism underlying the development of cancer in patients with congenital biliary malformation is not fully understood; however, theories suggest that biliary stasis, chronic inflammation, and deconjugated biliary contents may contribute to the development of cancer [32, 33].

Chemicals and Toxins Exposure

Several toxins are linked to the development of cholangiocarcinoma. Of these agents, thorotrast, a radiological contrast agent used prior to 1960, is reported to be strongly associated with the development of cholangiocarcinoma. The exposed population carries a 300-fold increased risk of developing cholangiocarcinoma years after exposure [34–36]. Other substances linked to the development of cholangiocarcinoma include nitrosamines asbestos, and rubber [37, 38].

Viral Hepatitis

Cirrhotic patients have an increased risk of developing cholangiocarcinoma [3, 39]. Although hepatitis B and C may result in cirrhosis, these viruses alone represent risk factors of cholangiocarcinoma [19, 25, 40]. Multiple meta-analyses have reported a 3.42–5.10 relative risk in hepatitis B patients to develop cholangiocarcinoma ($p < 0.05$), compared to a relative risk of 3.42–4.84 in hepatitis C patients ($p < 0.05$) [41–43]. The mechanism through which these viruses lead to cancer development is not clear, although chronic inflammation, increased cellular proliferation, and viral infection of the progenitor cells could possibly contribute to tumorigenesis [44, 45].

Others

Smoking, alcohol consumption, and/or the presence of inflammatory bowel disease are possible associations between PSC and cholangiocarcinoma [15, 46–48]. A recent meta-analysis revealed that diabetics and alcohol consumers have a higher risk of developing cholangiocarcinoma with a relative risk of 1.82 (95 % CI: 1.74–2.07) and 2.81 (95 %CI: 1.52–5.21), respectively [41]. Further studies are needed to evaluate the impact of these factors on the development of cholangiocarcinoma.

Clinical Presentation

Cholangiocarcinoma tends to be asymptomatic until later stages. In some patients, nonspecific symptoms of biliary obstruction may be present; the most common being jaundice, weight loss, abdominal pains, pruritus, and cholangitis [4, 49, 50]. The presence of right upper quadrant pain, fever, and rigors are suggestive of cholangitis. Incomplete biliary obstruction can delay the appearance of symptoms, while unilateral or segmental obstruction can occur without symptoms.

On physical examination, nonspecific findings may be present. Jaundice may be evident, and signs of multiple skins excoriations can be seen from the effect of pruritus. Occasionally, the liver may become palpable with a firm consistency. In cases with intrahepatic or hilar disease, the gallbladder is usually not palpated, and its palpation indicates a more distal obstruction (Courvoisier's sign). Long-standing biliary obstruction and/or portal vein obstruction may result in portal hypertension, with caput medusa, spider angiomas, hemorrhoids, and/or ascites. Less commonly, the disease is suspected based on abnormal imaging or laboratory results.

Investigations

Abdominal ultrasound is usually the initial investigation for patients presenting with biliary symptoms. Dilatation of the intrahepatic ducts should raise the suspicion of cholangiocarcinoma. Cases with dilated intrahepatic bile ducts and normal-caliber extrahepatic ducts may have a hilar cancer. On ultrasound, hilar tumors may appear as isoechoic (65 %), hypoechoic (21 %), or hyperechoic (15 %) masses. In patients presenting with IHCC, a mass may be visualized, although the lack of distinctive IHCC imaging features on ultrasound makes it difficult to definitively diagnose cholangiocarcinoma [51]. In EHCC cases, tumor detection may be challenging as air inside intestinal loops can conceal a discrete lesion, though signs of ductal dilatation and/or ductal wall thickening are suggestive of EHCC. Ultrasound is also used to examine for choledocholithiasis, and color-Doppler ultrasound can evaluate portal vein and/or hepatic artery for occlusion/compression. Further cross-sectional imaging with CT scan is typically required before establishing the diagnosis of cholangiocarcinoma, and can assist with surgical planning.

Endoscopic ultrasound (EUS) allows better visualization of the extrahepatic biliary tree, vascular structures, surrounding lymph nodes, and is useful in obtaining a tissue diagnosis in suspicious cases [52, 53]. The potential risk of seeding following EUS-biopsy is very low, and it should not prohibit a biopsy when necessary [54, 55]. EUS is credited with an 88 % sensitivity and 90 % specificity in diagnosing biliary obstruction, although less accurate for cancer than for choledocholithiasis [56].

Cross sectional imaging with Computed tomography (CT) usually follows ultrasound in cases suspicious for malignancy. CT scans provide information regarding tumor localization, hepatic parenchymal involvement, vascular invasion and the presence of distant metastasis [57, 58]. On CT, a mass forming lesion may be seen in IHCC, with intrahepatic ductal dilatation, capsular retraction, parenchymal atrophy, and/or vascular invasion [59]. In patients presenting with hilar tumors, CT predicts resectability in 60–90 % of cases and provides 80 % accuracy when assessing horizontal tumor spread and 100 % accuracy in detecting vertical tumor spread [58, 60]. The utilization of CT angiography and cholangiography for assessment improves resectability rates to 95.7 % [61]. Similar to HiCC, CT scans are more accurate in evaluating vertical extension of EHCC, while it may underestimate the longitudinal spread [62, 63]. CT angiography is able to detect small metastases that may be missed with routine CT as well as diagnose portal vein and hepatic artery invasion with an accuracy of 92.9 % and 93.3 %, respectively [61, 64].

Magnetic resonance imaging (MRI): MRI represents an ideal investigation in cases suspicious for cholangiocarcinoma, delineating liver parenchyma, biliary ducts, and vasculature. MRI can differentiate between benign and malignant causes of biliary obstruction with a sensitivity of 91 % and a specificity of 94 % [65]. Combined with magnetic resonance cholangiopancreatography (MRCP), these modalities are highly effective for diagnosing cholangiocarcinoma. Further advantages include the ability to identify intrahepatic lesions, and 3D construction of the pancreatico-biliary tree [66]. Romagnuolo et al. reported an 88 % sensitivity and 95 % specificity of MRCP in detecting malignancy, and a 98 % sensitivity and 98 % specificity in detecting the level of obstruction [67].

Compared to endoscopic retrograde cholangiopancreatography (ERCP), MRCP provides a detailed image of the biliary tree above the level of obstruction, which is typically inaccessible to endoscopic contrast. [68] ERCP and PTC, however, allow for stent placement and brushings/biopsy. Though, a tissue diagnosis is not mandated in surgically resectable cases.

Positron emission tomography (PET) scans may provide valuable input regarding nodal involvement and disease metastases [69, 70]. In PSC cases, FDG-PET is useful in detecting small tumors (1 cm) and excluding malignancy; and therefore is suggested as a potential screening method for cholangiocarcinoma in patients undergoing evaluation for transplantation [71, 72].

Laboratory investigations: Cholangiocarcinoma typically presents with an elevation in bilirubin, alkaline phosphatase, and gamma-glutamyl transferase. Tumor markers CEA and CA19-9 can aid in the diagnosis and follow-up. CA19-9 is elevated in 85 % of patients, although it could also be elevated in pancreatic cancer, gastric malignancies, PSC, and other causes of biliary obstruction. Following biliary decompression, persistent elevation of CA19-9 points to possible malignancy [11]. CEA is of more limited benefit as it is elevated in only 30 % of the cases [73]. A 100 % sensitivity and 78 % specificity have been reported upon the combination of a CEA cutoff >5.2 ng/ml and CA19-9 of 180U/ml [74]. As a result, the diagnosis of cholangiocarcinoma remains a combination of clinical imaging and laboratory investigations.

Hilar Strictures: Bismuth Classification

Bismuth and Corlette provided a useful classification for cholangiocarcinoma arising at the confluence of the right and left hepatic duct, that is based on the location and extent of ductal involvement (Fig. 2) [75]. This classification is utilized to predict the resectability of cholangiocarcinoma and does not correlate directly with survival.

- Type I tumors below the confluence of the left and right hepatic ducts
- Type II tumors occlude the confluence
- Type IIIa tumors occlude the common hepatic duct and the right hepatic duct
- Type IIIb tumors occlude the common hepatic duct and the left hepatic duct
- Type IV tumors are either multifocal or involves the confluence and both the right or left hepatic duct

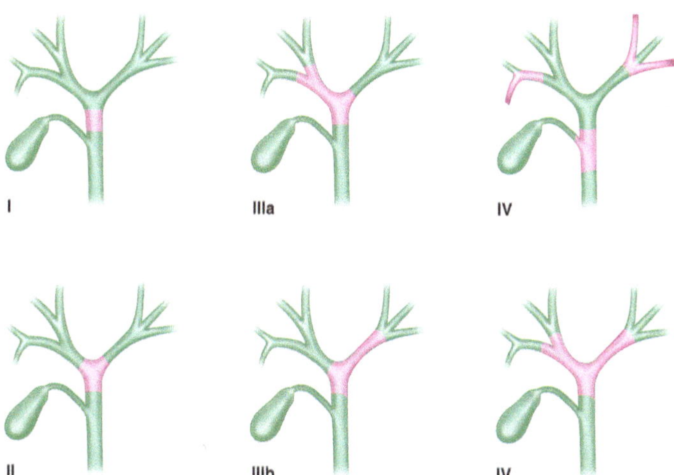

FIG. 2 Bismuth–Corlette classification of biliary strictures; Type I: tumors below the confluence of the left and right hepatic ducts. Type II: tumors reaching the confluence but not involving left or right hepatic ducts. Type III: tumors occluding the common hepatic duct and either the right (IIIa) or the left (IIIb) hepatic duct. Type IV: tumors that are multicentric or involving both right and left hepatic ducts

Bile duct tumors that involve the common hepatic duct bifurcation are referred to as Klatskin tumors or hilar cholangiocarcinoma regardless of whether they arise from the intrahepatic or extrahepatic portion of the biliary tree [76].

Staging

Cholangiocarcinoma staging is based on the TNM staging system (Tumor-Node-Metastasis). Previously, AJCC staging manual 6th edition utilized a staging system for IHCC and HiCC based on hepatocellular carcinoma (HCC). In 2010, the AJCC 7th edition staging manual introduced a separate staging system for IHCC. Staging for IHCC, EHCC and HiCC is shown in Tables 1, 2, and 3.

Treatment

Surgical Management

Patients with cholangiocarcinoma generally have a poor prognosis with 5-year survival of 5–10 % [77]. Treatment varies according to the location of the cancer, where surgical resection with negative (R0) margins represents the only curative option [49, 78]. Unfortunately, few patients presenting with the disease are eligible for surgical resection; thus, careful selection of those approached surgically is essential. Staging laparoscopy immediately preceding intended resection is suggested to assess the resectability of the disease and its accuracy can be improved by the addition of laparoscopic ultrasound [79–82].

For patients presenting with IHCC, a clear margin results in improved survival, with a median overall survival between 28 and 46 months following R0 resections [4, 83, 84]. Factors indicating unresectable disease include: bilateral hepatic duct involvement to secondary radicals, bilobar hepatic artery involvement, encasement of the portal vein proximal to its bifurcation, atrophy of one liver lobe with contralateral portal vein encasement, and/or contralateral biliary radical involvement or extrahepatic metastasis [85–87]. Negative prognostic factors of survival include vascular invasion, nodal involvement, tumor metastasis and/or >3 nodules [88]. Although nodal involvement represents an important prognostic factor, the performance of routine lymphadenectomy does not offer a survival benefit [84, 89, 90].

Similarly, surgical resection offers the best survival benefit for HiCC patients as well [88, 91, 92]. The Bismuth–Corlette classification is used to predict the resectability of hilar tumors based on the depth of tumor invasion. Bismuth type I, II and IIIa lesions usually require an en bloc resection of the gallbladder with the extrahepatic bile ducts and an extended right hepatic lobectomy. Patients with type IIIb typically require a left hepatectomy. Roux-en-Y hepaticojejunostomy reconstruction is necessary in these cases for biliary

TABLE I AJCC 7th edition staging system for intrahepatic duct cholangiocarcinoma

Stage	TNM Stage		
	T-stage	N-stage	M-stage
Stage 0	Tis	N0	M0
Stage I	T1	N0	M0
Stage II	T2	N0	M0
Stage III	T3	N0	M0
Stage IV A	T4	N0	M0
	Any T	N1	M0
Stage IV B	Any T	Any N	M1

Primary tumor (T)

TX	Primary tumor cannot be assessed
T0	No evidence of primary tumor
Tis	Carcinoma in situ (intraductal tumor)
T1	Solitary tumor without vascular invasion
T2a	Solitary tumor with vascular invasion
T2b	Multiple tumors, with or without vascular invasion
T3	Tumor perforating the visceral peritoneum or involving the local extrahepatic structures by direct invasion
T4	Tumor with periductal invasion

Regional Lymph Nodes (N)

NX	Regional lymph nodes cannot be assessed
N0	No regional lymph node metastasis
N1	Regional lymph node metastasis present

Distant Metastasis (M)

M0	No distant metastasis
M1	Distant metastasis

drainage. Caudate lobectomy should be routinely considered for patients with Bismuth type II, III, and IV, as it improves local recurrence rates and offers a survival benefit [93–95]. In patients with advanced disease and portal vein involvement, portal vein resection offers a survival benefit, and should not be considered a contraindication for surgery [96–98]. Patients with unresectable tumor may be eligible for liver transplant and should be considered for evaluation.

EHCC is the most resectable type of cholangiocarcinoma, with 91 % resectability rates compared to 60 % and 56 % for IHCC and HiCC, respectively [49]. Surgical resection of the disease often involves a pancreatoduodenectomy. T-stage and nodal involvement are important in determining the disease prognosis; thus careful assessment of the lymph nodes and T-stage is essential [78, 99, 100].

Liver Transplant

Early studies examined liver transplant as a potential cure for cholangiocarcinoma. Discouraging outcomes were frequently seen although patients presenting with smaller tumor size, earlier TNM stage, and lower CA19-9 values experienced better survival. Negative prognostic variables include multi-focal tumors of infiltrative pattern, perineural and/or vascular invasion, history of PSC, and lack of adjuvant/neoadjuvant therapy [101–104].

Mayo Clinic established a successful protocol for liver transplant and demonstrated a 5-year survival of 74 % [105]. Eligibility criteria included those with lesions ≤3 cm, no intrahepatic or extrahepatic metastasis, no prior receipt of radiation therapy, previous attempt of surgical resection or tumor biopsy. Neoadjuvant chemoradiotherapy is delivered prior to the liver transplant and is followed by a staging laparotomy. Negative predictors of survival in transplanted HiCC patients include elevated CA19-9, portal vein encasement and residual tumor on explant. Surprisingly, PSC, age, and waiting times were not reported as independent predictors

TABLE 2 AJCC 7th edition staging system for hilar cholangiocarcinoma

Stage	TNM Stage		
	T-stage	N-stage	M-stage
Stage 0	Tis	N0	M0
Stage I	T1	N0	M0
Stage II	T2a-b	N0	M0
Stage IIIA	T3	N0	M0
Stage IIIB	T1-3	N1	M0
Stage IVA	T4	N0-1	M0
Stage IVB	Any T	N2	M0
	Any T	Any N	M1

Primary tumor (T)

TX   Primary tumor cannot be assessed

T0   No evidence of primary tumor

Tis   Carcinoma in situ

T1   Tumor confined to the bile duct, with extension up to the muscle layer or fibrous tissue

T2a   Tumor invades beyond the wall of the bile duct to surrounding adipose tissue

T2b   Tumor invades adjacent hepatic parenchyma

T3   Tumor invades unilateral branches of the portal vein or hepatic artery

T4   Tumor invades main portal vein or its branches bilaterally; or the common hepatic artery; or the second-order biliary radicals bilaterally; or unilateral second-order biliary radicals with contralateral portal vein or hepatic artery involvement

Regional Lymph Nodes (N)

(continued)

Table 2 (continued)

Stage	TNM Stage		
	T-stage	N-stage	M-stage
NX	Regional lymph nodes cannot be assessed		
N0	No regional lymph node metastasis		
N1	Regional lymph node metastasis (including nodes along the cystic duct, common bile duct, hepatic artery, and portal vein)		
N2	Metastasis to periaortic, pericaval, superior mesenteric artery, and/or celiac artery lymph nodes		
Distant Metastasis (M)			
M0	No distant metastasis		
M1	Distant metastasis		

of survival [106]. Transplant centers utilizing these criteria for liver transplant experienced a 65 % rate of recurrence-free survival after 5 years compared to other centers [107]. Similarly, patients with PSC receiving neoadjuvant chemoradiation followed by liver transplant experienced a higher overall survival (82 %) with fewer recurrences, making liver transplant a possible alternative to resection for patients with HiCC [108].

In conclusion, promising survival rates can be seen following a thoughtful selection of cholangiocarcinoma patients with unresectable disease to receive neoadjuvant chemoradiation and liver transplant.

Chemotherapy

Chemotherapy is typically delivered for unresectable disease, as adjuvant therapy with surgery, or before liver transplant. Systemic therapies for patients with cholangiocarcinoma were originally fluoropyrimidine-based therapies. Earlier studies examined the combination of 5-fluorouracil (5-FU) and other chemotherapeutic agents, such as cisplatin, mitomycin, and

TABLE 3 AJCC 7th edition staging system for distal cholangiocarcinoma

Stage	TNM Stage		
	T-stage	N-stage	M-stage
Stage 0	Tis	N0	M0
Stage IA	T1	N0	M0
Stage IB	T2	N0	M0
Stage IIA	T3	N0	M0
Stage IIB	T1	N1	M0
	T2	N1	M0
	T3	N1	M0
Stage III	T4	Any N	M0
Stage IV	Any T	Any N	M1

Primary tumor (T)

TX   Primary tumor cannot be assessed

T0   No evidence of primary tumor

Tis   Carcinoma in situ

T1   Tumor confined to the bile duct histologically

T2   Tumor invades beyond the wall of the bile duct

T3   Tumor invades the gallbladder, pancreas, duodenum, or other adjacent organs without involvement of the celiac axis, or the superior mesenteric artery

T4   Tumor involves the celiac axis, or the superior mesenteric artery

Regional Lymph Nodes (N)

NX   Regional lymph nodes cannot be assessed

N0   No regional lymph node metastasis

N1   Regional lymph node metastasis

(continued)

Table 3 (continued)

Stage	T-stage	N-stage	M-stage
	TNM Stage		
Distant Metastasis (M)			
M0	No distant metastasis		
M1	Distant metastasis		

etoposide for advanced biliary tract cancers (BTC). These studies reported superior overall survival and disease free progression compared to 5-FU alone [109–111]. Due to the relatively low response to these combinations, gemcitabine was investigated, showing an overall survival of 30–56 weeks [112–114]. Subsequent trials revealed that gemcitabine combined with capecitabine or oxaliplatin result in better disease control and more favorable survival outcomes [115–118].

In 2010, the ABC-02 trial established the benefit of the gemcitabine–cisplatin regimen for biliary tract cancers, showing a median overall survival of 11.7 months and a median progression-free survival of 8 months [119]. A similar study from Japan reported a median overall survival of 11.2 months and a median progression-free survival of 5.8 months [120]. In a recent meta-analysis, patients receiving gemcitabine–cisplatin experienced a better survival outcomes, higher response rate and a longer progression free survival [121]. Currently, gemcitabine–cisplatin is a standard therapeutic approach for patients presenting with biliary tract cancers including cholangiocarcinoma.

Adjuvant chemotherapy has been shown to prolong survival following surgical intervention [122]. Dumitrascu et al. reported improved median overall and disease-free survival in patients receiving adjuvant gemcitabine following HiCC resection [123]. Subsequent studies showed a survival benefit in patients receiving adjuvant therapy, that is most noticeable in those with positive resection margins and/or lymph nodes positive disease [124, 125].

Radiation Therapy

Radiotherapy is utilized in cholangiocarcinoma as a neoadjuvant therapy, or occasionally combined with chemotherapy in the adjuvant setting. Earlier studies showed that adjuvant radiotherapy following R0 resections did not have any effect on patient's survival [126, 127]; although a survival benefit was recognized for patients with unresectable disease or those with R1 margins [128–130].

In patients with non-metastatic disease that are not eligible for surgical intervention, radiotherapy may serve as a palliative measure. Ben-Josef et al. reported a median survival of 15.8 months and a 17 % 3-year survival for a cohort of 128 patients with intrahepatic malignancies [131]. Kopek et al. reported a similar finding in a cohort of 27 patients with unresectable cholangiocarcinoma, showing an overall survival of 10.6 months following radiotherapy [132].

Palliative Biliary Drainage

A large population of cholangiocarcinoma patients will have biliary obstruction at presentation. The obstruction leads to liver congestion, jaundice, nausea, pruritus, and an increased risk of cholangitis [133, 134]. Palliative interventions include surgical bypass, percutaneous or endoscopic biliary drainage. Surgical drainage includes choledochojejunostomy and/or hepaticojejunostomy. The limitations to surgical palliation include biliary leaks following surgical bypass (6–21 %), and substantial procedure-related mortality (6–12 %) [135, 136]. Minimally invasive bypass operations have been suggested as a possible alternative, though satisfactory outcomes following PTC or ERCP drainage make the necessity of surgical bypass uncommon [137].

Endoscopic palliation represents the most widely utilized option for patients with obstructive symptoms. Typically, endoscopic retrograde cholangiography (ERCP) is performed, followed by wire-guided plastic/metal stent insertion. In early studies, metal stents placement was debated due to associated cost. However, the frequent need to change plastic stents due to their early occlusion by sludge resulted in metal stents being more cost-effective in patients with life expectancy greater than 6 months [138, 139]. The introduction of the self-expanding metal stents (SEMS) allowed a more successful drainage with longer patency rates and fewer procedures compared to plastic stents [140, 141]. A recent meta-analysis confirmed better patency, lower occlusion rates, and fewer adverse effects associated with SEMS for distal and hilar biliary obstructions [142].

Percutaneous drainage typically follows a failed endoscopic approach to stent. Paik et al. reported that percutaneous placement of SEMS in HiCC is associated with higher success rates and lower risk of procedure-related cholangitis than endoscopic stent placement [143]. The lower risk of cholangitis following percutaneous biliary drainage makes this modality favorable in patients with hilar disease [144].

Unilateral vs. bilateral stenting: In hilar cholangiocarcinoma patients, unilateral stent insertion is easier and associated with fewer complications rates [145]. However, reinterventions are frequent due to stent occlusion or stent migration [146]. Conversely, bilateral stenting provides longer patency times allowing extended drainage [147]. In a recent meta-analysis, Sawas et al. reported similar occlusion rates and 30-day mortality between unilateral and bilateral stent groups [142]. A more successful insertion rate in the unilateral stent group (odds ratio: 3.17 [95%CI: 1.49–6.74]) coupled with the higher rate of adverse effects in the bilateral stenting group makes the use of unilateral stenting for biliary drainage of malignant hilar lesions advisable.

Photodynamic Therapy

Photodynamic therapy (PDT) involves the injection of a porphyrin photosensitizer followed by endoscopic illumination of the tumor bed to activate the injected substance and cause tumor death. Early reports showed a possible efficacy of the modality in restoring biliary drainage and improving survival in patients with unresectable disease [148, 149]. In a recent study, PDT following endoscopic stenting resulted in extended patency and longer survival rates [18]. The side effects of this modality include cutaneous complications, as erythema and hyperpigmentation. The utilization of PDT is still limited due to availability.

Conclusion

Cholangiocarcinoma is a rare malignancy that arises from the biliary tract epithelial lining and carries a grave prognosis. Three types of the disease exist according to the tumor location: intrahepatic, hilar, and extrahepatic cholangiocarcinoma. Survival is limited due to late presentation of the disease; and surgical resection represents the mainstay of treatment. In patients not eligible for surgical resection, liver transplantation provides satisfactory 5-year survival rates in carefully selected candidates. Radiotherapy and/or chemotherapy in the form of combined gemcitabine–cisplatin provide palliation for patients. In cases presenting with symptoms of biliary congestions, self-expanding metal stents relieve the congestion and improve the patients' quality of life.

References

1. Vauthey JN, Blumgart LH. Recent advances in the management of cholangiocarcinomas. Semin Liver Dis. 1994; 14(2):109–14.
2. Shaib Y, El-Serag HB. The epidemiology of cholangiocarcinoma. Semin Liver Dis. 2004;24(2):115–25.
3. Shaib YH, El-Serag HB, Davila JA, Morgan R, McGlynn KA. Risk factors of intrahepatic cholangiocarcinoma in the United States: a case-control study. Gastroenterology. 2005;128(3):620–6.
4. DeOliveira ML, Cunningham SC, Cameron JL, Kamangar F, Winter JM, Lillemoe KD, et al. Cholangiocarcinoma: thirty-one-year experience with 564 patients at a single institution. Ann Surg. 2007;245(5):755–62.

5. Khan SA, Davidson BR, Goldin R, Pereira SP, Rosenberg WM, Taylor-Robinson SD, et al. Guidelines for the diagnosis and treatment of cholangiocarcinoma: consensus document. Gut. 2002;51 Suppl 6:VI1–9.

6. Khan SA, Taylor-Robinson SD, Toledano MB, Beck A, Elliott P, Thomas HC. Changing international trends in mortality rates for liver, biliary and pancreatic tumours. J Hepatol. 2002;37(6):806–13.

7. Jepsen P, Vilstrup H, Tarone RE, Friis S, Sørensen HT. Incidence rates of intra- and extrahepatic cholangiocarcinomas in Denmark from 1978 through 2002. J Natl Cancer Inst. 2007;99(11):895–7.

8. West J, Wood H, Logan RF, Quinn M, Aithal GP. Trends in the incidence of primary liver and biliary tract cancers in England and Wales 1971-2001. Br J Cancer. 2006;94(11):1751–8.

9. Patel T. Worldwide trends in mortality from biliary tract malignancies. BMC Cancer. 2002;2:10.

10. Strom BL, Hibberd PL, Soper KA, Stolley PD, Nelson WL. International variations in epidemiology of cancers of the extrahepatic biliary tract. Cancer Res. 1985;45(10):5165–8.

11. Khan SA, Davidson BR, Goldin RD, Heaton N, Karani J, Pereira SP, et al. Guidelines for the diagnosis and treatment of cholangiocarcinoma: an update. Gut. 2012;61(12):1657–69.

12. Siegel RL, Miller KD, Jemal A. Cancer statistics, 2015. CA Cancer J Clin. 2015;65(1):5–29.

13. Lee YM, Kaplan MM. Primary sclerosing cholangitis. N Engl J Med. 1995;332(14):924–33.

14. Rosen CB, Nagorney DM, Wiesner RH, Coffey RJ, LaRusso NF. Cholangiocarcinoma complicating primary sclerosing cholangitis. Ann Surg. 1991;213(1):21–5.

15. Bergquist A, Ekbom A, Olsson R, Kornfeldt D, Lööf L, Danielsson A, et al. Hepatic and extrahepatic malignancies in primary sclerosing cholangitis. J Hepatol. 2002;36(3):321–7.

16. Burak K, Angulo P, Pasha TM, Egan K, Petz J, Lindor KD. Incidence and risk factors for cholangiocarcinoma in primary sclerosing cholangitis. Am J Gastroenterol. 2004;99(3):523–6.

17. Boonstra K, Weersma RK, van Erpecum KJ, Rauws EA, Spanier BW, Poen AC, et al. Population-based epidemiology, malignancy risk, and outcome of primary sclerosing cholangitis. Hepatology. 2013;58(6):2045–55.

18. Cheon YK, Lee TY, Lee SM, Yoon JY, Shim CS. Longterm outcome of photodynamic therapy compared with biliary

stenting alone in patients with advanced hilar cholangiocarcinoma. HPB (Oxford). 2012;14(3):185–93.

19. Shin HR, Lee CU, Park HJ, Seol SY, Chung JM, Choi HC, et al. Hepatitis B and C virus, Clonorchis sinensis for the risk of liver cancer: a case-control study in Pusan. Korea Int J Epidemiol. 1996;25(5):933–40.

20. Watanapa P. Cholangiocarcinoma in patients with opisthorchiasis. Br J Surg. 1996;83(8):1062–4.

21. Watanapa P, Watanapa WB. Liver fluke-associated cholangiocarcinoma. Br J Surg. 2002;89(8):962–70.

22. Sripa B, Pairojkul C. Cholangiocarcinoma: lessons from Thailand. Curr Opin Gastroenterol. 2008;24(3):349–56.

23. Su CH, Shyr YM, Lui WY, P'Eng FK. Hepatolithiasis associated with cholangiocarcinoma. Br J Surg. 1997;84(7):969–73.

24. Chijiiwa K, Yamashita H, Yoshida J, Kuroki S, Tanaka M. Current management and long-term prognosis of hepatolithiasis. Arch Surg. 1995;130(2):194–7.

25. Donato F, Gelatti U, Tagger A, Favret M, Ribero ML, Callea F, et al. Intrahepatic cholangiocarcinoma and hepatitis C and B virus infection, alcohol intake, and hepatolithiasis: a case-control study in Italy. Cancer Causes Control. 2001;12(10):959–64.

26. Jan YY, Chen MF, Wang CS, Jeng LB, Hwang TL, Chen SC. Surgical treatment of hepatolithiasis: long-term results. Surgery. 1996;120(3):509–14.

27. Scott J, Shousha S, Thomas HC, Sherlock S. Bile duct carcinoma: a late complication of congenital hepatic fibrosis. Case report and review of literature. Am J Gastroenterol. 1980;73(2):113–9.

28. Lipsett PA, Pitt HA, Colombani PM, Boitnott JK, Cameron JL. Choledochal cyst disease. A changing pattern of presentation. Ann Surg. 1994;220(5):644–52.

29. Ohtsuka T, Inoue K, Ohuchida J, Nabae T, Takahata S, Niiyama H, et al. Carcinoma arising in choledochocele. Endoscopy. 2001;33(7):614–9.

30. Goto N, Yasuda I, Uematsu T, Kanemura N, Takao S, Ando K, et al. Intrahepatic cholangiocarcinoma arising 10 years after the excision of congenital extrahepatic biliary dilation. J Gastroenterol. 2001;36(12):856–62.

31. Dayton MT, Longmire WP, Tompkins RK. Caroli's Disease: a premalignant condition? Am J Surg. 1983;145(1):41–8.

32. Khan SA, Thomas HC, Davidson BR, Taylor-Robinson SD. Cholangiocarcinoma. Lancet. 2005;366(9493):1303–14.

33. Chapman RW. Risk factors for biliary tract carcinogenesis. Ann Oncol. 1999;10 Suppl 4:308–11.

34. Sahani D, Prasad SR, Tannabe KK, Hahn PF, Mueller PR, Saini S. Thorotrast-induced cholangiocarcinoma: case report. Abdom Imaging. 2003;28(1):72–4.

35. Rubel LR, Ishak KG. Thorotrast-associated cholangiocarcinoma: an epidemiologic and clinicopathologic study. Cancer. 1982;50(7):1408–15.

36. Lipshutz GS, Brennan TV, Warren RS. Thorotrast-induced liver neoplasia: a collective review. J Am Coll Surg. 2002;195(5):713–8.

37. Mitacek EJ, Brunnemann KD, Hoffmann D, Limsila T, Suttajit M, Martin N, et al. Volatile nitrosamines and tobacco-specific nitrosamines in the smoke of Thai cigarettes: a risk factor for lung cancer and a suspected risk factor for liver cancer in Thailand. Carcinogenesis. 1999;20(1):133–7.

38. Szendröi M, Németh L, Vajta G. Asbestos bodies in a bile duct cancer after occupational exposure. Environ Res. 1983;30(2):270–80.

39. Sorensen HT, Friis S, Olsen JH, Thulstrup AM, Mellemkjaer L, Linet M, et al. Risk of liver and other types of cancer in patients with cirrhosis: a nationwide cohort study in Denmark. Hepatology. 1998;28(4):921–5.

40. Kobayashi M, Ikeda K, Saitoh S, Suzuki F, Tsubota A, Suzuki Y, et al. Incidence of primary cholangiocellular carcinoma of the liver in Japanese patients with hepatitis C virus-related cirrhosis. Cancer. 2000;88(11):2471–7.

41. Palmer WC, Patel T. Are common factors involved in the pathogenesis of primary liver cancers? A meta-analysis of risk factors for intrahepatic cholangiocarcinoma. J Hepatol. 2012;57(1):69–76.

42. Zhou Y, Zhao Y, Li B, Huang J, Wu L, Xu D, et al. Hepatitis viruses infection and risk of intrahepatic cholangiocarcinoma: evidence from a meta-analysis. BMC Cancer. 2012;12:289.

43. Li M, Li J, Li P, Li H, Su T, Zhu R, et al. Hepatitis B virus infection increases the risk of cholangiocarcinoma: a meta-analysis and systematic review. J Gastroenterol Hepatol. 2012;27(10):1561–8.

44. Ralphs S, Khan SA. The role of the hepatitis viruses in cholangiocarcinoma. J Viral Hepat. 2013;20(5):297–305.

45. Bergquist A, von Seth E. Epidemiology of cholangiocarcinoma. Best Pract Res Clin Gastroenterol. 2015;29(2):221–32.

46. Chalasani N, Baluyut A, Ismail A, Zaman A, Sood G, Ghalib R, et al. Cholangiocarcinoma in patients with primary sclerosing cholangitis: a multicenter case-control study. Hepatology. 2000;31(1):7–11.
47. Bergquist A, Glaumann H, Persson B, Broomé U. Risk factors and clinical presentation of hepatobiliary carcinoma in patients with primary sclerosing cholangitis: a case-control study. Hepatology. 1998;27(2):311–6.
48. Welzel TM, Graubard BI, El-Serag HB, Shaib YH, Hsing AW, Davila JA, et al. Risk factors for intrahepatic and extrahepatic cholangiocarcinoma in the United States: a population-based case-control study. Clin Gastroenterol Hepatol. 2007;5(10): 1221–8.
49. Nakeeb A, Pitt HA, Sohn TA, Coleman J, Abrams RA, Piantadosi S, et al. Cholangiocarcinoma. A spectrum of intrahepatic, perihilar, and distal tumors. Ann Surg. 1996;224(4):463–73. discussion 73-5.
50. Washburn WK, Lewis WD, Jenkins RL. Aggressive surgical resection for cholangiocarcinoma. Arch Surg. 1995;130(3): 270–6.
51. Slattery JM, Sahani DV. What is the current state-of-the-art imaging for detection and staging of cholangiocarcinoma? Oncologist. 2006;11(8):913–22.
52. Abu-Hamda EM, Baron TH. Endoscopic management of cholangiocarcinoma. Semin Liver Dis. 2004;24(2):165–75.
53. Mohamadnejad M, DeWitt JM, Sherman S, LeBlanc JK, Pitt HA, House MG, et al. Role of EUS for preoperative evaluation of cholangiocarcinoma: a large single-center experience. Gastrointest Endosc. 2011;73(1):71–8.
54. El Chafic AH, Dewitt J, Leblanc JK, El Hajj II, Cote G, House MG, et al. Impact of preoperative endoscopic ultrasound-guided fine needle aspiration on postoperative recurrence and survival in cholangiocarcinoma patients. Endoscopy. 2013;45(11):883–9.
55. Strongin A, Singh H, Eloubeidi MA, Siddiqui AA. Role of endoscopic ultrasonography in the evaluation of extrahepatic cholangiocarcinoma. Endosc Ultrasound. 2013;2(2):71–6.
56. Garrow D, Miller S, Sinha D, Conway J, Hoffman BJ, Hawes RH, et al. Endoscopic ultrasound: a meta-analysis of test performance in suspected biliary obstruction. Clin Gastroenterol Hepatol. 2007;5(5):616–23.

57. Feydy A, Vilgrain V, Denys A, Sibert A, Belghiti J, Vullierme MP, et al. Helical CT assessment in hilar cholangiocarcinoma: correlation with surgical and pathologic findings. AJR Am J Roentgenol. 1999;172(1):73–7.

58. Soares KC, Kamel I, Cosgrove DP, Herman JM, Pawlik TM. Hilar cholangiocarcinoma: diagnosis, treatment options, and management. Hepatobiliary Surg Nutr. 2014;3(1):18–34.

59. Bridgewater J, Galle PR, Khan SA, Llovet JM, Park JW, Patel T, et al. Guidelines for the diagnosis and management of intrahepatic cholangiocarcinoma. J Hepatol. 2014;60(6):1268–89.

60. Unno M, Okumoto T, Katayose Y, Rikiyama T, Sato A, Motoi F, et al. Preoperative assessment of hilar cholangiocarcinoma by multidetector row computed tomography. J Hepatobiliary Pancreat Surg. 2007;14(5):434–40.

61. Chen HW, Lai EC, Pan AZ, Chen T, Liao S, Lau WY. Preoperative assessment and staging of hilar cholangiocarcinoma with 16-multidetector computed tomography cholangiography and angiography. Hepatogastroenterology. 2009;56(91-92):578–83.

62. Seo H, Lee JM, Kim IH, Han JK, Kim SH, Jang JY, et al. Evaluation of the gross type and longitudinal extent of extrahepatic cholangiocarcinomas on contrast-enhanced multidetector row computed tomography. J Comput Assist Tomogr. 2009;33(3):376–82.

63. Park MS, Lee DK, Kim MJ, Lee WJ, Yoon DS, Lee SJ, et al. Preoperative staging accuracy of multidetector row computed tomography for extrahepatic bile duct carcinoma. J Comput Assist Tomogr. 2006;30(3):362–7.

64. Bach AM, Hann LE, Brown KT, Getrajdman GI, Herman SK, Fong Y, et al. Portal vein evaluation with US: comparison to angiography combined with CT arterial portography. Radiology. 1996;201(1):149–54.

65. Materne R, Van Beers BE, Gigot JF, Jamart J, Geubel A, Pringot J, et al. Extrahepatic biliary obstruction: magnetic resonance imaging compared with endoscopic ultrasonography. Endoscopy. 2000;32(1):3–9.

66. Lomanto D, Pavone P, Laghi A, Panebianco V, Mazzocchi P, Fiocca F, et al. Magnetic resonance-cholangiopancreatography in the diagnosis of biliopancreatic diseases. Am J Surg. 1997;174(1):33–8.

67. Romagnuolo J, Bardou M, Rahme E, Joseph L, Reinhold C, Barkun AN. Magnetic resonance cholangiopancreatography: a meta-analysis of test performance in suspected biliary disease. Ann Intern Med. 2003;139(7):547–57.

68. Pavone P, Laghi A, Passariello R. MR cholangiopancreatography in malignant biliary obstruction. Semin Ultrasound CT MR. 1999;20(5):317–23.

69. Kim JY, Kim MH, Lee TY, Hwang CY, Kim JS, Yun SC, et al. Clinical role of 18F-FDG PET-CT in suspected and potentially operable cholangiocarcinoma: a prospective study compared with conventional imaging. Am J Gastroenterol. 2008;103(5):1145–51.

70. Kluge R, Schmidt F, Caca K, Barthel H, Hesse S, Georgi P, et al. Positron emission tomography with [(18)F]fluoro-2-deoxy-D-glucose for diagnosis and staging of bile duct cancer. Hepatology. 2001;33(5):1029–35.

71. Keiding S, Hansen SB, Rasmussen HH, Gee A, Kruse A, Roelsgaard K, et al. Detection of cholangiocarcinoma in primary sclerosing cholangitis by positron emission tomography. Hepatology. 1998;28(3):700–6.

72. Prytz H, Keiding S, Björnsson E, Broomé U, Almer S, Castedal M, et al. Dynamic FDG-PET is useful for detection of cholangiocarcinoma in patients with PSC listed for liver transplantation. Hepatology. 2006;44(6):1572–80.

73. Ustundag Y, Bayraktar Y. Cholangiocarcinoma: a compact review of the literature. World J Gastroenterol. 2008;14(42):6458–66.

74. Siqueira E, Schoen RE, Silverman W, Martin J, Rabinovitz M, Weissfeld JL, et al. Detecting cholangiocarcinoma in patients with primary sclerosing cholangitis. Gastrointest Endosc. 2002;56(1):40–7.

75. Bismuth H, Corlette MB. Intrahepatic cholangioenteric anastomosis in carcinoma of the hilus of the liver. Surg Gynecol Obstet. 1975;140(2):170–8.

76. Klatskin G. Adenocarcinoma of the hepatic duct at its bifurcation within the porta hepatis. An unusual tumor with distinctive clinical and pathological features. Am J Med. 1965;38:241–56.

77. Anderson CD, Pinson CW, Berlin J, Chari RS. Diagnosis and treatment of cholangiocarcinoma. Oncologist. 2004;9(1):43–57.

78. Wade TP, Prasad CN, Virgo KS, Johnson FE. Experience with distal bile duct cancers in U.S. Veterans Affairs hospitals: 1987-1991. J Surg Oncol. 1997;64(3):242–5.

79. Joseph S, Connor S, Garden OJ. Staging laparoscopy for cholangiocarcinoma. HPB (Oxford). 2008;10(2):116–9.

80. Connor S, Barron E, Wigmore SJ, Madhavan KK, Parks RW, Garden OJ. The utility of laparoscopic assessment in the preoperative staging of suspected hilar cholangiocarcinoma. J Gastrointest Surg. 2005;9(4):476–80.
81. Weber SM, DeMatteo RP, Fong Y, Blumgart LH, Jarnagin WR. Staging laparoscopy in patients with extrahepatic biliary carcinoma. Analysis of 100 patients. Ann Surg. 2002;235(3):392–9.
82. Barlow AD, Garcea G, Berry DP, Rajesh A, Patel R, Metcalfe MS, et al. Staging laparoscopy for hilar cholangiocarcinoma in 100 patients. Langenbecks Arch Surg. 2013;398(7):983–8.
83. Lang H, Sotiropoulos GC, Frühauf NR, Dömland M, Paul A, Kind EM, et al. Extended hepatectomy for intrahepatic cholangiocellular carcinoma (ICC): when is it worthwhile? Single center experience with 27 resections in 50 patients over a 5-year period. Ann Surg. 2005;241(1):134–43.
84. Endo I, Gonen M, Yopp AC, Dalal KM, Zhou Q, Klimstra D, et al. Intrahepatic cholangiocarcinoma: rising frequency, improved survival, and determinants of outcome after resection. Ann Surg. 2008;248(1):84–96.
85. Burke EC, Jarnagin WR, Hochwald SN, Pisters PW, Fong Y, Blumgart LH. Hilar Cholangiocarcinoma: patterns of spread, the importance of hepatic resection for curative operation, and a presurgical clinical staging system. Ann Surg. 1998;228(3):385–94.
86. Jarnagin WR, Fong Y, DeMatteo RP, Gonen M, Burke EC, Bodniewicz BSJ, et al. Staging, resectability, and outcome in 225 patients with hilar cholangiocarcinoma. Ann Surg. 2001;234(4):507–17. discussion 17-9.
87. Spolverato G, Vitale A, Cucchetti A, Popescu I, Marques HP, Aldrighetti L, et al. Can hepatic resection provide a long-term cure for patients with intrahepatic cholangiocarcinoma? Cancer. 2015;121(22):3998–4006.
88. Wang Y, Li J, Xia Y, Gong R, Wang K, Yan Z, et al. Prognostic nomogram for intrahepatic cholangiocarcinoma after partial hepatectomy. J Clin Oncol. 2013;31(9):1188–95.
89. Shirabe K, Shimada M, Harimoto N, Sugimachi K, Yamashita Y, Tsujita E, et al. Intrahepatic cholangiocarcinoma: its mode of spreading and therapeutic modalities. Surgery. 2002;131(1 Suppl):S159–64.
90. de Jong MC, Nathan H, Sotiropoulos GC, Paul A, Alexandrescu S, Marques H, et al. Intrahepatic cholangiocarcinoma: an international multi-institutional analysis of prognostic factors and lymph node assessment. J Clin Oncol. 2011;29(23):3140–5.

91. Regimbeau JM, Fuks D, Le Treut YP, Bachellier P, Belghiti J, Boudjema K, et al. Surgery for hilar cholangiocarcinoma: a multi-institutional update on practice and outcome by the AFC-HC study group. J Gastrointest Surg. 2011;15(3):480–8.

92. Nguyen KT, Steel J, Vanounou T, Tsung A, Marsh JW, Geller DA, et al. Initial presentation and management of hilar and peripheral cholangiocarcinoma: is a node-positive status or potential margin-positive result a contraindication to resection? Ann Surg Oncol. 2009;16(12):3308–15.

93. Parikh AA, Abdalla EK, Vauthey JN. Operative considerations in resection of hilar cholangiocarcinoma. HPB (Oxford). 2005;7(4):254–8.

94. Dinant S, Gerhards MF, Busch OR, Obertop H, Gouma DJ, Van Gulik TM. The importance of complete excision of the caudate lobe in resection of hilar cholangiocarcinoma. HPB (Oxford). 2005;7(4):263–7.

95. Kow AW, Wook CD, Song SC, Kim WS, Kim MJ, Park HJ, et al. Role of caudate lobectomy in type III A and III B hilar cholangiocarcinoma: a 15-year experience in a tertiary institution. World J Surg. 2012;36(5):1112–21.

96. Wu XS, Dong P, Gu J, Li ML, Wu WG, Lu JH, et al. Combined portal vein resection for hilar cholangiocarcinoma: a meta-analysis of comparative studies. J Gastrointest Surg. 2013;17(6):1107–15.

97. de Jong MC, Marques H, Clary BM, Bauer TW, Marsh JW, Ribero D, et al. The impact of portal vein resection on outcomes for hilar cholangiocarcinoma: a multi-institutional analysis of 305 cases. Cancer. 2012;118(19):4737–47.

98. Hemming AW, Mekeel K, Khanna A, Baquerizo A, Kim RD. Portal vein resection in management of hilar cholangiocarcinoma. J Am Coll Surg. 2011;212(4):604–13. discussion 13-6.

99. Ito K, Ito H, Allen PJ, Gonen M, Klimstra D, D'Angelica MI, et al. Adequate lymph node assessment for extrahepatic bile duct adenocarcinoma. Ann Surg. 2010;251(4):675–81.

100. Hong SM, Pawlik TM, Cho H, Aggarwal B, Goggins M, Hruban RH, et al. Depth of tumor invasion better predicts prognosis than the current American Joint Committee on Cancer T classification for distal bile duct carcinoma. Surgery. 2009; 146(2):250–7.

101. Shimoda M, Farmer DG, Colquhoun SD, Rosove M, Ghobrial RM, Yersiz H, et al. Liver transplantation for cholangiocellular

carcinoma: analysis of a single-center experience and review of the literature. Liver Transpl. 2001;7(12):1023–33.

102. Fu BS, Zhang T, Li H, Yi SH, Wang GS, Xu C, et al. The role of liver transplantation for intrahepatic cholangiocarcinoma: a single-center experience. Eur Surg Res. 2011;47(4):218–21.

103. Robles R, Figueras J, Turrión VS, Margarit C, Moya A, Varo E, et al. Spanish experience in liver transplantation for hilar and peripheral cholangiocarcinoma. Ann Surg. 2004;239(2):265–71.

104. Friman S, Foss A, Isoniemi H, Olausson M, Höckerstedt K, Yamamoto S, et al. Liver transplantation for cholangiocarcinoma: selection is essential for acceptable results. Scand J Gastroenterol. 2011;46(3):370–5.

105. Gores GJ, Nagorney DM, Rosen CB. Cholangiocarcinoma: is transplantation an option? For whom? J Hepatol. 2007;47(4):455–9.

106. Darwish Murad S, Kim WR, Therneau T, Gores GJ, Rosen CB, Martenson JA, et al. Predictors of pretransplant dropout and posttransplant recurrence in patients with perihilar cholangiocarcinoma. Hepatology. 2012;56(3):972–81.

107. Darwish Murad S, Kim WR, Harnois DM, Douglas DD, Burton J, Kulik LM, et al. Efficacy of neoadjuvant chemoradiation, followed by liver transplantation, for perihilar cholangiocarcinoma at 12 US centers. Gastroenterology. 2012;143(1):88–98. e3; quiz e14.

108. Rea DJ, Heimbach JK, Rosen CB, Haddock MG, Alberts SR, Kremers WK, et al. Liver transplantation with neoadjuvant chemoradiation is more effective than resection for hilar cholangiocarcinoma. Ann Surg. 2005;242(3):451–8. discussion 8-61.

109. Rao S, Cunningham D, Hawkins RE, Hill ME, Smith D, Daniel F, et al. Phase III study of 5FU, etoposide and leucovorin (FELV) compared to epirubicin, cisplatin and 5FU (ECF) in previously untreated patients with advanced biliary cancer. Br J Cancer. 2005;92(9):1650–4.

110. Ducreux M, Van Cutsem E, Van Laethem JL, Gress TM, Jeziorski K, Rougier P, et al. A randomised phase II trial of weekly high-dose 5-fluorouracil with and without folinic acid and cisplatin in patients with advanced biliary tract carcinoma: results of the 40955 EORTC trial. Eur J Cancer. 2005;41(3):398–403.

111. Hezel AF, Zhu AX. Systemic therapy for biliary tract cancers. Oncologist. 2008;13(4):415–23.

112. Gallardo JO, Rubio B, Fodor M, Orlandi L, Yáñez M, Gamargo C, et al. A phase II study of gemcitabine in gallbladder carcinoma. Ann Oncol. 2001;12(10):1403–6.

113. Kubicka S, Rudolph KL, Tietze MK, Lorenz M, Manns M. Phase II study of systemic gemcitabine chemotherapy for advanced unresectable hepatobiliary carcinomas. Hepatogastroenterology. 2001;48(39):783–9.

114. Tsavaris N, Kosmas C, Gouveris P, Gennatas K, Polyzos A, Mouratidou D, et al. Weekly gemcitabine for the treatment of biliary tract and gallbladder cancer. Invest New Drugs. 2004;22(2):193–8.

115. Androulakis N, Aravantinos G, Syrigos K, Polyzos A, Ziras N, Tselepatiotis E, et al. Oxaliplatin as first-line treatment in inoperable biliary tract carcinoma: a multicenter phase II study. Oncology. 2006;70(4):280–4.

116. André T, Tournigand C, Rosmorduc O, Provent S, Maindrault-Goebel F, Avenin D, et al. Gemcitabine combined with oxaliplatin (GEMOX) in advanced biliary tract adenocarcinoma: a GERCOR study. Ann Oncol. 2004;15(9):1339–43.

117. Knox JJ, Hedley D, Oza A, Feld R, Siu LL, Chen E, et al. Combining gemcitabine and capecitabine in patients with advanced biliary cancer: a phase II trial. J Clin Oncol. 2005;23(10):2332–8.

118. Cho JY, Paik YH, Chang YS, Lee SJ, Lee DK, Song SY, et al. Capecitabine combined with gemcitabine (CapGem) as first-line treatment in patients with advanced/metastatic biliary tract carcinoma. Cancer. 2005;104(12):2753–8.

119. Valle J, Wasan H, Palmer DH, Cunningham D, Anthoney A, Maraveyas A, et al. Cisplatin plus gemcitabine versus gemcitabine for biliary tract cancer. N Engl J Med. 2010;362(14): 1273–81.

120. Okusaka T, Nakachi K, Fukutomi A, Mizuno N, Ohkawa S, Funakoshi A, et al. Gemcitabine alone or in combination with cisplatin in patients with biliary tract cancer: a comparative multicentre study in Japan. Br J Cancer. 2010;103(4):469–74.

121. Yang R, Wang B, Chen YJ, Li HB, Hu JB, Zou SQ. Efficacy of gemcitabine plus platinum agents for biliary tract cancers: a meta-analysis. Anticancer Drugs. 2013;24(8):871–7.

122. Murakami Y, Uemura K, Sudo T, Hashimoto Y, Nakashima A, Kondo N, et al. Prognostic factors after surgical resection for intrahepatic, hilar, and distal cholangiocarcinoma. Ann Surg Oncol. 2011;18(3):651–8.

123. Dumitrascu T, Chirita D, Ionescu M, Popescu I. Resection for hilar cholangiocarcinoma: analysis of prognostic factors and the impact of systemic inflammation on long-term outcome. J Gastrointest Surg. 2013;17(5):913–24.
124. Horgan AM, Amir E, Walter T, Knox JJ. Adjuvant therapy in the treatment of biliary tract cancer: a systematic review and meta-analysis. J Clin Oncol. 2012;30(16):1934–40.
125. Miura JT, Johnston FM, Tsai S, George B, Thomas J, Eastwood D, et al. Chemotherapy for Surgically Resected Intrahepatic Cholangiocarcinoma. Ann Surg Oncol. 2015;22(11):3716–23.
126. Cameron JL, Pitt HA, Zinner MJ, Kaufman SL, Coleman J. Management of proximal cholangiocarcinomas by surgical resection and radiotherapy. Am J Surg. 1990;159(1):91–7. discussion 7-8.
127. Pitt HA, Nakeeb A, Abrams RA, Coleman J, Piantadosi S, Yeo CJ, et al. Perihilar cholangiocarcinoma. Postoperative radiotherapy does not improve survival. Ann Surg. 1995;221(6):788–97. discussion 97-8.
128. Kamada T, Saitou H, Takamura A, Nojima T, Okushiba SI. The role of radiotherapy in the management of extrahepatic bile duct cancer: an analysis of 145 consecutive patients treated with intraluminal and/or external beam radiotherapy. Int J Radiat Oncol Biol Phys. 1996;34(4):767–74.
129. Todoroki T, Ohara K, Kawamoto T, Koike N, Yoshida S, Kashiwagi H, et al. Benefits of adjuvant radiotherapy after radical resection of locally advanced main hepatic duct carcinoma. Int J Radiat Oncol Biol Phys. 2000;46(3):581–7.
130. Gerhards MF, van Gulik TM, González González D, Rauws EA, Gouma DJ. Results of postoperative radiotherapy for resectable hilar cholangiocarcinoma. World J Surg. 2003;27(2):173–9.
131. Ben-Josef E, Normolle D, Ensminger WD, Walker S, Tatro D, Ten Haken RK, et al. Phase II trial of high-dose conformal radiation therapy with concurrent hepatic artery floxuridine for unresectable intrahepatic malignancies. J Clin Oncol. 2005;23(34):8739–47.
132. Kopek N, Holt MI, Hansen AT, Høyer M. Stereotactic body radiotherapy for unresectable cholangiocarcinoma. Radiother Oncol. 2010;94(1):47–52.
133. Polydorou AA, Cairns SR, Dowsett JF, Hatfield AR, Salmon PR, Cotton PB, et al. Palliation of proximal malignant biliary obstruction by endoscopic endoprosthesis insertion. Gut. 1991;32(6):685–9.

134. Goenka MK, Goenka U. Palliation: Hilar cholangiocarcinoma. World J Hepatol. 2014;6(8):559–69.
135. Blumgart LH, Hadjis NS, Benjamin IS, Beazley R. Surgical approaches to cholangiocarcinoma at confluence of hepatic ducts. Lancet. 1984;1(8368):66–70.
136. Singhal D, van Gulik TM, Gouma DJ. Palliative management of hilar cholangiocarcinoma. Surg Oncol. 2005;14(2):59–74.
137. Lai EC, Tang CN. Robot-assisted laparoscopic hepaticojejunostomy for advanced malignant biliary obstruction. Asian J Surg. 2015.
138. Davids PH, Groen AK, Rauws EA, Tytgat GN, Huibregtse K. Randomised trial of self-expanding metal stents versus polyethylene stents for distal malignant biliary obstruction. Lancet. 1992;340(8834-8835):1488–92.
139. Prat F, Chapat O, Ducot B, Ponchon T, Pelletier G, Fritsch J, et al. A randomized trial of endoscopic drainage methods for inoperable malignant strictures of the common bile duct. Gastrointest Endosc. 1998;47(1):1–7.
140. Raju RP, Jaganmohan SR, Ross WA, Davila ML, Javle M, Raju GS, et al. Optimum palliation of inoperable hilar cholangiocarcinoma: comparative assessment of the efficacy of plastic and self-expanding metal stents. Dig Dis Sci. 2011;56(5):1557–64.
141. Levy MJ, Baron TH, Gostout CJ, Petersen BT, Farnell MB. Palliation of malignant extrahepatic biliary obstruction with plastic versus expandable metal stents: An evidence-based approach. Clin Gastroenterol Hepatol. 2004;2(4):273–85.
142. Sawas T, Al Halabi S, Parsi MA, Vargo JJ. Self-expandable metal stents versus plastic stents for malignant biliary obstruction: a meta-analysis. Gastrointest Endosc. 2015.
143. Paik WH, Park YS, Hwang JH, Lee SH, Yoon CJ, Kang SG, et al. Palliative treatment with self-expandable metallic stents in patients with advanced type III or IV hilar cholangiocarcinoma: a percutaneous versus endoscopic approach. Gastrointest Endosc. 2009;69(1):55–62.
144. Nomura T, Shirai Y, Hatakeyama K. Cholangitis after endoscopic biliary drainage for hilar lesions. Hepatogastroenterology. 1997;44(17):1267–70.
145. De Palma GD, Galloro G, Siciliano S, Iovino P, Catanzano C. Unilateral versus bilateral endoscopic hepatic duct drainage in patients with malignant hilar biliary obstruction: results of a prospective, randomized, and controlled study. Gastrointest Endosc. 2001;53(6):547–53.

146. Ridtitid W, Rerknimitr R, Janchai A, Kongkam P, Treeprasertsuk S, Kullavanijaya P. Outcome of second interventions for occluded metallic stents in patients with malignant biliary obstruction. Surg Endosc. 2010;24(9):2216–20.
147. Liberato MJ, Canena JM. Endoscopic stenting for hilar cholangiocarcinoma: efficacy of unilateral and bilateral placement of plastic and metal stents in a retrospective review of 480 patients. BMC Gastroenterol. 2012;12:103.
148. Ortner MA, Liebetruth J, Schreiber S, Hanft M, Wruck U, Fusco V, et al. Photodynamic therapy of nonresectable cholangiocarcinoma. Gastroenterology. 1998;114(3):536–42.
149. Ortner ME, Caca K, Berr F, Liebetruth J, Mansmann U, Huster D, et al. Successful photodynamic therapy for nonresectable cholangiocarcinoma: a randomized prospective study. Gastroenterology. 2003;125(5):1355–63.

Chapter 14
Autoimmune Liver Diseases: Primary Sclerosing Cholangitis

José Franco

Abbreviations

AIDS	Acquired immune deficiency syndrome
ALT	Alanine aminotransferase
AST	Aspartate aminotransferase
CT	Computerized tomography
DEXA	Dual energy X-ray absorptiometry
ERC	Endoscopic retrograde cholangiography
FISH	Fluorescent in situ hybridization
IBD	Inflammatory bowel disease
IgG4	Immunoglobulin G4
MELD	Model for end-stage liver disease
MRC	Magnetic resonance cholangiography
MRI	Magnetic resonance imaging
P-ANCA	Perinuclear antineutrophil cytoplasmic antibodies
PSC	Primary sclerosing cholangitis
PTC	Percutaneous transhepatic cholangiography
SAM-E	S-adenosylmethionine

J. Franco (✉)
Division of Gastroenterology and Hepatology,
Medical College of Wisconsin, 8700 West Wisconsin Avenue,
Milwaukee, WI 53226, USA
e-mail: jfranco@mcw.edu

© Springer International Publishing Switzerland 2016
K. Dua, R. Shaker (eds.), *Pancreas and Biliary Disease*,
DOI 10.1007/978-3-319-28089-9_14

TIPS   Transjugular intrahepatic portosystemic shunt
UDCA   Ursodeoxycholic acid
UNOS   United Network for Organ Sharing

Patient Questions and Answers

What Is Primary Sclerosing Cholangitis and How Did I Get It?

Primary sclerosing cholangitis, or PSC for short, is a chronic liver disease that leads to strictures or narrowing of the large and small bile ducts in the liver. The bile ducts are the plumbing of the liver and serve to move products produced in the liver to the small intestine, where they perform functions necessary for survival. While the exact cause of PSC remains unclear, it is frequently classified as an autoimmune disease. This means that it may be the result of an overactive or abnormal immune system. Patients with PSC frequently have other autoimmune disorders with the most common being inflammation of the colon, or colitis. Unfortunately, there is no effective therapy that prevents the progression of PSC and many patients will develop advanced liver disease and possibly cirrhosis which is severe, irreversible scarring of the liver. It is important to recognize that PSC is not associated with alcohol use, specific diets or behaviors. Primary sclerosing cholangitis is not the result of an infection or exposure to other individuals. You cannot transmit PSC to other individuals.

What Can I Do to Treat Primary Sclerosing Cholangitis?

It is important to remember that your PSC is not the result of anything you have done wrong. While not related to alcohol, it is important to avoid alcohol as regular alcohol use can by itself lead to liver damage. As with all chronic liver diseases, you should be checked for immunity or protection to hepatitis A and B. If tests show that you are not protected, you should undergo vaccination. Both of these vaccines are safe and effective. It is important to maintain a healthy diet as patients who are able to accomplish this are better able to tolerate chronic illnesses, including PSC. Because of the strong association with colitis (inflammation of the colon), you should undergo a colonoscopy (a test to examine your colon) unless you have already had one. Primary sclerosing cholangitis can also lead to difficulty absorbing certain vitamins such as vitamin D. When patients have low vitamin D levels it can lead to thinning of the bones, osteoporosis and possible bone fractures. Because of this, you should undergo a test known as a bone densitometry to determine whether you are at risk for developing bone disease.

There is no specific medicine that has been shown to be effective in slowing the progression of PSC. While it is classified as an autoimmune disorder, it does not respond to medications that are effective against other autoimmune conditions. While you may want to explore alternative or natural therapies such as herbal therapies, I would discourage you from using these substances as they are frequently not regulated by the Food and Drug Administration and in some cases have also been shown to be harmful to the liver. You should always let all of your doctors know of any medicine you are taking, as some medicines may not be as well tolerated by patients with liver disease such as PSC.

Will I Need a Liver Transplant?

The natural history of PSC is highly variable. Some patients present at a young age and have an aggressive course leading to the need for liver transplantation, while others will carry a diagnosis of PSC for many years and not require liver transplantation or die from this condition. Since PSC is a progressive disease and there is no known effective medical therapy, it will be important that you follow-up with a hepatologist or liver doctor on a regular basis even if you do not have any symptoms. During these visits you will be asked about symptoms as well as undergo a physical exam and blood tests that will allow your hepatologist to determine the overall status of the PSC and when a liver transplant evaluation should be considered. Your hepatologist may determine that a repeat examination of your bile ducts is necessary, particularly if there is suspicion that a cancer has developed in the bile ducts. Cancer of the bile ducts is known as cholangiocarcinoma. You should have an ultrasound of the liver and gallbladder every year as there in an increased risk of developing both liver and gallbladder cancer. You should contact your physicians immediately if you experience symptoms including jaundice or yellowing of the eyes and skin, worsening itching throughout your body which is most noticeable at night, fever, weight loss, and abdominal pain which most commonly occurs in the area over your liver.

Autoimmune Liver Diseases: Primary Sclerosing Cholangitis

Summary

Primary sclerosing cholangitis (PSC) is a chronic condition characterized by inflammation, fibrosis and obliteration involving the intra as well as extrahepatic bile ducts. Initially described in 1924 and once considered a rare condition, the condition can no longer be considered rare as advancements in cholangiography have led to more frequent diagnosis. While the etiology remains elusive, it is commonly classified as an autoimmune liver disease and other immune-mediated conditions, most notably inflammatory bowel disease, are frequently concurrently encountered. Genetic predisposition also appears to play a contributory role based on the finding of associated as well as protective haplotypes. Complications of PSC are both nonspecific and associated with chronic cholestatic liver disease as well as those specific to PSC. The natural history is highly variable with the potential for progression to cirrhosis, end-stage liver disease and the need for liver transplantation. Patients with PSC are also at an increased risk for the development of cholangiocarcinoma as well as colorectal, gallbladder and hepatocellular carcinoma. Despite the evaluations of multiple pharmacologic agents, there is currently no medical therapy that has been shown to alter the timeline to death or the need for liver transplantation. Liver transplantation is the only effective therapy for long-term survival in those who develop complications of end-stage liver disease and is associated with excellent long-term results. Variants of PSC include small-duct PSC, overlap PSC and autoimmune hepatitis and immunoglobulin G cholangiopathy.

Epidemiology

Various epidemiological studies have placed the incidence of PSC from 0.9 to 1.31 cases per 100,000 person-years and the prevalence at 8.5 to 13.6 cases per 100,000 persons [1, 2]. There is however, significant regional variability which supports the theory of genetic predisposition playing a role. Sixty to 70 % of affected patients have underlying inflammatory bowel disease (IBD), more frequently chronic Ulcerative Colitis than Crohn Disease with colonic involvement [3, 4]. The IBD is typically diagnosed several years prior to PSC [5]. In addition, while associated with IBD, the two disorders' activity level and progression do not necessarily correlate. Approximately two-thirds of those affected with PSC are male with the median age at diagnosis of approximately 37 [2].

Etiology

While the exact etiology of PSC remains unknown, it appears that both genetic and immunologic factors play prominent roles.

Genetics

Evidence supporting a genetic cause includes strong familial patterns as well as a strong association with specific haplotypes, most notably B8DR3, B8DR13, and B8DR15. Conversely, haplotypes DRB1*040, DRB1*070, and MICA*002 are associated with a decreased risk of developing PSC [6–9].

Immune-Mediated

An immune mechanism is supported by the findings of serum autoantibodies in a large number of those with PSC, the most common being perinuclear antineutrophil cytoplasmic antibodies (p-ANCA) which are found in up to two-thirds of patients. Other autoantibodies occasionally encountered include antinuclear and anti-smooth muscle antibodies [10]. Additionally, hypergammaglobulinemia is common as is the association with other autoimmune disorders, most notably inflammatory bowel disease.

Other potential etiologies that may play minor roles in PSC include infectious causes, toxin exposure and vascular complications.

Infectious

The association of PSC with IBD has led to the theory that damaged colonic mucosa leads to translocation of bacteria that enter the blood stream and bile ducts. The failure to identify specific organisms, the absence of portal phlebitis, failure of antibiotics or colectomy to alter the natural history and the fact that not all patients with PSC have IBD argues against an infectious etiology.

Toxin-mediated

Toxin exposure as a cause of PSC is based on the theory that imbalances between hydrophilic and hydrophobic bile acids, such as lithocolic acid, can lead to biliary epithelial damage and strictures. Other toxic agents that have been evaluated include iron and copper, both of which are shown to be elevated in many patients with PSC. Elevated iron and copper levels however, are nonspecific findings and can be associated with both hepatocellular and cholestatic disorders.

Vascular Injury

Vascular injury to the hepatic artery has long been associated with biliary strictures in liver transplant recipients; however, examination of the hepatic vasculature in PSC has failed to demonstrate damage to the hepatic artery, portal vein, or hepatic vein.

Clinical Presentation

The clinical presentation of patients affected by PSC is highly variable. At one end of the spectrum is the asymptomatic patient who is diagnosed based on cholestatic hepatic biochemistries obtained in the setting of IBD. The majority of patients with PSC will be diagnosed when presenting with symptoms that lead to further investigation. The most common presenting symptoms are pruritus, jaundice, right upper quadrant abdominal pain and acute cholangitis. Unfortunately, some patients will present with advanced liver disease manifested by weight loss, ascites, hepatic encephalopathy, portal hypertensive bleeding, or cholangiocarcinoma.

Diagnosis

Laboratories

The majority of patients with PSC will demonstrate cholestasis on hepatic biochemistries. Alkaline phosphatase values greater than 2.5-fold normal values are seen in the majority of patients. As a result, elevated alkaline phosphatase values which are confirmed to be of biliary origin should result in a thorough evaluation and consideration for PSC. Total bilirubin values are elevated in over 50 % of affected patients and 90 % demonstrate a two- to threefold elevation in alanine aminotransferase (ALT) and aspartate aminotransferase (AST). Serum iron and copper values are frequently elevated, but as previously mentioned, are nonspecific and therefore not helpful for diagnostic purposes. Despite the finding of p-ANCA autoantibodies in the majority of PSC patients, their presence is nonspecific and should not be utilized to make a diagnosis of PSC. This is in contrast to other autoimmune hepatic disorders such as autoimmune hepatitis and primary biliary cirrhosis where serum autoantibodies play a pivotal role in diagnosis.

Cholangiography

The diagnosis of PSC is made based on the classic cholangiographic findings of diffuse strictures with intervening areas of normal appearing bile ducts leading to the so-called "beading." Seventy-five percent of strictures involve both the intra and extrahepatic bile ducts, with 15 % having strictures limited to the extrahepatic system. The cystic duct and gallbladder are involved in approximately 15 % of patients and a smaller number have pancreatic duct involvement [11–13]. Dominant strictures, defined as a diameter less than 1.5 mm in the common bile duct and less than 1.0 mm in the hepatic duct, are present in approximately half of PSC patients. Pseudodiverticula, particularly in the common bile duct, are occasionally seen. While initially used as exclusionary criteria in PSC patients, the presence of biliary stones are now well-recognized as a common finding and frequent cause of cholangitis. There are three current modalities that can be used to image the biliary system. Endoscopic retrograde cholangiography (ERC) allows direct biliary visualization as well as also providing the opportunity to perform cytologic analysis, stricture dilation, removal of stones and biliary stenting. Potential complications of ERC include bleeding, cholangitis and pancreatitis [14]. Percutaneous hepatic cholangiography (PTC) also allows direct access to the biliary system but has similar complications to ERC and requires experienced radiologists as intrahepatic bile ducts are generally not dilated in PSC. The test of choice when attempting to make a diagnosis of PSC is the magnetic resonance cholangiography (MRC). The noninvasive nature of MRC limits complications and is more cost-effective than ERC or PTC. These advantages must be weighed against the fact that MRC unlike ERC and PTC does not offer the opportunity to perform biliary brushings for cytology nor intervene therapeutically. Magnetic resonance cholangiography also lacks sensitivity compared to ERC when assessing for peripheral bile duct changes. Once a diagnosis of PSC is established, there is no indication for further instrumentation of the biliary system unless there is a change in the patient's clinical status.

Histology

Liver biopsy at the present is not felt to be necessary to establish a diagnosis of PSC, nor to determine disease severity. Liver biopsy should be considered in all patients suspected of having small-duct PSC or overlap syndrome with autoimmune hepatitis. The classic finding when a liver biopsy is performed in PSC patients is the concentric fibrosis (onion-skinning) involving the periductal region. This lesion however is observed in only a minority of patients [12].

Additionally, biopsy sampling variation may fail to detect these lesions in patients who otherwise have classic cholangiographic findings.

Natural History

The natural history of PSC is highly variable and while it is a progressive disease, the rate of progression per year varies significantly in individual patients. Multiple studies have attempted to determine the time period from diagnosis to the need for liver transplantation or death and estimates range from 7 to 18 years from presentation [4, 15, 16]. Much of this variability is associated with the fact that some patients present early in their disease course without symptoms but have abnormal liver biochemistries, while others' initial presentation may be a complication of advanced disease with portal hypertension or cholangiocarcinoma.

Various prognostic models have been utilized in an attempt to predict future outcomes but their value is questionable in this clinical setting due the highly variable nature of PSC. The most common employed of these prognostic models is one proposed by the Mayo Clinic and utilizes the following variables: total bilirubin, age, presence or absence of variceal bleeding, serum albumin and aspartate aminotransferase values [17].

Primary Sclerosing Cholangitis Variants

Small-Duct Primary Sclerosing Cholangitis

Small-duct PSC is characterized by cholestatic biochemistries with a normal cholangiogram. Liver biopsy is essential in this group for diagnostic purposes and may demonstrate the periductal damage and onion-skinning previously described. Small-duct PSC represents approximately 10 % of all PSC cases. Small-duct PSC patients may have symptoms but a greater percentage are asymptomatic when compared to large-duct PSC. Approximately 10–15 % of those with small-duct PSC will progress to large-duct PSC, typically over 5–10 years. Patients with small-duct PSC have a better long-term prognosis with fewer complications when compared to their large-duct counterparts [18, 19].

Overlap Syndrome with Autoimmune Hepatitis

Between 1 and 17 % of patients with PSC will also have an overlap syndrome with autoimmune hepatitis [20–22]. These patients will present with a hepatocellular injury as well as cholestasis and have detectable antinuclear antibodies and anti-smooth muscle antibodies. Immunoglobulin G elevations, as in classical autoimmune hepatitis, are typically seen. Liver biopsy should therefore be performed in all patients with PSC who have aminotransferase values greater than five times the upper limit of normal or IgG values greater than two times the upper limit of normal. Liver biopsy demonstrates histologic findings of both conditions; the periductal "onion-skinning" damage seen in PSC and the interface hepatitis and prominent plasma cell infiltration which is classically described in autoimmune hepatitis. The autoimmune hepatitis component unlike the PSC component is responsive to immunosuppression, with the most common agents utilized being corticosteroids and azathioprine. Patients with overlap PSC and autoimmune hepatitis may progress more rapidly than those affected by PSC alone due to the combination of the hepatocellular and cholestatic components.

Primary Sclerosing Cholangitis in Association with Autoimmune Pancreatitis

Autoimmune pancreatitis is a manifestation of a systemic disorder affecting multiple organs and is associated with an elevated serum immunoglobulin G4 (IgG4). Histology of the pancreas shows a predominantly lymphocyte and plasma cell infiltrate. Pancreatic abnormalities include lesions that are frequently difficult to differentiate from malignancy as well as pancreatic duct strictures. A subset of these patients will have biliary strictures similar to those seen in PSC occasionally in the absence of pancreatic abnormalities, a condition occasionally referred to as IgG4 cholangiopathy. Those with IgG4 cholangiopathy tend to have a more aggressive disease course compared to those with PSC and normal IgG4 values [23, 24]. Primary sclerosing cholangitis associated with elevated IgG4 levels are frequently responsive to corticosteroid therapy and it is recommended to measure IgG4 levels in all newly diagnosed PSC patients [25].

Secondary Sclerosing Cholangitis

There are various conditions that can affect the biliary system and produce findings that mimic the strictures seen in PSC. Prior to making a diagnosis of PSC these secondary causes must be carefully looked for and eliminated as potential etiologies. Secondary causes include congenital biliary tract disorders such as biliary atresia and Caroli's Disease, AIDS cholangiopathy, ischemic strictures, biliary malignancies such as cholangiocarcinoma not associated with PSC, previous biliary injuries as a result of surgery and chemical exposure to toxins such as floxuridine, a pyrimidine analogue infused via the hepatic artery in patients with metastatic colon cancer to the liver [26].

Complications of Primary Sclerosing Cholangitis

Complications of PSC can be classified as those that are related to the cholestatic nature of the disorder and those that are unique to PSC.

Complications of Cholestatic Liver Disease

Cholestasis-related complications include pruritus, bone disease, fat soluble vitamin deficiency and portal hypertension.

Pruritus

Pruritus can be one of the most disabling complications of cholestatic liver diseases with failure to respond to therapy frequently leading to frustration in both patients and clinicians. While much attention has been focused on the accumulation of biliary compounds in various tissues, the exact mechanism remains unknown [27]. There does not appear to be a strong correlation with the severity of liver disease and patients with mild to moderate biliary strictures may have the most severe symptoms. The subjective nature of pruritus makes accurate measurement difficult and while multiple tools including visual aids are available, they are not generally utilized in clinical practice. The treatment of pruritus generally involves a stepwise approach. First line therapy typically involves anion exchange resins such as cholestyramine initially at four grams twice daily (before and after breakfast if the gallbladder is present) and increasing to four times daily as necessary [28]. Patients must communicate with their pharmacist in order to ensure that cholestyramine does not interfere with the absorption of other medications or fat-soluble vitamins. Side effects include mild constipation, diarrhea, abdominal pain, flatulence, nausea, and vomiting. If the pruritus remains refractory, rifampin at doses of 150 mg to 300 mg twice daily can be added with careful monitoring of serum liver and renal biochemistries [29]. Additional first line agents include Sertraline, a selective serotonin uptake inhibitor, at 100 mg daily and nighttime antihistamines due to their sedative side-effect profile. Second line therapies include naltrexone, an opioid antagonist, at 50 mg daily and phenobarbital at doses of 60 mg to 100 mgs nightly [30]. Third line therapies include plasmapheresis which is effective but cumbersome. Therapies that have been proposed but lack supporting data include dronabinol, ondansetron, ultraviolet light, and S-adenosylmethionine (SAM-E). Liver transplant has been proposed for patients with severe, refractory pruritus despite low Model for End Stage Liver Disease (MELD) scores. Exception points for patients with low MELD scores can be requested due to refractory pruritus but the subjective nature of this complication has led to few exceptions being granted.

Bone Disease

Bone disease in the setting of chronic liver diseases is frequently referred to as hepatic osteodystrophy and includes osteopenia and osteoporosis. Both are now recognized as a frequent finding in all patients with chronic liver diseases but are most pronounced in those with cholestasis [31]. The mechanism for bone disease in PSC is likely multifactorial and includes decreased formation and increased resorption. Vitamin D deficiency may play a minor role. Longer duration of IBD, older age, female gender and low body weight are other contributing factors. All patients with newly diagnosed PSC should undergo bone mineral density assessment (DEXA) and at intervals of 2–3 years based on initial results [32, 33]. Treatment includes calcium 1200 mg daily and vitamin D 1000 IU supplementation. This supplementation should be in conjunction with a regular exercise regimen. Hormone replacement while effective is not generally employed due to the side-effect profile. Bisphosphonate therapy is beneficial in patients with osteoporosis and primary biliary cirrhosis and is also indicated for those with osteoporosis and PSC [34]. Bisphosphonates should be avoided in those patients with esophageal varices as they have been shown to increase the risk of bleeding due to esophageal ulcerations. Intravenous bisphosphonates are effective options in those with osteoporosis who have contraindications to oral therapy due to esophageal varices.

Fat-Soluble Vitamin Deficiency

Patients with cholestatic hepatic disorders including PSC are at risk for developing malabsorption and deficiency of vitamins A, D, E and K due to decrease in the availability of bile salts [35]. While bile salt production from cholesterol and bile acids is normal, the impaired flow of bile salts due to biliary strictures results in a relative deficiency in bile salt function in the small intestine. Vitamin A deficiency is rarely of clinical consequence. Levels can be measured and effective supplementation is available. Care must be taken to avoid vitamin A toxicity from over-supplementation. Vitamin D deficiency is the most clinically significant of all the fat-soluble vitamin deficiencies. As previously mentioned, by itself it is not responsible for bone disease, but likely plays a contributing role. Vitamin D levels are also easily measured and supplemented. Vitamin E deficiency is rare and can be supplemented if serum levels are decreased. Vitamin K deficiency can lead to elevated prothrombin times and typically responds well to supplementation.

Portal Hypertension

Patients with PSC frequently progress to cirrhosis and develop portal hypertension complicated by esophageal and gastric varices, ascites and hepatic encephalopathy. These patients should be treated similar to non-PSC cirrhotic patients. While current recommendations are for all patients with cirrhosis to undergo an upper endoscopy to evaluate for varices, those affected by PSC are also at risk for the development of pre-cirrhotic, pre-sinusoidal portal hypertension and should therefore undergo endoscopic evaluation. Non-selective beta blockade for primary prophylaxis of documented varices is effective with band ligation utilized in those intolerant of beta blockers. Sodium restricted diets in combination with diuretics, most commonly spironolactone and furosemide, are the standard of care in patients with ascites. Beta blockers should be avoided in PSC patients with refractory ascites due to concerns for the development of acute kidney injury. Avoidance of factors that precipitate hepatic encephalopathy including intravascular volume depletion, infections, gastrointestinal bleeding and electrolyte disturbances are paramount. Minimal hepatic encephalopathy, as well as overt encephalopathy, should be treated with lactulose and if necessary the addition of rifaximin as a second agent.

Complications Specific to Primary Sclerosing Cholangitis

Disease specific complications associated with PSC include IBD and colorectal cancer, peristomal varices, dominant strictures, biliary stones, gallbladder carcinoma, and cholangiocarcinoma.

Inflammatory Bowel Disease and Colorectal Carcinoma

The majority of patients with PSC will have concurrent IBD, more frequently ulcerative colitis than Crohn Disease with colonic involvement. Up to 7.5 % of IBD patients will be affected by PSC [3, 4]. The IBD is typically diagnosed prior to PSC in the majority of patients, but can vary with some patients' first symptoms of IBD being years after the diagnosis of PSC or even following liver transplantation. Inflammatory Bowel Disease in the setting of PSC differs from those not affected by PSC with more rectal sparing, greater right-sided disease, more backwash ileitis and more quiescent disease in those with PSC [36, 37]. While all patients with chronic colitis are at increased risk for the development of colorectal cancer, those IBD patients with PSC are at a much greater risk [38]. Current recommendations include colonoscopy every 1–2 years in those IBD patients who also carry a diagnosis of PSC. Colon biopsies should always be obtained to evaluate for dysplastic changes. The use of ursodeoxycholic acid (UDCA) has been advocated by some as decreasing the risk of colonic dysplasia and colorectal carcinoma based on two small studies [39, 40], but subsequent studies have not supported its effectiveness. Patients with PSC and IBD who undergo liver transplant have been shown as a group to have more difficult to manage IBD despite the fact that their post-transplant medical regimen includes one or more immunosuppressive agents.

Peristomal Varices

Patients with concurrent IBD and PSC have frequently undergone proctocolectomy with ileostomy formation due to refractory colitis or colorectal cancer. These patients will occasionally develop peristomal varices. While not associated with the mortality seen in patients with esophageal or gastric variceal bleeding, the morbidity and impact on quality of life can be significant. Local temporizing measures have been of limited efficacy with transjugular intrahepatic portosystemic shunt (TIPS) proving to be beneficial in refractory cases if no contraindications exist.

Dominant Biliary Strictures

Dominant strictures, defined as a diameter less than 1.5 mm in the common bile duct and less than 1 mm in the hepatic duct, are seen in up to half of all PSC patients [41, 42]. The length of these strictures varies but are typically short. Dominant strictures can result in deterioration of previously stable disease and lead to worsening jaundice, pruritus and cholangitis. Strictures should be promptly addressed with endoscopic therapy being the preferred method. Following sphincterotomy, balloon dilation of the stricture with stent placement is frequently necessary. The need for stents, their associated exchanges and instrumentation increases the risk of cholangitis and mandates the need for pre and post-procedure antibiotics. Unfortunately, strictures in the intrahepatic region are not always accessible endoscopically and may require a percutaneous approach. Finally, it is imperative to perform brush cytology of dominant strictures whether by endoscopic or percutaneous approaches to differentiate dominant non-malignant strictures from cholangiocarcinoma.

Biliary Stones

As previously mentioned, biliary stones, once considered exclusionary for PSC, are now recognized as a common finding. Strictures, in particular dominant strictures, and impaired bile flow play key roles in stone formation. Complications include pain, cholangitis, and clinical deterioration. Aggressive antibiotic use particularly for biliary pathogens and prompt endoscopic stone retrieval are indicated. While there may be a role for UDCA to prevent stone formation and improve bile flow, little data currently exists.

Gallbladder Disease Including Adenocarcinoma

Primary sclerosing cholangitis involves the gallbladder as well as the cystic duct in 15 % of patients. Gallstones, which are common in the general population, are seen in up to 26 % of PSC patients [13]. Patients with PSC are also at risk for the development of mass lesions. Gallbladder polyps in particular are common and can lead to dysplasia and adenocarcinoma [43]. Current recommendations include performing annual gallbladder ultrasounds to evaluate for mass lesions and if present for the patients to undergo cholecystectomy regardless of the size of the lesion unless contraindications exists [32].

Cholangiocarcinoma

One of the most feared complications of PSC is the development of cholangiocarcinoma. Approximately 50 % of patients diagnosed with cholangiocarcinoma will be diagnosed within one year of their PSC diagnosis. Afterwards the annual risk is 0.5–1.0 % with a 10-year risk of 7–10 % [44–47]. Unfortunately, a large number have advanced disease including locoregional as well as distant disease at the time of diagnosis. It remains unclear as to what specific factors in PSC patients predispose them to develop cholangiocarcinoma. The differentiation between benign strictures and cholangiocarcinoma, particularly in dominant strictures, remains a challenge. Biochemical testing with CA19-9 is limited by the fact that it is nonspecific and can be elevated from benign strictures and cholangitis. Patients who lack the Lewis antigen will not demonstrate detectable CA19-9 even in the presence of cholangiocarcinoma. Imaging studies with computerized tomography, ultrasound, MRC, and ERC fail to consistently differentiate benign from malignant strictures. Biliary brushing done at the time of ERC have long been recognized to have good specificity but sensitivities under 50 %. Newer approaches to aid in the diagnosis of cholangiocarcinoma include fluorescent in situ hybridization (FISH). This technique evaluates cells obtained from suspicious lesions by brush cytology and evaluates for polysomy (the duplication of two or more chromosomes) in greater than five cells [48]. At the present time, there are no formal recommendations from any society regarding cholangiocarcinoma screening and surveillance with CA19-9, MRC, cholangioscopy during ERC or other imaging modalities.

Treatment of cholangiocarcinoma has traditionally been limited. The diffuse biliary nature of PSC has made surgical resection an option for a limited few and chemotherapy has not been shown to be of significant benefit. More recently, liver transplant in a highly selected group of patients with hilar lesions less than three cm in diameter and without evidence of spread has been evaluated. These patients undergo external beam as well as brachytherapy in conjunction with chemotherapy. Percutaneous transhepatic cholangiography should be avoided in these patients for fear of seeding the peritoneum with malignant cells. Some centers are reporting 5-year survival comparable to non-cholangiocarcinoma patients [49]. Transplant centers with an active protocol in place can petition regional review boards for MELD exception points for these patients.

Hepatocellular Carcinoma

While not unique to cholestatic liver diseases or PSC, patients with established cirrhosis are at risk for developing hepatocellular carcinoma (HCC). Screening and surveillance for HCC is indicated in all cirrhotic patients regardless of age and involves ultrasound examination every 6 months with suspicious lesions warranting further evaluation with a dynamic study such as CT or MRI [50]. The role of alpha fetoprotein for screening of HCC remains controversial and no recommendations can be made at this time.

Medical Therapy in Primary Sclerosing Cholangitis

Numerous agents have been evaluated in the treatment of PSC and there is no evidence to suggest that there is effective medical therapy. Agents that have been evaluated in small trials include corticosteroids, cyclosporine, tacrolimus, azathioprine, methotrexate, penicillamine, and colchicine. Antibiotics while indicated for invasive procedures and for episodes of cholangitis, do not alter the natural history of PSC. The most studied of all agents is ursodeoxycholic acid (UDCA) which has been shown to slow disease progression and alter the natural history in patients with primary biliary cirrhosis (PBC) at doses ranging from 13 to 15 mg/kg/day [51]. Similar doses in PSC patients resulted in biochemical improvement but failed to alter the natural history [52]. Due to the large bile duct involvement in PSC relative to PBC, it was theorized that greater doses would be necessary for a benefit to be seen. Despite increasing doses, this benefit did not materialize and a multicenter trial evaluating doses of 28 to 30 mg/kg/day was terminated due to an increased frequency of decompensation, need for transplant and death in the treatment group [53]. As previously mentioned, corticosteroid therapy is indicated in patients with IgG4-associated cholangitis and in combination with azathioprine in those with PSC-AIH overlap.

Liver Transplantation for Primary Sclerosing Cholangitis

Liver transplantation has been shown to be the only effective therapy that alters the natural history of PSC with approximately 250 transplants performed annually in the USA for PSC. Listing for liver transplantation is overseen and regulated by the United Network for Organ Sharing (UNOS) and utilizes the MELD score to determine listing priority. Refractory pruritus, recurrent bacterial cholangitis, and cholangiocarcinoma are PSC-specific complications that will be considered by regional review boards for MELD exception points [54]. Due to the diffuse biliary strictures associated with PSC as well as the risk of future cholangiocarcinoma in the recipient remnant bile duct, the biliary anastomosis performed at the time of transplantation is a Roux-Y-choledochojejunostomy. Overall results following liver transplant for PSC are excellent with 5-year survival of approximately 85 %. Recurrent PSC in the transplant liver occurs in approximately 20 % of patients and will occasionally result in the need for retransplantation [55, 56]. Biliary strictures which can be due to other factors including ischemia and hepatic artery injury are frequently difficult to differentiate from recurrent PSC strictures. Biliary access for interventional purposes following liver transplant typically involves a percutaneous approach due to the Roux-Y-choledochojejunostomy biliary anastomosis.

Future Trends

There are three major areas in PSC that will require greater attention if we are to make significant impact on morbidity and mortality.

First, there is no effective medical therapy and this requires immediate attention. Large, multicenter, randomized controlled trials are urgently needed. Without medical therapy, physicians are forced to address complications while taking a wait and see approach regarding liver transplantation.

Second, consensus recommendations regarding cholangiocarcinoma screening and surveillance need to be developed. Imaging studies and/or biomarkers that are both cost-effective and have acceptable sensitivity and specificity are currently lacking. This has resulted in multiple imaging modalities usually in combination with CA 19-9 being employed despite lack of supporting data.

Finally, once a lesion that is suspicious for cholangiocarcinoma develops, current diagnostic testing including brush cytology and FISH are suboptimal. While the negative predictive value for the combination of brush cytology and FISH is 90 %, the positive predictive value is only 50 % [48]. Liver transplantation is now an effective therapy in selected patients with cholangiocarcinoma. It is essential that patients with cholangiocarcinoma be identified as early as possible in order to undergo transplant evaluation at centers with established protocols.

References

1. Bambha K, Kim WR, Tawalkar J, Torgensen H, Benson J, Therneau T, et al. Incidence, clinical spectrum, and outcomes of primary sclerosing cholangitis in a United States community. Gastroenterology. 2003;125(5):1364–9.
2. Boberg KM, Aadland E, Jahnsen J, Raknerud M, Stiris H. Incidence and prevalence of primary biliary cirrhosis, primary sclerosing cholangitis, and autoimmune hepatitis in a Norwegian population. Scand J Gastroenterol. 1999;33(1):99–103.

3. Schrumpf E, Fausa O, Elgio K, Kolmannskog F. Hepatobiliary complications of inflammatory bowel disease. Semin Liver Dis. 1988;8:201–9.
4. Wiesner R, Grambsch P, Dickson E, Ludwig J, MacCarty R, Hunter E, et al. Primary sclerosing cholangitis: natural history, prognostic factors and survival analysis. Hepatology. 1989;10:430–6.
5. Loftus E, Harewood G, Loftus C, Tremaine W, Harmsen W, Zeinsmeister A, et al. PSC-IBD: a unique form of inflammatory bowel disease associated with primary sclerosing cholangitis. Gut. 2005;54:91–6.
6. Jorge A, Esley C, Ahamuda J. Family incidence of primary sclerosing cholangitis associated with immunologic diseases. Endoscopy. 1987;19:114–7.
7. Donaldson P, Farrant J, Wilkinson M, et al. Dual association of HLA DR2 and DR3 with primary sclerosing cholangitis. Hepatology. 1991;13:129–33.
8. Donaldson P, Doherty D, Haylar K, et al. Susceptibility to autoimmune chronic active hepatitis: human leukocyte antigens DR4 and A1-B8-DR3 are independent risk factors. Hepatology. 1991;13:701–6.
9. Norris S, Elli K, Collins R, Stephens H, Harrison P, Vaughan R, et al. Mapping MHC-encoded susceptibility and resistance in primary sclerosing cholangitis: the role of MICA polymorphism. Gastroenterology. 2001;120(6):1475–82.
10. Hov J, Boberg K, Karlsen T. Autoantibodies in primary sclerosing cholangitis. World J Gastroenterol. 2008;14:3781–91.
11. MacCarty R, LaRusso N, Wiesner R, Ludwig J. Primary sclerosing cholangitis: findings on cholangiography and pancreatography. Radiology. 1983;149:39–44.
12. Lee Y, Kaplan M. Primary sclerosing cholangitis. N Engl J Med. 1995;332:924–33.
13. Brandt D, MacCarty R, Charboneau J, LaRusso N, Wiesner R, Ludwig J. Gallbladder disease in patients with primary sclerosing cholangitis. Am J Roentgenol. 1988;150:571–4.
14. Navaneethan U, Jegadeesan R, Nayak S, Vennisavanth L, Madhusushan R, Vargo J, et al. ERCP-related adverse events in patients with primary sclerosing cholangitis. Gastrointest Endosc. 2015;81:410–9.
15. Aadland E, Schrumpf E, Fausa O, Heilo A, Aakhus T, Gjone E. Primary sclerosing cholangitis: a long-term follow-up study. Scand J Gastroenterol. 1987;22:655–64.

16. Farrant J, Hayllar K, Wilkinson M, et al. Natural history and prognostic variables in primary sclerosing cholangitis. Gastroenterology. 1991;100:1710–7.
17. http://www.mayoclinic.org/gi-rst/mayomodel3.html.
18. Wee A, Ludwig J. Pericholangitis in chronic ulcerative colitis; primary sclerosing cholangitis of the small bile ducts? Ann Intern Med. 1985;102:581–7.
19. Chapman R. Small duct primary sclerosing cholangitis. J Hepatol. 2002;36:692–4.
20. Van Buuren H, Hoogstraten H, Terkivatan T, Schalm S, Vleggaar F. High prevalence of autoimmune hepatitis among patients with primary sclerosing cholangitis. J Hepatol. 2000;33:543–8.
21. Kaya M, Angulo P, Lindor K. Overlap of autoimmune hepatitis and primary sclerosing cholangitis: an evaluation of a modified scoring system. J Hepatol. 2000;33:537–42.
22. Floreani A, Rizzotto E, Ferrerra F, et al. Clinical course and outcome of autoimmune hepatitis/primary sclerosing cholangitis overlap syndrome. Am J Gastroenterol. 2005;100:1516–22.
23. Bjornsson E, Chari S, Smyrk T, Lindor K. Immunoglobulin G4 associated cholangitis: description an emerging clinical entity based on review of the literature. Hepatology. 2007;45:1547–54.
24. Mendes F, Jorgensen R, Keach J, et al. Elevated serum IgG4 concentration in patients with primary sclerosing cholangitis. Am J Gastroenterol. 2006;101:2070–5.
25. Hamano H, Kawa S, Horiuchi A, Unno H, Furuya N, Akamatso T, et al. High serum IgG4 concentrations in patients with sclerosing pancreatitis. N Engl J Med. 2001;344:732–8.
26. Iman M, Talwalkar J, Lindor K. Secondary sclerosing cholangitis; pathogenesis, diagnosis and management. Clin Liver Dis. 2013;17:269–77.
27. Jones E, Vergasa N. The pruritus of cholestasis and the opioid system. JAMA. 1992;268:3359–62.
28. Datta D, Sherlock S. Treatment of pruritus of obstructive jaundice with cholestyramine. Br Med J. 1963;1:216–9.
29. Bachs L, Pares A, Elena M, et al. Effects of long-term rifampicin administration in primary biliary cirrhosis. Gastroenterology. 1992;102:2077–80.
30. Bloomer J, Boyer J. Phenobarbital effects in cholestatic liver diseases. Ann Intern Med. 1975;82:310–7.
31. Sokhi R, Anantharaju A, Kondaveeti R, Creech S, Islam K, Van Thiel D. Bone mineral density among cirrhotic patients awaiting liver transplantation. Liver Transpl. 2004;10:648–53.

32. Chapman R, Fevery J, Kalloo A, Nagorney D, Boberg K, Shneider B. Diagnosis and management of primary sclerosing cholangitis. AASLD practice guidelines. Hepatology. 2010;51:660–78.
33. Crippin J, Jorgensen R, Dickson E, et al. Hepatic osteodystrophy in primary biliary cirrhosis; effects of medical treatment. Am J Gastroenterol. 1994;89:47–50.
34. Zein C, Lindor K, Angulo P. Alendronate improves bone mineral density in primary biliary cirrhosis: a randomized placebo-controlled trial. Hepatology. 2005;42:62–771.
35. Phillips J, Angulo P, Petterson T, et al. Fat-soluble vitamin levels in patients with primary biliary cirrhosis. Am J Gastroenterol. 2001;96:2745–50.
36. Broome U, Bergquist A. Primary sclerosing cholangitis, inflammatory bowel disease, and colon cancer. Semin Liver Dis. 2006;26:31–41.
37. Schrumpf E, Elgio K, Fausa O, et al. Sclerosing cholangitis in ulcerative colitis. Scand J Gastroenterol. 1980;15:689–97.
38. Broome U, Lofberg R, Veress B, Eriksson L. Primary sclerosing cholangitis and ulcerative colitis: evidence for increased neoplastic potential. Hepatology. 1995;22:1404–8.
39. Pardi D, Loftus E, Kremers W, Keach J, Lindor K. Ursodeoxycholic acid as a chemopreventive agent in patients with ulcerative colitis and primary sclerosing cholangitis. Gastroenterology. 2003;124:889–93.
40. Tung B, Edmond M, Haggitt R, Bronner M, Kimmey B, Krowdley K, et al. Ursodiol use is associated with lower prevalence of colonic neoplasia in patients with ulcerative colitis and primary sclerosing cholangitis. Ann Intern Med. 2001;134:89–95.
41. Stiehl A, Rudolph G, Kloters-Plachky P, Sauer P, Siegfried W. Development of dominant bile duct stenosis in patients with primary sclerosing cholangitis treated with ursodeoxycholic acid: outcome after endoscopic treatment. J Hepatol. 2002;36:151–6.
42. Bjornsson E, Lindqvist-Ottosson J, Asztely M, et al. Dominant strictures in patients with primary sclerosing cholangitis. Am J Gastroenterol. 2004;99:502–8.
43. Lewis J, Talwalkar J, Rosen C, Smyrk T, Abraham S. Prevalence and risk factors for gallbladder neoplasia in patients with primary sclerosing cholangitis; evidence for a metaplasia-dysplasia-carcinoma sequence. Am J Surg Pathol. 2007;31:907–13.
44. Boberg K, Lind G. Primary sclerosing cholangitis and malignancy. Best Pract Res Clin Gastroenterol. 2011;25:753–64.

45. Bergquist A, Ekborn A, Olsson R, Kornfeldt D, Loof L, Danielsson A. Hepatic and extrahepatic malignancies in primary sclerosing cholangitis. J Hepatol. 2002;36:321–7.
46. Burak K, Angulo P, Pasha T, et al. Incidence and risk factors for cholangiocarcinoma in primary sclerosing cholangitis. Am J Gastroenterol. 2004;99:523–6.
47. Boberg K, Bergquist A, Mitchell S, Pares A, Broome U, Chapman R, et al. Cholangiocarcinoma in primary sclerosing cholangitis: risk factors and clinical presentation. Scand J Gastroenterol. 2003;37:1205–11.
48. Moreno L, Kipp B, Halling K, Sebo T, Kremer W, Roberts L, et al. Advanced cytologic techniques for the detection of malignant pancreatobiliary strictures. Gastroenterology. 2006;131:1064–72.
49. Rea D, Heimbach J, Rosen C, Haddock M, Alberts S, Kremers W, et al. Liver transplantation with neoadjuvant chemoradiation is more effective than resection for hilar cholangiocarcinoma. Ann Surg. 2005;242:451–8.
50. Bruix J, Sherman M. Management of hepatocellular carcinoma; an update. AASLD practice guidelines. Hepatology. 2005;42:1208–36.
51. Coperchot C, Carrat F, Bahr A, Chretien Y, Poupon R-E, Poupon R. The effect of ursodeoxycholic acid therapy on the natural history of primary biliary cirrhosis. Gastroenterology. 2005;128:297–303.
52. Lindor K. Ursodiol for primary sclerosing cholangitis. Mayo Primary Sclerosing Cholangitis–Ursodeoxycholic Acid Study Group. N Engl J Med. 1997;336:691–5.
53. Lindor K, Kowdley K, Velimir A, Harrison E, McCashland T, Befeler A, et al. High-dose ursodeoxycholic acid for the treatment of primary sclerosing cholangitis. Hepatology. 2008;50:808–14.
54. Gores G, Nagorney D, Rosen C. Cholangiocarcinoma: is transplantation an option? For whom? Hepatology. 2007;47:455–9.
55. Graziadei I, Wiesner R, Marotta P, Porayko M, Hay J, Charlton M, et al. Long-term results of patients undergoing liver transplantation for primary sclerosing cholangitis. Hepatology. 1999;30:1121–7.
56. Campsen J, Zimmerman M, Trotter J, Wachs M, Bak T, Steinberg T, et al. Clinically recurrent primary sclerosing cholangitis following liver transplantation; a time course. Liver Transpl. 2008;14:181–5.

Part 6
Clinical Scenario: Painless Jaundice

Chapter 15
Point-of-Care Clinical Guide: Gallbladder Cancer

Abdulrahman Y. Hammad, Natesh Shivakumar, and T. Clark Gamblin

Patient's Perspective: Questions on Gallbladder Cancer

What Are the Main Risk Factors for Gallbladder Cancer? Is My Family at Increased Risk?

Gallbladder cancer affects women more than men with a ratio of 3:1. The disease has a geographical distribution with very high rates in Bolivia, Chili, Ecuador, followed by Asian countries such as China and Japan.

There is a strong association between gallstones and gallbladder cancer. Gallstones are present in up to 75 % of people affected with gallbladder cancer. Porcelain gallbladder and large adenomatous polyps signify higher risk. A higher incidence of gallbladder cancer is also present in patients with gallbladder infections such as typhoid bacillus.

A.Y. Hammad, M.D. • N. Shivakumar
• T.C. Gamblin, M.D., M.S. (✉)
Division of Surgical Oncology, Medical College of Wisconsin,
9200 West Wisconsin Avenue, Milwaukee, WI 53226-3596, USA
e-mail: tcgamblin@mcw.edu

© Springer International Publishing Switzerland 2016
K. Dua, R. Shaker (eds.), *Pancreas and Biliary Disease,*
DOI 10.1007/978-3-319-28089-9_15

There is an increased risk of GC among first degree relatives with studies showing a relative risk of 4.8 (95 % CI: 2.4–8.5). However, gall bladder cancer is such a rare cancer the overall risk that family members will be affected is still very low.

I Was Diagnosed with a Stage II Disease, What Are My Options? Will I Need to Receive Chemotherapy or Radiation After My Surgery for Gallbladder Cancer?

Surgical resection represents the core of gallbladder cancer management. Patients with stage II disease typically receive a laparoscopic evaluation of their disease followed by the removal of their gallbladder, gallbladder bed, and a part of the adjacent liver tissue. Clear resection margins signify a more successful operation, with a higher chance of survival.

Generally radiation and chemotherapy are not used postoperatively for gallbladder cancer. Scarce reports show that radiotherapy may provide benefit for patients with stage≥2. As for chemotherapy, there is no evidence to support its delivery following a successful operation. However, chemotherapy can be used for those with advanced diseases as evidence suggests that a combination of gemcitabine and cisplatin provides a survival advantage.

Gall Bladder Cancer and Cholangiocarcinoma

Overview

Gallbladder cancer is an uncommon disease that carries a high mortality rate due to its often late presentation. The disease follows a slow steady asymptomatic growth, and may be discovered incidentally at an earlier stage during a cholecystectomy. Gallbladder cancer possesses an infiltrating growth pattern towards the neighboring portal vasculature.

Historically, in 1924 Alfred Blalock stated that "no operation should be performed" following the diagnosis of gallbladder cancer, as surgery will only shorten the patient's life [1]. This nihilistic view was carried for years due to patients' limited survival. Recent studies report a decline in mortality rates in several parts of the world, although survival remains dismal for advanced stages. Gallbladder cancer is more commonly seen in South American countries such as Chile, Bolivia, and Ecuador, followed by Eastern Asian Countries such as Japan and South Korea. Lower incidence of the disease is reported in Europe; and the North American continent is considered a low risk area. No clear factors are associated with the development of gallbladder cancer; yet some risk factors are frequently linked to it. In the next sections, possible risk factors are discussed followed by clinical presentation, investigations, and treatment considerations for patients with gallbladder cancer.

Epidemiology

Gallbladder cancer (GBC) is the most common biliary tract neoplasm and the fourth most common upper gastrointestinal malignancy worldwide. The disease shows a predilection for females older than 65 years [2, 3]. The female–male (F/M) ratio of the disease varies worldwide and is typically around 2.5/1. Higher F/M ratios exist in countries with high risk such as Pakistan, Columbia, and Spain, while countries such as Japan, Korea, and China approach a 1:1 ratio.

Worldwide, the highest incidence of GBC is reported in Bolivia and Chile (15/100,000), followed by eastern Asian countries such as South Korea, and Japan. Eastern European countries exhibit intermediate incidence rates, while lower rates (<3/100,000) are reported in the US, the UK, and New Zealand. Reports show different incidence rates in ethnic groups, suggesting a possible contribution of ethnicity towards the risk of disease [4].

In the US, the incidence of the disease is lower than other parts of the world. A previous analysis of the Surveillance,

Epidemiology and End Results (SEER) database revealed an overall incidence of 1–2 cases/100,000 [5]. The Caucasian population exhibit a 50 % increased likelihood of diagnosis compared to the African American population. Hispanic women in California and New Mexico has the highest incidence among all US ethnic groups (8.2/100,000 and 5.4/100,000, respectively) [4]. Subsequent reports show a decline in the incidence of the disease that is more noticeable in American Indians followed by Hispanics and non-Hispanics [6].

Analysis of mortality trends worldwide indicated minimal mortality changes in countries with low risk of the disease, such as Spain and Italy, although other countries such as Australia, Canada, and the UK displayed a declining mortality rate. Countries with high risk of the disease, such as Chile or Japan, have experienced an increase in GBC mortality [3]. In the USA, a decrease in cancer-related mortality was seen for the period between 1980 and 1995 [3].

Nihilism associated with gallbladder cancer has recently begun to change. An analysis of the SEER demonstrated a median survival of 19 months for patients with stage I disease, 7 months for stage II, 4 months for stage III and 2 months for patients presenting with stage IV disease, representing an improvement from previous reports [7, 8]. The wide geographical and ethnic variability associated with gallbladder cancer suggests multifactorial causes and is the focus of future strategies.

Etiology

Cholelithiasis (Gallstones)

Gallstones are an established risk factor for gallbladder cancer, and up to 90 % of patients with GBC have a history of gallstones [9–11]. Previous studies reported signs of epithelial hyperplasia, atypical hyperplasia and carcinoma in situ in cholecystectomy specimens of patients having a history of cholelithiasis [12]. Patients with gallstones carry a relative risk (RR) of 3.6–4.4 for GBC [4, 13]. A positive correlation exists between the size of gall stones and the cancer risk. Patients with stones ≥3 cm have a 9.2–10.1 RR of GBC compared to those with stones <3 cm [14, 15].

Larger stones are associated with epithelial inflammation of greater duration and intensity, and may promote dysplasia, inducing carcinoma [3]. Furthermore, the bacterial breakdown of some bile components and the subsequent production of endogenous carcinogen may add to the inflammatory process [3]. This theory is challenged by the fact that only a minority of patients with gallstones actually develop cancer (1–3 %), suggesting that other genetic and environmental risk factors contribute [16, 17].

Porcelain Gallbladder

Gallbladder wall calcification may occur as a consequence of long standing inflammation. The term "porcelain gallbladder" refers to the pathological presence of widespread calcifications, in association with discoloration and brittle consistency of the gallbladder wall [18]. The disease is associated with cholelithiasis in more than 95 % of the case and is more prevalent starting in the sixth decade of life, with a female predominance (female to male ratio of 3–5:1) [19, 20]. The condition is typically asymptomatic and is often diagnosed incidentally on abdominal imaging or following the discovery of a palpable right upper quadrant abdominal mass. Recent studies report cancer development in 15 % of the cases; a lower incidence compared to previous reports [21, 22]. The different incidences may be due to different ethnic populations studied [23]. Yet the causality relationship between porcelain gallbladder and gallbladder cancer remains unproven. Prophylactic laparoscopic cholecystectomy for this pathology is not mandatory and remains debated [22, 24, 25].

Polyps

Gallbladder polyps represent mucosal outgrowth and can be benign or malignant. Benign gallbladder polyps include adenomas, adenomyomas, inflammatory polyps and cholesterol polyps. Cholesterol is the most common type of polyps, accounting for more than 50 % of all identified [26]. Adenocarcinoma compromises most of the malignant polyps; in addition to less frequent squamous cell carcinoma, angiosarcoma, clear cell cancer, and metastatic disease. Several studies have investigated the association between size, shape (sessile vs. pedunculated), number of polyps, and gallbladder cancer. Typically, polyp size >10 mm and sessile morphology in ages >50 years represent a high risk with malignancy [27, 28]. Endoscopic ultrasound (EUS) and computed tomography (CT) can differentiate benign from malignant polypoid lesion with high sensitivity [29, 30]. Transabdominal ultrasound is reported as a superior imaging modality compared to EUS in differentiating smaller neoplastic versus non-neoplastic lesions [31]. At present, it is widely acceptable that patients with a polyp ≤10 mm can be safely observed while those >10 mm should be considered for cholecystectomy due to malignancy risk [32–36].

Anomalous Pancreaticobiliary Duct Junction

Anomalous pancreaticobiliary duct junction (APBDJ) is an abnormal anatomic variation of the pancreatic duct and the common bile duct, resulting from embryologic ducts migration failure. This anomaly occurs outside the duodenal wall and results in the formation of a long common channel (usually longer than 15 mm). The shared channel prior to the duodenal wall is not controlled by the sphincter of Oddi, and thus leads to free flow of pancreatic juice into the bile tract. Subsequent activation of proteolytic enzymes, inflammation and bile stasis may lead to precancerous changes in the gallbladder mucosa. The condition is most prevalent in the Asian population and in females and is reported in 4.6–12.9 % of

GBC patients [37–41]. Hu et al. reported a strong association of APBDJ with GBC (odds ratio: 50.7, $p<0.001$). Due to the high frequency of malignancy reported in patients with APBDJ, prophylactic cholecystectomy is considered [38, 42].

Carcinogens

Different carcinogens are suggested as causal agents of gallbladder cancer. Increased risk has been reported in workers of oil, paper, chemical, shoe, textile, and cellulose acetate plants. Miners exposed to radon also carry a higher risk, signifying another potential occupational hazard [3]. Exposure to wood or coal dust has also been proposed as independent risk factors for gallbladder cancer [43]. Furthermore, some studies report that gallbladder cancer is more prevalent in smokers [44, 45]. A dose-dependent relationship exists between smoking and gallbladder cancer, although the mechanism by which smoking affects the gallbladder is unknown.

Other Factors

Possible associations also exist between typhoid infection and gallbladder cancer [16, 46, 47]. Eradication of the carrier state and elective cholecystectomy has been suggested as possible management strategies for patients with typhoid [48, 49]. Other studies examining the association of some drugs and biliary tract cancer suggested that methyl dopa, and isoniazid might also represent risk factor in cancer pathogenesis [50–52].

Clinical Presentation

Patients with GBC tend to present with one of four different clinical presentations; (1) GBC suspected based on symptoms, (2) GBC discovered incidentally on abdominal imaging, (3) GBC discovered intraoperatively during cholecystectomy, or lastly (4) GBC discovered on pathological examination of a cholecystectomy specimen. The disease is most commonly discovered intra- and/or post-operatively on pathological examination of surgical specimens. In a study examining 435 gallbladder cancer cases from Memorial Sloan Kettering Cancer Center, 47 % of all cases were discovered incidentally during a laparoscopic cholecystectomy [53]. In general, GBC is reported in 0.27–2.1 % of all laparoscopic cholecystectomy cases [25, 54, 55]. This mode of presentation stresses the importance of surgeon-directed mucosal examination of the gallbladder specimens following cholecystectomy and frozen section examination for any suspicious lesion [56, 57].

Patients with GBC tend to remain asymptomatic in the earlier stages, and thus often present at an advanced stage. However, symptoms, if present, are usually nonspecific and their presence for an extended period of time should raise suspicion of GBC. Symptom wise, pain is reported as the most common complaint in GBC patients, followed by weight loss, anorexia, nausea, and vomiting [58]. If jaundice is the presenting sign, it signifies the presence of advanced disease that is often unresectable [59, 60]. Similarly, the presence of a palpable mass in the RUQ may predict an advanced unresectable gallbladder malignancy [61].

Investigations

Ultrasound: Ultrasound is typically the first imaging modality in the gallbladder examination due to its high availability, low cost and easy handling. Intraluminal growths and suspicious polyps can often be detected by ultrasound. Identification of asymmetric thickening of the gallbladder wall and mucosal irregularity are also possible [62]. Ultrasound can additionally detect the presence of a mass lesion replacing the gallbladder or invading the gallbladder bed at the interface with the liver. Findings that increase the likelihood of GBC include gallbladder wall calcifications (porcelain gallbladder), mural thickening, and large gallbladder stones. Color sonography may further facilitate the process by showing an increased blood flow velocity within gallbladder lesions, which is associated with GBC [63, 64]. Overall, ultrasound is valuable in diagnosing gallbladder cancer; however, its ability to identify nodal involvement or peritoneal metastasis is limited, making it less useful in disease staging [65–68]. Ultrasound is also limited by the body habitus of the patient and is also operator dependent.

Endoscopic ultrasound (EUS) has been proposed as a possible adjunct imaging for further evaluation of suspicious lesions [65]. Findings such as gallbladder wall thickening beyond 10 mm, disruption of the normal two-layered gallbladder wall and hypoechoic internal echogenicity are independent predictors of GBC [69, 70]. EUS is useful in investigating the depth of gallbladder wall invasion, T-stage of GBC, and involvement of surrounding lymph nodes in the porta hepatis and peripancreatic area [71, 72]. Additionally, EUS allows for ultrasound directed biopsy of suspicious lymph nodes. The collective functions of EUS make it one of the most recommended modalities to differentiate benign and malignant portal nodes.

Cross sectional imaging of the abdomen utilizing computed tomography (CT) and magnetic resonance imaging (MRI) can provide valuable information about the extent of the disease and its proximity to the surrounding structures. CT scans can detect the presence of polypoid lesions bulging into the gallbladder lumen as well as characterize the pattern of wall thickening. The presence of asymmetrical wall thickening on CT with 3D reconstruction is a strong predictor of malignancy [73, 74]. Other findings suspicious of malignancy include a thick enhancing inner layer of the gallbladder ≥ 2.6 mm, with a thin outer layer ≤ 3.4 mm, strong enhancement of the inner wall and irregular wall contour [75]. CT scan images also allow for the detection of lymph node metastasis, vascular invasion, or local involvement of the liver with an overall accuracy of 71–83.9 % for GBC staging [76, 77].

MRI is an essential part of the diagnostic work-up for GBC cases, and a useful tool for staging. MRI is able to examine gallbladder wall thickening, depict soft tissue invasion, and detect some benign entities, such as adenomas and adenomyomatosis. Studies suggest that MRI in combination with MRA (magnetic resonance angiography) or MRCP (magnetic resonance cholangiopancreatography) is valuable in preoperative evaluation of GBC. Combined MRI and MRCP depict the depth of hepatic invasion, lymph node metastasis, and vascular or biliary tract invasion, allowing for accurate assessment of disease resectability [78, 79].

Positron emission tomography (PET) scan with 18F-flurodeoxyglucose (FDG) is commonly used in cases of suspected malignancy. FDG-PET is useful in differentiating benign from malignant lesions, for staging purposes, and/or for the detection of disease recurrence [80, 81]. The combined FDG-PET is credited with sensitivity of 75–80 % and specificity of 82–100 % for GBC [82, 83]. However, PET scans can show a false positive result when evaluating benign inflammatory conditions [83, 84].

Laboratory Investigations

Various laboratory abnormalities and tumor markers are seen in GBC. Alkaline phosphatase (ALP) and bilirubin levels are typically elevated in cases of bile duct obstruction. Tumor markers, carcinoembryonic antigen (CEA) and carbonic anhydrase (CA19-9) are commonly elevated in GBC, although not diagnostic. CA19-9 at 20.0 units/ml or higher provides a specificity of 79.2 % and a sensitivity of 79.4 % for GBC, while a CEA level of ≥4.0 ng/ml carries a specificity of 92.7 % and a sensitivity of 50 % [85]. These markers play a valuable role in patient follow-up and assessment of response to therapy [86].

Differential Diagnosis

Gallbladder masses include a large spectrum of pathologies beside gallbladder cancers. Other mass-causing lesions include gallbladder adenomyomatosis, found in approximately 1–8 %

of cholecystectomy specimens [87]. Less frequent lesions include tumefactive sludge, and xanthogranulomatous cholecystitis. Metastases, most commonly from melanoma, followed by hepatocellular carcinoma and renal cell carcinoma, are also a part of the differential diagnoses. In the case of diagnostic dilemma, surgical intervention with laparoscopic cholecystectomy and pathological examination is recommended.

Staging Systems

Different staging systems have been proposed for GBC staging based on pathologic factors. One of the most commonly used staging systems is the one developed by the American Joint Committee on Cancer (AJCC); (Table 15.1). The AJCC staging utilizes TNM (tumor, lymph node, metastases) staging for gallbladder cancer and was adopted in 2002. Other commonly used staging systems include the Japanese Biliary Surgical Society system [88], the Nevin system [89], and the modified Nevin system [90] (Table 15.2).

A study performed by Fong et al. examined the AJCC 6th edition accuracy in 10,705 GBC cases diagnosed between 1989 and 1996 from the National Cancer Database (NCDB). The study reported that utilizing the 6th edition staging system provided no discrimination between Stage III and Stage IV patients following 3-year and 5-year survival analyses [91]. The authors proposed a modified staging system, where stage III disease should be divided into stage IIIA encompassing T3N0M0 patients and Stage IIIB consisting of T1-T3N1M0 patients. This suggestion was based on the understanding that lymph node metastases represent different cancer biology. Patients with Stage IVA and stage IVB were also regrouped, where stage IVA contained T4N0M0 patients while stage IVB contained those with nodal metastasis. Recent changes introduced to the AJCC 7th edition in 2010 sought to address the previous edition shortcomings, and provide a better correlation with resectability and patient outcomes (Table 15.3).

TABLE 15.1 American Joint Committee on cancer staging for gallbladder cancers, 7th edition

	TNM stage		
Stage	T-stage	N-stage	M-stage
Stage 0	Tis	N0	M0
Stage I	T1	N0	M0
Stage II	T2	N0	M0
Stage IIIA	T3	N0	M0
Stage IIIB	T1-3	N1	M0
Stage IVA	T4	N0-1	M0
Stage IVB	Any T	N2	M0
	Any T	Any N	M1

Primary tumor (T)

TX	Primary tumor cannot be assessed
T0	No evidence of primary tumor
Tis	Carcinoma in situ
T1a	Tumor invades lamina propria
T1b	Tumor invades muscle layer
T2	Tumor invades perimuscular connective tissue; no extension beyond serosa or into liver
T3	Tumor perforates the serosa (visceral peritoneum) and/or directly invades the liver and/or 1 adjacent organ/structure
T4	Tumor invades main portal vein or hepatic artery or invades two or more extrahepatic organs or structures

Regional lymph nodes (N)

NX	Regional lymph nodes cannot be assessed

(continued)

TABLE 15.1 (continued)

Stage	T-stage	N-stage	M-stage
	TNM stage		
N0	No regional lymph node metastasis		
N1	Metastasis to nodes along the cystic duct, common bile duct, hepatic artery, and/or portal vein		
N2	Metastasis to periaortic, pericaval, superior mesenteric artery, and/or celiac lymph nodes.		
Distant metastasis (M)			
M0	No distant metastasis		
M1	Distant metastasis		

Treatment

Surgical Management

Surgical resection remains the mainstay of GBC management and the only potentially curative therapy. Unfortunately, most patients present with an unresectable disease at the time of diagnosis. Although a laparoscopic approach for early stage GBC resection has been proposed, open surgery remains generally recommended due to the risk of gallbladder perforation and subsequent peritoneal seeding in laparoscopic operations [92–94]. Usually, a staging laparoscopy is performed immediately preceding open surgery to exclude peritoneal carcinomatosis. Benefits of laparoscopy include less associated pain, hospital stay and morbidity. Staging laparoscopy is able to identify 23–48 % of unresectable cases, thus reducing the number of nontherapeutic open operations [95, 96].

Patients with stage 1 disease are generally categorized as T1a and T1b based on the tumor invasion into the muscular layer. T1a patients can achieve cure from a simple cholecystectomy [97, 98]. In most instances, these tumors are discovered postoperatively on histological examination of a cholecystectomy specimen, and require no further intervention. However, patients with a T1b tumor usually present with a high rate of locoregional recurrence if treated with simple cholecystectomy, and thus are managed with an extended cholecystectomy (gallbladder is removed en bloc with liver gallbladder bed). Extended cholecystectomy is reported to improve survival compared to simple cholecystectomy for patients with T1b tumors, although associated with higher perioperative mortality [99].

Stage II tumors invade the perimuscular connective tissue, and have typically received a radical cholecystectomy with liver resection [100–103]. Regional lymphadenectomy is performed as it provides a survival benefit for stage II disease patients [104]. Current management no longer mandates a formal segmentectomy but rather a negative hepatic resection margin.

Patients with Stage III disease have direct tumor invasion into the liver through the gallbladder serosa or lymph node metastasis. Treatment involves radical resection of the gallbladder en bloc with a portion of liver segments IVb and V, and regional lymphadenectomy [103]. Tumor extension to the adjacent structures (colon, duodenum, or stomach) necessities en bloc resection based on anatomic involvement. Patients with disease extending to the cystic and/or bile duct require common duct resection. Frozen section of the cystic duct stump guides the necessity of common duct removal.

Stage IV disease is often unresectable due to extension to surrounding organs and/or vasculature. Major resections are associated with increased morbidity without noticeable survival benefit [101]. For cases with distal nodal involvement (N2 disease), the curative role of resection becomes futile, and referral to palliative treatment should occur.

Management of Incidentally Discovered GBC

Due to the large number of cancer cases discovered intraoperatively or on the postoperative pathologic report, a high index of suspicion should be maintained. Suspicion should be higher in patients with characteristics such as porcelain gallbladder, large polyps of the gallbladder, long standing gall

TABLE 15.2 Comparison between different staging systems used in gallbladder cancer

Stage	AJCC; 7th edition	Japanese classification	Modified Nevin classification
I	Carcinoma invading mucosal or muscular layer; T1N0M0	Carcinoma confined to gallbladder beyond the capsule	Carcinoma in situ
II	Transmural invasion, no extension beyond the serosa; T2N0M0	Suspicious liver or bile duct invasion + N1	Mucosal or muscular layer invasion
III	Local invasion of nearby organ; T1-T3, N0-N1, M0	Marked hepatic or bile duct invasion + N2 or N3	Transmural and direct liver invasion
IV	Major vascular invasion or invasion of nearby organs or distant metastasis T4, N0-N1, M0; Any T, N2, M0-M1	Extensive hepatic and bile duct invasion, liver and peritoneal metastasis	Lymph node metastasis
V			Distant metastases

stones and/or recurrent gallbladder infection. If a suspicious lesion was discovered intraoperatively, frozen section examination should guide subsequent management. In cases diagnosed postoperatively requiring further surgical management beyond simple cholecystectomy, or if the surgeon is unfamiliar with complex liver resections, referral to an experienced center should occur [102, 105].

Stenting

A large number of GBC patients tend to present with unresectable disease. In these patients, palliative measures are employed to alleviate pain and other symptoms, such as jaundice, pruritus, gastrointestinal obstruction, and cholangitis. Cases presenting with obstructive symptoms were previously

TABLE 15.3 Comparison between AJCC 6th and 7th edition

Difference between AJCC 6th edition and AJCC 7th edition		
Sixth edition		Seventh edition
Tis=Carcinoma in situ T1=Tumor invades lamina propria (T1a) or muscle layer (T1b) T2=Tumor invades perimuscular connective tissue T3=Tumor perforates serosa and/or invades the liver or adjacent organs T4=Tumor invades main portal vein or hepatic artery, or multiple extrahepatic organs	T-stage	Tis=Carcinoma in situ T1=Tumor invades lamina propria (T1a) or muscle layer (T1b) T2=Tumor invades perimuscular connective tissue T3=Tumor perforates serosa and/or invades the liver and/or one adjacent organ T4=Tumor invades main portal vein or hepatic artery or multiple extrahepatic organs
N0=No regional nodal metastases N1=Positive regional nodal metastases	N-stage	N0=No regional nodal metastases N1=Metastases to nodes along cystic duct, hepatic artery, common bile duct, and/or portal vein N2=Metastases to pericaval, periaortic, superior mesenteric artery, and/or celiac artery nodes
M0=No distant metastases M1=Distant metastases	M-stage	M0=No distant metastases M1=Distant metastases

considered for bypass surgery to provide adequate drainage [106]. However, the development of percutaneous interventions and advances in endoscopic procedures provide valuable alternatives that carry less morbidity [107, 108]. Palliative interventions aim to improve symptoms although a recent study questioned their impact on patients' quality of life [108].

Nonsurgical Management

Chemotherapy may provide potential survival benefit for patients with unresectable disease. Recent studies reported a potential benefit of gemcitabine, alone or in combination with other regimens, for patients with advanced biliary tract cancers [109–111]. Following the results of the ABC-02 trial from the UK, current practice often focuses on gemcitabine with cisplatin in the treatment of biliary tract disease including gallbladder cancer [112].

Radiation therapy (RT) efficacy in patients with unresectable GBC and CC has been reported. Houry et al. suggested that an intraoperative "boost" of 15Gy of radiation followed by 40–50Gy of external radiation postoperatively might provide a survival benefit [113]. A study examining a cohort of 4180 GBC patients from the SEER database reported that RT provided a survival benefit for patients with stage $\geq$T2 stage disease with nodal metastases [114]. The 2-year survival rates improved from 17 to 33 % and the median survival from 9 months to 14 months following the delivery of RT. The impact of combination RT and chemotherapy for GBC is unknown [115].

Conclusion

In conclusion, gallbladder cancer is a disease with a poor prognosis. Risk factors are not well understood, and are largely centered on gallstones, porcelain gallbladder, and polyps. Current imaging advances have allowed the identification of patients that would benefit most from surgical intervention. Laparoscopy is usually performed to assess the extent of disease and guide the operative decision. Surgery remains the only curative option and provides promising results in patients with early disease. Stenting through a percutaneous or endoscopic approach may palliate symptoms in advanced stages. While radiotherapy may provide survival benefit for patients with disease stage $\geq$T2, patients with widespread disease currently benefit most from chemotherapy regimen of gemcitabine and cisplatin.

References

1. Blalock AA. A statistical study of 888 cases of biliary tract disease. Johns Hopkins Hosp Bull. 1924;35:391–409.
2. Tada M, Yokosuka O, Omata M, Ohto M, Isono K. Analysis of ras gene mutations in biliary and pancreatic tumors by polymerase chain reaction and direct sequencing. Cancer. 1990;66(5):930–5.
3. Lazcano-Ponce EC, Miquel JF, Muñoz N, Herrero R, Ferrecio C, Wistuba II, et al. Epidemiology and molecular pathology of gallbladder cancer. CA Cancer J Clin. 2001;51(6):349–64.
4. Randi G, Franceschi S, La Vecchia C. Gallbladder cancer worldwide: geographical distribution and risk factors. Int J Cancer. 2006;118(7):1591–602.
5. Carriaga MT, Henson DE. Liver, gallbladder, extrahepatic bile ducts, and pancreas. Cancer. 1995;75(1 Suppl):171–90.
6. Barakat J, Dunkelberg JC, Ma TY. Changing patterns of gallbladder carcinoma in New Mexico. Cancer. 2006;106(2): 434–40.
7. Henson DE, Albores-Saavedra J, Corle D. Carcinoma of the gallbladder. Histologic types, stage of disease, grade, and survival rates. Cancer. 1992;70(6):1493–7.
8. Perpetuo MD, Valdivieso M, Heilbrun LK, Nelson RS, Connor T, Bodey GP. Natural history study of Gallbladder cancer (GBC): a review of 36 years experience at M. D. Anderson Hospital and Tumor Institute. Cancer. 1978;42(1):330–5.
9. Graham EA. The prevention of carcinoma of the gall-bladder. Ann Surg. 1931;93(1):317–22.
10. Hart J, Modan B, Shani M. Cholelithiasis in the aetiology of gallbladder neoplasms. Lancet. 1971;1(7710):1151–3.
11. Hsing AW, Gao YT, Han TQ, Rashid A, Sakoda LC, Wang BS, et al. Gallstones and the risk of biliary tract cancer: a population-based study in China. Br J Cancer. 2007;97(11):1577–82.
12. Albores-Saavedra J, Alcántra-Vazquez A, Cruz-Ortiz H, Herrera-Goepfert R. The precursor lesions of invasive gallbladder carcinoma. Hyperplasia, atypical hyperplasia and carcinoma in situ. Cancer. 1980;45(5):919–27.
13. Chow WH, Johansen C, Gridley G, Mellemkjaer L, Olsen JH, Fraumeni JF. Gallstones, cholecystectomy and risk of cancers of the liver, biliary tract and pancreas. Br J Cancer. 1999; 79(3–4):640–4.

14. Diehl AK. Gallstone size and the risk of gallbladder cancer. JAMA. 1983;250(17):2323–6.
15. Lowenfels AB, Walker AM, Althaus DP, Townsend G, Domellöf L. Gallstone growth, size, and risk of Gallbladder cancer (GBC): an interracial study. Int J Epidemiol. 1989;18(1):50–4.
16. Strom BL, Soloway RD, Rios-Dalenz JL, Rodriguez-Martinez HA, West SL, Kinman JL, et al. Risk factors for gallbladder cancer. An international collaborative case-control study. Cancer. 1995;76(10):1747–56.
17. Wenckert A, Robertson B. The natural course of gallstone disease: eleven-year review of 781 nonoperated cases. Gastroenterology. 1966;50(3):376–81.
18. Berk RN, Armbuster TG, Saltzstein SL. Carcinoma in the porcelain gallbladder. Radiology. 1973;106(1):29–31.
19. Ashur H, Siegal B, Oland Y, Adam YG. Calcified ballbladder (porcelain gallbladder). Arch Surg. 1978;113(5):594–6.
20. Pandey M, Shukla VK. Lifestyle, parity, menstrual and reproductive factors and risk of gallbladder cancer. Eur J Cancer Prev. 2003;12(4):269–72.
21. Stephen AE, Berger DL. Carcinoma in the porcelain gallbladder: a relationship revisited. Surgery. 2001;129(6):699–703.
22. Khan ZS, Livingston EH, Huerta S. Reassessing the need for prophylactic surgery in patients with porcelain gallbladder: case series and systematic review of the literature. Arch Surg. 2011;146(10):1143–7.
23. Cunningham SC, Alexander HR. Porcelain gallbladder and cancer: ethnicity explains a discrepant literature? Am J Med. 2007;120(4):e17–8.
24. Brown KM, Geller DA. Porcelain gallbladder and risk of gallbladder cancer. Arch Surg. 2011;146(10):1148.
25. Kwon AH, Inui H, Matsui Y, Uchida Y, Hukui J, Kamiyama Y. Laparoscopic cholecystectomy in patients with porcelain gallbladder based on the preoperative ultrasound findings. Hepatogastroenterology. 2004;51(58):950–3.
26. Terzi C, Sökmen S, Seçkin S, Albayrak L, Uğurlu M. Polypoid lesions of the gallbladder: report of 100 cases with special reference to operative indications. Surgery. 2000;127(6):622–7.
27. Ishikawa O, Ohhigashi H, Imaoka S, Nakaizumi A, Kitamura T, Sasaki Y, et al. The difference in malignancy between pedunculated and sessile polypoid lesions of the gallbladder. Am J Gastroenterol. 1989;84(11):1386–90.

28. Pilgrim CHC, Groeschl RT, Christians KK, Gamblin TC. Modern perspectives on factors predisposing to the development of gallbladder cancer. HPB. 2013;15(11):839–44.
29. Sugiyama M, Xie XY, Atomi Y, Saito M. Differential diagnosis of small polypoid lesions of the gallbladder: the value of endoscopic ultrasonography. Ann Surg. 1999;229(4):498–504.
30. Furukawa H, Kosuge T, Shimada K, Yamamoto J, Kanai Y, Mukai K, et al. Small polypoid lesions of the gallbladder: differential diagnosis and surgical indications by helical computed tomography. Arch Surg. 1998;133(7):735–9.
31. Cheon YK, Cho WY, Lee TH, Cho YD, Moon JH, Lee JS, et al. Endoscopic ultrasonography does not differentiate neoplastic from non-neoplastic small gallbladder polyps. World J Gastroenterol. 2009;15(19):2361–6.
32. Ito H, Hann LE, D'Angelica M, Allen P, Fong Y, Dematteo RP, et al. Polypoid lesions of the gallbladder: diagnosis and followup. J Am Coll Surg. 2009;208(4):570–5.
33. Yang HL, Sun YG, Wang Z. Polypoid lesions of the gallbladder: diagnosis and indications for surgery. Br J Surg. 1992;79(3):227–9.
34. Kubota K, Bandai Y, Noie T, Ishizaki Y, Teruya M, Makuuchi M. How should polypoid lesions of the gallbladder be treated in the era of laparoscopic cholecystectomy? Surgery. 1995;117(5):481–7.
35. Anderson MA, Appalaneni V, Ben-Menachem T, Decker GA, Early DS, Evans JA, et al. The role of endoscopy in the evaluation and treatment of patients with biliary neoplasia. Gastrointest Endosc. 2013;77(2):167–74.
36. Sarkut P, Kilicturgay S, Ozer A, Ozturk E, Yilmazlar T. Gallbladder polyps: factors affecting surgical decision. World J Gastroenterol. 2013;19(28):4526–30.
37. Hu B, Gong B, Zhou DY. Association of anomalous pancreaticobiliary ductal junction with gallbladder carcinoma in Chinese patients: an ERCP study. Gastrointest Endosc. 2003;57(4):541–5.
38. Chijiiwa K, Kimura H, Tanaka M. Malignant potential of the gallbladder in patients with anomalous pancreaticobiliary ductal junction. The difference in risk between patients with and without choledochal cyst. Int Surg. 1995;80(1):61–4.
39. Roukounakis NE, Kuhn JA, McCarty TM. Association of an abnormal pancreaticobiliary junction with biliary tract cancers. Proc (Bayl Univ Med Cent). 2000;13(1):11–3.

40. Hasumi A, Matsui H, Sugioka A, Uyama I, Komori Y, Fujita J, et al. Precancerous conditions of biliary tract cancer in patients with pancreaticobiliary maljunction: reappraisal of nationwide survey in Japan. J Hepatobiliary Pancreat Surg. 2000;7(6): 551–5.
41. Kang CM, Kim KS, Choi JS, Lee WJ, Kim BR. Gallbladder carcinoma associated with anomalous pancreaticobiliary duct junction. Can J Gastroenterol. 2007;21(6):383–7.
42. Elnemr A, Ohta T, Kayahara M, Kitagawa H, Yoshimoto K, Tani T, et al. Anomalous pancreaticobiliary ductal junction without bile duct dilatation in gallbladder cancer. Hepatogastroenterology. 2001;48(38):382–6.
43. Jain K, Sreenivas V, Velpandian T, Kapil U, Garg PK. Risk factors for Gallbladder cancer (GBC): a case-control study. Int J Cancer. 2013;132(7):1660–6.
44. Yagyu K, Kikuchi S, Obata Y, Lin Y, Ishibashi T, Kurosawa M, et al. Cigarette smoking, alcohol drinking and the risk of gallbladder cancer death: a prospective cohort study in Japan. Int J Cancer. 2008;122(4):924–9.
45. Scott TE, Carroll M, Cogliano FD, Smith BF, Lamorte WW. A case-control assessment of risk factors for gallbladder carcinoma. Dig Dis Sci. 1999;44(8):1619–25.
46. Dutta U, Garg PK, Kumar R, Tandon RK. Typhoid carriers among patients with gallstones are at increased risk for carcinoma of the gallbladder. Am J Gastroenterol. 2000;95(3): 784–7.
47. Shukla VK, Singh H, Pandey M, Upadhyay SK, Nath G. Carcinoma of the gallbladder—is it a sequel of typhoid? Dig Dis Sci. 2000;45(5):900–3.
48. Nagaraja V, Eslick GD. Systematic review with meta-analysis: the relationship between chronic Salmonella typhi carrier status and gall-bladder cancer. Aliment Pharmacol Ther. 2014;39(8):745–50.
49. Nath G, Singh H, Shukla VK. Chronic typhoid carriage and carcinoma of the gallbladder. Eur J Cancer Prev. 1997; 6(6):557–9.
50. Ellis EF, Gordon PR, Gottlieb LS. Oral contraceptives and cholangiocarcinoma. Lancet. 1978;1(8057):207.
51. Lowenfels AB, Norman J. Isoniazid and bile duct cancer. JAMA. 1978;240(5):434–5.
52. Brodén G, Bengtsson L. Biliary carcinoma associated with methyldopa therapy. Acta Chir Scand Suppl. 1980;500:7–12.

53. Duffy A, Capanu M, Abou-Alfa GK, Huitzil D, Jarnagin W, Fong Y, et al. Gallbladder cancer (GBC): 10-year experience at Memorial Sloan-Kettering Cancer Centre (MSKCC). J Surg Oncol. 2008;98(7):485–9.

54. Darmas B, Mahmud S, Abbas A, Baker AL. Is there any justification for the routine histological examination of straightforward cholecystectomy specimens? Ann R Coll Surg Engl. 2007;89(3):238–41.

55. Frauenschuh D, Greim R, Kraas E. How to proceed in patients with carcinoma detected after laparoscopic cholecystectomy. Langenbecks Arch Surg. 2000;385(8):495–500.

56. Miller G, Jarnagin WR. Gallbladder carcinoma. Eur J Surg Oncol. 2008;34(3):306–12.

57. Matthyssens LE, Ziol M, Barrat C, Champault GG. Routine surgical pathology in general surgery. Br J Surg. 2006; 93(3):362–8.

58. Misra S, Chaturvedi A, Misra NC, Sharma ID. Carcinoma of the gallbladder. Lancet Oncol. 2003;4(3):167–76.

59. Hawkins WG, DeMatteo RP, Jarnagin WR, Ben-Porat L, Blumgart LH, Fong Y. Jaundice predicts advanced disease and early mortality in patients with gallbladder cancer. Ann Surg Oncol. 2004;11(3):310–5.

60. Malik IA. Clinicopathological features and management of gallbladder cancer in Pakistan: a prospective study of 233 cases. J Gastroenterol Hepatol. 2003;18(8):950–3.

61. Thorbjarnarson B, Glenn F. Carcinoma of the gallbladder. Cancer. 1959;12:1009–15.

62. Joo I, Lee JY, Kim JH, Kim SJ, Kim MA, Han JK, et al. Differentiation of adenomyomatosis of the gallbladder from early-stage, wall-thickening-type gallbladder cancer using high-resolution ultrasound. Eur Radiol. 2013;23(3):730–8.

63. Komatsuda T, Ishida H, Konno K, Hamashima Y, Naganuma H, Sato M, et al. Gallbladder carcinoma: color Doppler sonography. Abdom Imaging. 2000;25(2):194–7.

64. Ueno N, Tomiyama T, Tano S, Wada S, Kimura K. Diagnosis of gallbladder carcinoma with color Doppler ultrasonography. Am J Gastroenterol. 1996;91(8):1647–9.

65. Chijiiwa K, Sumiyoshi K, Nakayama F. Impact of recent advances in hepatobiliary imaging techniques on the preoperative diagnosis of carcinoma of the gallbladder. World J Surg. 1991;15(3):322–7.

66. Jang JY, Kim SW, Lee SE, Hwang DW, Kim EJ, Lee JY, et al. Differential diagnostic and staging accuracies of high resolution ultrasonography, endoscopic ultrasonography, and multidetector computed tomography for gallbladder polypoid lesions and gallbladder cancer. Ann Surg. 2009;250(6):943–9.

67. Pandey M, Sood BP, Shukla RC, Aryya NC, Singh S, Shukla VK. Carcinoma of the gallbladder: role of sonography in diagnosis and staging. J Clin Ultrasound. 2000;28(5):227–32.

68. Bach AM, Loring LA, Hann LE, Illescas FF, Fong Y, Blumgart LH. Gallbladder cancer (GBC): can ultrasonography evaluate extent of disease? J Ultrasound Med. 1998;17(5):303–9.

69. Kim HJ, Park JH, Park DI, Cho YK, Sohn CI, Jeon WK, et al. Clinical usefulness of endoscopic ultrasonography in the differential diagnosis of gallbladder wall thickening. Dig Dis Sci. 2012;57(2):508–15.

70. Mizuguchi M, Kudo S, Fukahori T, Matsuo Y, Miyazaki K, Tokunaga O, et al. Endoscopic ultrasonography for demonstrating loss of multiple-layer pattern of the thickened gallbladder wall in the preoperative diagnosis of gallbladder cancer. Eur Radiol. 1997;7(8):1323–7.

71. Sadamoto Y, Kubo H, Harada N, Tanaka M, Eguchi T, Nawata H. Preoperative diagnosis and staging of gallbladder carcinoma by EUS. Gastrointest Endosc. 2003;58(4):536–41.

72. Fujita N, Noda Y, Kobayashi G, Kimura K, Yago A. Diagnosis of the depth of invasion of gallbladder carcinoma by EUS. Gastrointest Endosc. 1999;50(5):659–63.

73. Kalra N, Suri S, Gupta R, Natarajan SK, Khandelwal N, Wig JD, et al. MDCT in the staging of gallbladder carcinoma. Am J Roentgenol. 2006;186(3):758–62.

74. Kim SJ, Lee JM, Lee JY, Kim SH, Han JK, Choi BI, et al. Analysis of enhancement pattern of flat gallbladder wall thickening on MDCT to differentiate gallbladder cancer from cholecystitis. Am J Roentgenol. 2008;191(3):765–71.

75. Pilgrim CHC, Groeschl RT, Pappas SG, Gamblin TC. An often overlooked diagnosis: imaging features of gallbladder cancer. J Am Coll Surg. 2013;216(2):333–9.

76. Kim BS, Ha HK, Lee IJ, Kim JH, Eun HW, Bae IY, et al. Accuracy of CT in local staging of gallbladder carcinoma. Acta Radiol. 2002;43(1):71–6.

77. Kim SJ, Lee JM, Lee JY, Choi JY, Kim SH, Han JK, et al. Accuracy of preoperative T-staging of gallbladder carcinoma using MDCT. Am J Roentgenol. 2008;190(1):74–80.

78. Schwartz LH, Black J, Fong Y, Jarnagin W, Blumgart L, Gruen D, et al. Gallbladder carcinoma: findings at MR imaging with MR cholangiopancreatography. J Comput Assist Tomogr. 2002;26(3):405–10.

79. Kim JH, Kim TK, Eun HW, Kim BS, Lee MG, Kim PN, et al. Preoperative evaluation of gallbladder carcinoma: efficacy of combined use of MR imaging, MR cholangiography, and contrast-enhanced dual-phase three-dimensional MR angiography. J Magn Reson Imaging. 2002;16(6):676–84.

80. Delbeke D, Martin WH, Sandler MP, Chapman WC, Wright JK, Pinson CW. Evaluation of benign vs malignant hepatic lesions with positron emission tomography. Arch Surg. 1998;133(5):510–5. discussion 5–6.

81. Corvera CU, Blumgart LH, Akhurst T, DeMatteo RP, D'Angelica M, Fong Y, et al. 18F-fluorodeoxyglucose positron emission tomography influences management decisions in patients with biliary cancer. J Am Coll Surg. 2008;206(1):57–65.

82. Rodriguez-Fernandez A, Gomez-Rio M, Llamas-Elvira JM, Ortega-Lozano S, Ferron-Orihuela JA, Ramia-Angel JM, et al. Positron-emission tomography with fluorine-18-fluoro-2-deoxy-D-glucose for gallbladder cancer diagnosis. Am J Surg. 2004;188(2):171–5.

83. Oe A, Kawabe J, Torii K, Kawamura E, Higashiyama S, Kotani J, et al. Distinguishing benign from malignant gallbladder wall thickening using FDG-PET. Ann Nucl Med. 2006;20(10):699–703.

84. Hansen N, Brown RK, Khan A, Frey KA, Orringer M. False positive diagnosis of metastatic esophageal carcinoma on positron emission tomography: a case report of cholecystitis simulating a hepatic lesion. Clin Nucl Med. 2010;35(6):409–12.

85. Strom BL, Maislin G, West SL, Atkinson B, Herlyn M, Saul S, et al. Serum CEA and CA 19-9: potential future diagnostic or screening tests for gallbladder cancer? Int J Cancer. 1990;45(5):821–4.

86. Ritts RE, Nagorney DM, Jacobsen DJ, Talbot RW, Zurawski VR. Comparison of preoperative serum CA19-9 levels with results of diagnostic imaging modalities in patients undergoing laparotomy for suspected pancreatic or gallbladder disease. Pancreas. 1994;9(6):707–16.

87. Ching BH, Yeh BM, Westphalen AC, Joe BN, Qayyum A, Coakley FV. CT differentiation of adenomyomatosis and gallbladder cancer. Am J Roentgenol. 2007;189(1):62–6.

88. Onoyama H, Yamamoto M, Tseng A, Ajiki T, Saitoh Y. Extended cholecystectomy for carcinoma of the gallbladder. World J Surg. 1995;19(5):758–63.
89. Nevin JE, Moran TJ, Kay S, King R. Carcinoma of the gallbladder: staging, treatment, and prognosis. Cancer. 1976;37(1):141–8.
90. Donohue JH, Nagorney DM, Grant CS, Tsushima K, Ilstrup DM, Adson MA. Carcinoma of the gallbladder. Does radical resection improve outcome? Arch Surg. 1990;125(2):237–41.
91. Fong Y, Wagman L, Gonen M, Crawford J, Reed W, Swanson R, et al. Evidence-based gallbladder cancer staging: changing cancer staging by analysis of data from the National Cancer Database. Ann Surg. 2006;243(6):767–71. discussion 71–4.
92. Cho JY, Han HS, Yoon YS, Ahn KS, Kim YH, Lee KH. Laparoscopic approach for suspected early-stage gallbladder carcinoma. Arch Surg. 2010;145(2):128–33.
93. Sarli L, Pietra N, Costi R, Grattarola M. Gallbladder perforation during laparoscopic cholecystectomy. World J Surg. 1999;23(11):1186–90.
94. Weiland ST, Mahvi DM, Niederhuber JE, Heisey DM, Chicks DS, Rikkers LF. Should suspected early gallbladder cancer be treated laparoscopically? J Gastrointest Surg. 2002;6(1):50–6. discussion 6–7.
95. Agarwal AK, Kalayarasan R, Javed A, Gupta N, Nag HH. The role of staging laparoscopy in primary gall bladder cancer—an analysis of 409 patients: a prospective study to evaluate the role of staging laparoscopy in the management of gallbladder cancer. Ann Surg. 2013;258(2):318–23.
96. Weber SM, DeMatteo RP, Fong Y, Blumgart LH, Jarnagin WR. Staging laparoscopy in patients with extrahepatic biliary carcinoma. Analysis of 100 patients. Ann Surg. 2002;235(3):392–9.
97. Yamaguchi K, Chijiiwa K, Ichimiya H, Sada M, Kawakami K, Nishikata F, et al. Gallbladder carcinoma in the era of laparoscopic cholecystectomy. Arch Surg. 1996;131(9):981–4. discussion 5.
98. Ootani T, Shirai Y, Tsukada K, Muto T. Relationship between gallbladder carcinoma and the segmental type of adenomyomatosis of the gallbladder. Cancer. 1992;69(11):2647–52.
99. Abramson MA, Pandharipande P, Ruan D, Gold JS, Whang EE. Radical resection for T1b Gallbladder cancer (GBC): a decision analysis. HPB (Oxford). 2009;11(8):656–63.

100. Wakai T, Shirai Y, Sakata J, Nagahashi M, Ajioka Y, Hatakeyama K. Mode of hepatic spread from gallbladder carcinoma: an immunohistochemical analysis of 42 hepatectomized specimens. Am J Surg Pathol. 2010;34(1):65–74.
101. D'Angelica M, Dalal KM, DeMatteo RP, Fong Y, Blumgart LH, Jarnagin WR. Analysis of the extent of resection for adenocarcinoma of the gallbladder. Ann Surg Oncol. 2009;16(4):806–16.
102. Pawlik TM, Gleisner AL, Vigano L, Kooby DA, Bauer TW, Frilling A, et al. Incidence of finding residual disease for incidental gallbladder carcinoma: implications for re-resection. J Gastrointest Surg. 2007;11(11):1478–86. discussion 86–7.
103. Ito H, Ito K, D'Angelica M, Gonen M, Klimstra D, Allen P, et al. Accurate staging for Gallbladder cancer (GBC): implications for surgical therapy and pathological assessment. Ann Surg. 2011;254(2):320–5.
104. Downing SR, Cadogan KA, Ortega G, Oyetunji TA, Siram SM, Chang DC, et al. Early-stage gallbladder cancer in the surveillance, epidemiology, and end results database: effect of extended surgical resection. Arch Surg. 2011;146(6):734–8.
105. Shih SP, Schulick RD, Cameron JL, Lillemoe KD, Pitt HA, Choti MA, et al. Gallbladder cancer (GBC): the role of laparoscopy and radical resection. Ann Surg. 2007;245(6):893–901.
106. Kapoor VK, Pradeep R, Haribhakti SP, Singh V, Sikora SS, Saxena R, et al. Intrahepatic segment III cholangiojejunostomy in advanced carcinoma of the gallbladder. Br J Surg. 1996;83(12):1709–11.
107. Saluja SS, Gulati M, Garg PK, Pal H, Pal S, Sahni P, et al. Endoscopic or percutaneous biliary drainage for Gallbladder cancer (GBC): a randomized trial and quality of life assessment. Clin Gastroenterol Hepatol. 2008;6(8):944–50.e3.
108. Robson PC, Heffernan N, Gonen M, Thornton R, Brody LA, Holmes R, et al. Prospective study of outcomes after percutaneous biliary drainage for malignant biliary obstruction. Ann Surg Oncol. 2010;17(9):2303–11.
109. Iyer RV, Gibbs J, Kuvshinoff B, Fakih M, Kepner J, Soehnlein N, et al. A phase II study of gemcitabine and capecitabine in advanced cholangiocarcinoma and carcinoma of the gallbladder: a single-institution prospective study. Ann Surg Oncol. 2007;14(11):3202–9.
110. Riechelmann RP, Townsley CA, Chin SN, Pond GR, Knox JJ. Expanded phase II trial of gemcitabine and capecitabine for advanced biliary cancer. Cancer. 2007;110(6):1307–12.

111. Verderame F, Russo A, Di Leo R, Badalamenti G, Santangelo D, Cicero G, et al. Gemcitabine and oxaliplatin combination chemotherapy in advanced biliary tract cancers. Ann Oncol. 2006;17 Suppl 7:vii68–72.
112. Valle J, Wasan H, Palmer DH, Cunningham D, Anthoney A, Maraveyas A, et al. Cisplatin plus gemcitabine versus gemcitabine for biliary tract cancer. N Engl J Med. 2010; 362(14):1273–81.
113. Houry S, Barrier A, Huguier M. Irradiation therapy for gallbladder carcinoma: recent advances. J Hepatobiliary Pancreat Surg. 2001;8(6):518–24.
114. Wang SJ, Fuller CD, Kim JS, Sittig DF, Thomas CR, Ravdin PM. Prediction model for estimating the survival benefit of adjuvant radiotherapy for gallbladder cancer. J Clin Oncol. 2008;26(13):2112–7.
115. Lin LL, Picus J, Drebin JA, Linehan DC, Solis J, Strasberg SM, et al. A phase II study of alternating cycles of split course radiation therapy and gemcitabine chemotherapy for inoperable pancreatic or biliary tract carcinoma. Am J Clin Oncol. 2005;28(3):234–41.

Part 7
Clinical Scenario: "Biliary" Pain With or Without Intermittent Elevation of LFTs/Lipase

Chapter 16
Motility Disorders

Jennifer A. Cahill and Walter J. Hogan

Questions

1. *Will removing my gallbladder improve my symptoms if there are no stones?*

   Possibly—but only if your pain is related to disordered motility of the gallbladder.

2. *My gallbladder was removed and I'm still having similar pain—how is this possible?*

   Possibly you could have a sphincter of Oddi disorder; however, this is uncommon.

3. *If this isn't my gallbladder, what is it?*

   There exists a broad differential for abdominal pain, even if it localizes to the RUQ or epigastrium. Further investigation may be warranted.

J.A. Cahill, M.D.
Department of Medicine, Medical College of Wisconsin, CLCC, 5th Floor, 9200 West Wisconsin Avenue, Milwaukee, WI, USA
e-mail: JENNIFER.CAHILL@lumc.edu

W.J. Hogan, M.D. (⊠)
Department of Gastroenterology, Froedtert and the Medical College of Wisconsin, Froedtert Specialty Clinics, 4 FEC, 9200 West Wisconsin Avenue, Milwaukee, WI 53226, USA
e-mail: whogan@mcw.edu

© Springer International Publishing Switzerland 2016
K. Dua, R. Shaker (eds.), *Pancreas and Biliary Disease,*
DOI 10.1007/978-3-319-28089-9_16

Gallbladder

- Physiology.
  - The biliary system consists of the numerous ducts originating in the liver, which eventually form the right hepatic duct and left hepatic duct. These empty into the common hepatic duct. As the common hepatic duct emerges from the liver it joins with the cystic duct, which communicates with the gallbladder. These ducts combine to form the common bile duct, which merges distally with the pancreatic duct prior to emptying into the duodenum through the papilla of Vater, which incorporates the sphincter of Oddi (Fig. 16.1). Cholecystokinin is the primary enteric hormone influencing gallbladder function. It is released from the walls of the duodenum during eating. It causes contraction of the gallbladder and relaxation of the sphincter of Oddi in a healthy individual, thus promoting bile and pancreatic enzyme release for the digestion of fat and protein.

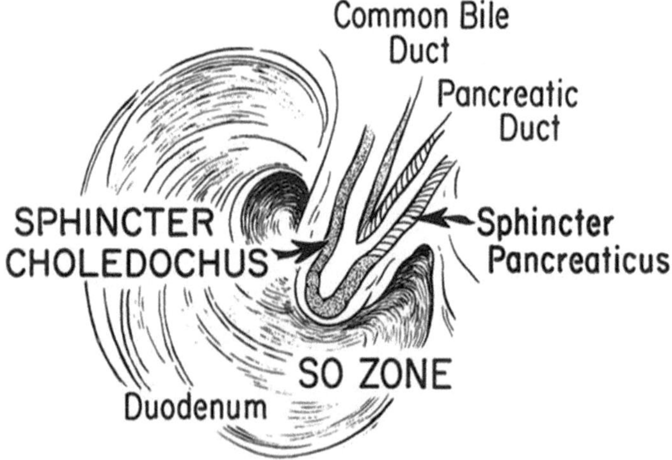

Fig. 16.1 Schema of distal anatomy of common bile duct and pancreatic duct, emptying into the duodenum via the sphincter of Oddi

- The primary function of the gallbladder is concentration and storage of bile, and eventual delivery into the duodenum in response to meals. Nestled beneath the liver in Hartmann's pouch, 80 % of bile is stored in the gallbladder during fasting; its capacity approximates 30–50 mL. There is receptive relaxation of the gallbladder between meals in unison with tonic contractions of the sphincter of Oddi (SO), which creates a pressure gradient directing flow of bile into the gallbladder. The change in gallbladder volume over time can be used to calculate the gallbladder ejection fraction (GBEF) (Fig. 16.2).
- Gallbladder emptying through the common bile duct occurs as a coordinated effort of contraction stimulated by the release of the hormone cholecystokinin in response to meals and relaxation of basal SO pressure. The gallbladder empties 50–70 % of its contents in

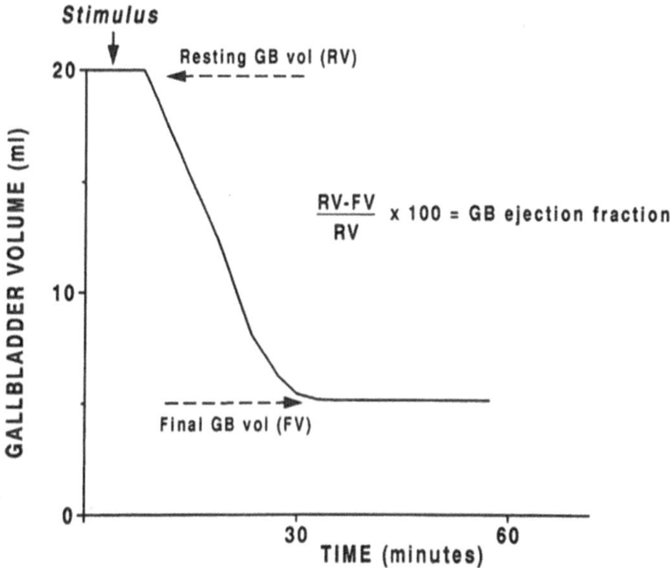

$$\frac{RV\text{-}FV}{RV} \times 100 = GB\ \text{ejection fraction}$$

FIG. 16.2 Schema of change in gallbladder volume during CCK infusion and the calculation of GBEF

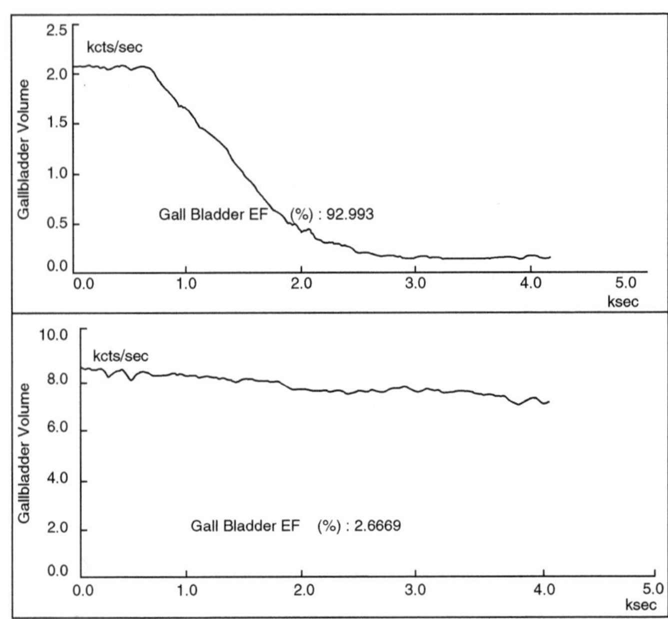

Fɪɢ. 16.3 Normal (*top*) and reduced (*bottom*) GBEF, as demonstrated by change in volume over time

30–40 min with eating; it refills in 60–90 min. Reduction of GBEF results in failure of the gallbladder to empty its volume (Fig. 16.3).

- Gallbladder Dyskinesia.
    - Patients with recurrent pain located in the epigastrium and/or right upper quadrant without evidence of gallstones should first undergo a diagnostic work-up to exclude structural alterations in the pancreaticobiliary tract. Ultrasound (US) of the biliary tract and liver should be obtained. The Rome III criteria provide diagnostic criteria for functional gallbladder and sphincter of Oddi disorders (Table 16.1). If patients meet these criteria for functional gallbladder disorders, further testing is indicated to determine whether they may benefit from appropriate therapy.

TABLE 16.1 Rome III criteria for functional biliary disorders

	Diagnostic criteria	Supportive criteria
Functional gallbladder and sphincter of Oddi disorders	Episodes lasting 30 min or longer	Associated with nausea and vomiting
	Recurrent symptoms occurring at different intervals (not daily)	
	The pain builds up to a steady level	
	The pain is moderate to severe enough to interrupt the patient's daily activities or lead to an emergency department visit	Radiates to the back and/or right infra subscapular region
	The pain is not relieved by bowel movements	
	The pain is not relieved by bowel movements	
	The pain is not relieved by antacids	Awakens from sleep in the middle of the night
	Exclusion of other structural disease that would explain the symptoms	
Functional gallbladder disorder	Gallbladder is present	
	Normal liver enzymes, conjugated bilirubin, and amylase/lipase	
Functional biliary sphincter of Oddi disorder	Normal amylase/lipase	Elevated serum transaminases, alkaline phosphatase, or conjugated bilirubin temporarily related to at least two pain episodes
Functional pancreatic sphincter of Oddi disorder	Elevated amylase/lipase	

- Imaging tests have been developed in the past to evaluate biliary dynamics. A noninvasive test has been devised to quantify gallbladder function, i.e., the gallbladder ejection fraction (GBEF). The GBEF can be measured following a cholecystokinin (CCK)-stimulated hepatobiliary iminodiacetic acid (HIDA) excretion study. The basis of testing is providing stimulation and evaluating subsequent change in the percent emptying over time.
- The HIDA scan follows the transit of a radioisotope as it passes from the hilum of the liver down the biliary tract to the duodenum. If there is a delay in transit, it suggests functional gallbladder or sphincter of Oddi dysfunction (Figs. 16.4 and 16.5).

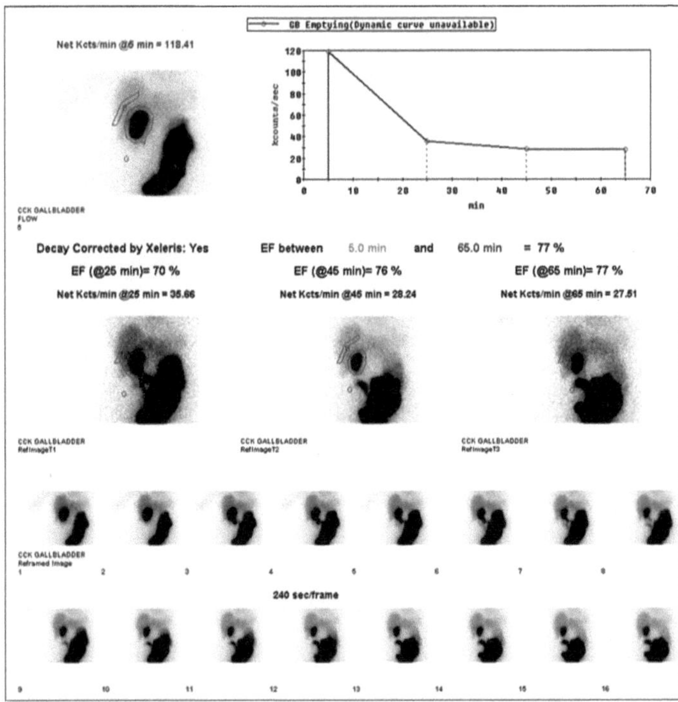

FIG. 16.4 Cholecystokinin (CCK)-stimulated hepatobiliary iminodiacetic acid (HIDA) study with normal GBEF (76 %)

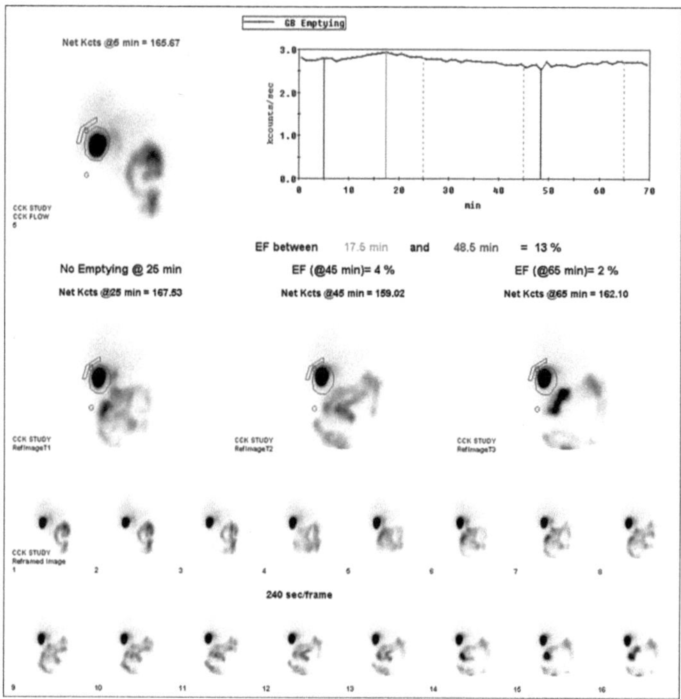

FIG. 16.5 Cholecystokinin (CCK)-stimulated hepatobiliary iminodiacetic acid (HIDA) study with abnormal GBEF (4 %)

HIDA (Cholescintigraphy) Methodology

This test monitors hepatic excretion of a radionucle-
otide technetium 99m (Tc(99m)) labeled iminodiacetic acid analog in the bile and measures
radioactivity of the gallbladder. Gallbladder emptying is calculated by computer-generated time–activity
curves in response to a cholecystokinin (CCK-8)
stimulus. The details of the procedure are outlined in
Table 16.2.

In normal individuals the GBEF at 15 min following
a 45-min infusion is 75 %. The response of the GBEF
to CCK-8 slow infusion is quite reproducible and
mimics the normal response of the gallbladder to
ingestion of a meal. The lowest possible false-positive

TABLE 16.2 Procedural description for evaluation of GBEF

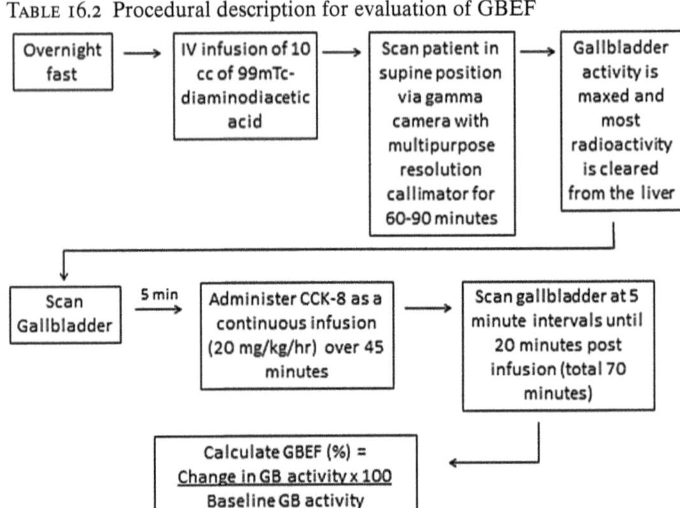

rates using this test depend upon the proper use of the study, i.e., optimal methodology in performing CCK cholescintigraphy, extensive experience using this test and interpreting results, and the clinical perspective involving the patient.

– Not all investigators have found the CCK-stimulated cholescintigraphy test to be useful. In one study a group of 57 patients with gallstones had a GBEF in effort to identify patients with "real biliary distress" versus those with "non-biliary" symptoms. Despite results of the GBEF, surgeons were unsuccessful in accurately separating those patients who benefited from cholecystectomy from those patients who improved without [1]. However, the method of infusion of CCK differed in this study from previous studies and the presence of gallstones is a complicating issue.

• Management.
   – If patients demonstrate significantly low GBEF (<35 %), symptoms may be improved or eliminated with gallbladder removal. Cholecystectomy is the treatment of choice if dyskinesia is confirmed by testing.

- Yap et al. in a randomized controlled trial described a group of patients with gallbladder EF <40 %, who improved after cholecystectomy [2]. After CCK infusion, 21 of 103 patients were found to have GBEF <40 %. After randomization to either cholecystectomy or no cholecystectomy, they were followed up symptomatically for 13–54 months. Of the patients who underwent cholecystectomy [3], 91 % of the patients lost their symptoms and 1 improved. All of the patients who did not undergo cholecystectomy [4] had persistent symptoms. Of the 13 gallbladders obtained from surgery, 12 showed evidence of chronic cholecystitis, muscle hypertrophy, and/or narrowed cystic duct. Dave et al. examined 100 consecutive patients with EF <35 % undergoing laparoscopic cholecystectomy, and 84 % reported symptomatic improvement post-operatively [5]. In another retrospective study, 53 patients with suspected biliary dyskinesia based on an abnormal GBEF <35 % were followed over a 5-year period. Twenty-seven patients had a cholecystectomy. Twenty-four of these patients (89 %) significantly improved. Two patients reported partial improvement while one patient was only minimally helped [6]. In another report, 69 patients with biliary-type symptoms (and no stones) had a GBEF test. Twenty-nine patients had a GBEF <35 % and 17 patients underwent cholecystectomy. Fifteen patients (88 %) had chronic cholecystitis on pathology, eight patients (47 %) had no symptoms, six patients (35 %) had significant improvement, and three patients were unimproved or worse [7].
- Medical therapies for suspected gallbladder dyskinesia are frequently ineffective. Non-narcotic pain medications and lifestyle modifications are usually implemented. If the patients have persistent symptoms following cholecystectomy, a consideration at this point would be evaluation of possible sphincter of Oddi dysfunction using the Rome III criteria (Table 16.1) and Milwaukee criteria (Table 16.3).

TABLE 16.3 Milwaukee criteria for sphincter of Oddi dysfunction

Milwaukee criteria for SOD	Biliary pain	LFT elevation 1.5× upper limit normal	Dilated CBD ≥ 8 mm	Delayed bile clearance
Type I	+	+	+	+
Type II	+	One of two of above		
Type III	+	None of the above		

- Differential Diagnosis.
    - In order to parse out the origin of a patient's symptoms a meticulous history must first be obtained. This will aid the clinician in directing further work-up and treatment. A wide differential diagnosis is indicated at the onset, despite the location of a patient's pain. Functional biliary and pancreatic disorders are not easily distinguishable from GERD, irritable bowel syndrome, and functional dyspepsia. These disorders need to be excluded or empirically treated prior to an evaluation for a functional biliary or pancreatic disorder. To reinforce this clinical problem, Kingham and Dawson described 22 patients with chronic RUQ pain for a decade, which was reproducible by balloon distension of the jejunum, ileum, right colon, and duodenum [8]. Utilization of the Rome III criteria (Table 16.1) may be useful in determining what is or is not biliary type pain.

Sphincter of Oddi (SO)

- Anatomic Location.
    - During emptying of radiocontrast from the common bile duct (CBD), careful observation can disclose a distal contracting segment on fluoroscopic imaging (Fig. 16.6). This is the SO zone, an 8–10 mm smooth muscle structure which encompasses the distal portion of the CBD and the pancreatic duct (PD) at their exit into the duodenum through the papilla of Vater.

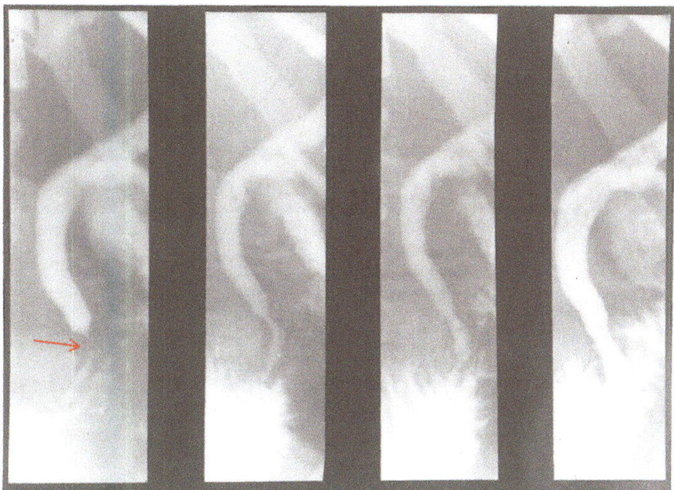

FIG. 16.6 Radiographic sequence over a 20 s period of time showing a contracting segment of distal common bile duct (*arrow*)

- Classification of Dysfunction.
  - Dysfunction of the SO has been characterized as a stenosis (structural alteration) or dyskinesia (functional alteration). SO manometry was developed in an effort to help distinguish between these two entities. Dyskinesia can be caused by an atypical response to CCK (contraction vs. relaxation), or the sphincter maintaining a persistently elevated tone. Stenosis refers more to a structural narrowing of the anatomic Sphincter versus a muscular dysfunction.
- SO Motility and Physiology.
  - The motor activity of the SO is recorded by endoscopic placement of a pressure recording catheter through the sphincter zone into the CBD or PD (Fig. 16.7). The SO provides a pressure gradient between the duodenum and respective ductal systems.
  - The SO is a sphincteric mechanism possessing both a basal pressure (tone) and a phasic activity (contraction), which control filling and emptying of the gallbladder

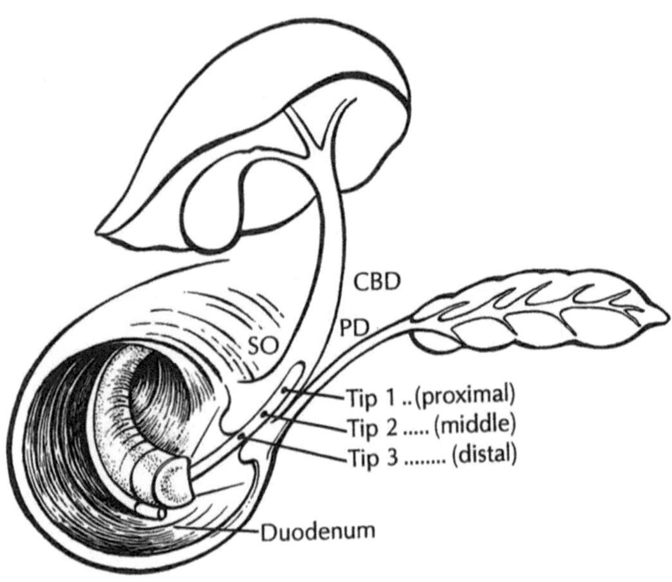

Fig. 16.7 Schema of sphincter of Oddi zone with pressure catheter in place

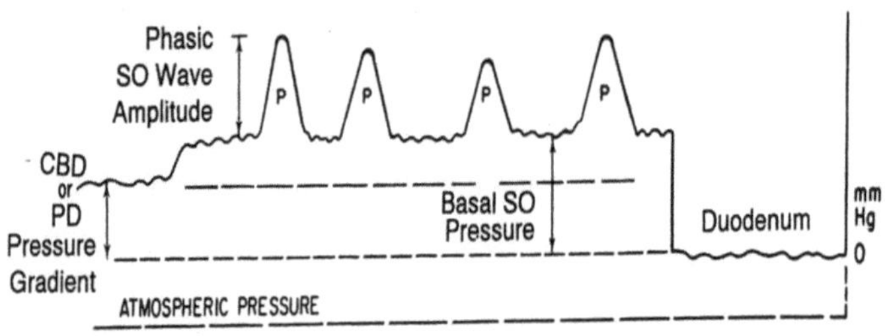

Fig. 16.8 Sphincter of Oddi pressure profile, exhibiting both basal pressure (tone) and a phasic activity (contractions)

(Fig. 16.8). The normal basal pressure averages 20 mmHg above resting duodenal pressure, thus preventing release of contents from the duct. Superimposed on the basal pressure are phasic contractions, which occur approximately 4 times per minute and have a mean amplitude of 150 mmHg. During periods of fasting the basal tone is intermittently elevated and phasic contractions occur in unison with the migrating myoelectrical contractions (MMC) in the intestine. During mealtime SO basal pressure decreases and phasic contractile activity accelerates to enhance delivery of bile and pancreatic secretion into the duodenum to intermingle with digestive contents (Fig. 16.9). These pressures are measured using a triple lumen catheter to obtain a circumferential pattern in the SO zone.

– SO recording technique.

SO manometric pressure recording catheters initially were water-perfused by a hydraulic pneumocapillary pump system. With improved technology, microtransducer catheters have become the preferred instrument, eliminating the infusion of water into the ductal structures. The manometry catheter is inserted by a side-viewing endoscope over a wire guide placed into the appropriate duct. The guidewire is removed subsequently because it will otherwise cause trace artifacts during the recording period. The manometry catheter is initially "stationed" in the duct for 2–3 min to allow a stabilization period. Subsequently the catheter is gradually withdrawn across the SO zone in 2 min increments using the circumferential depth markers on the catheter as reference points relative to catheter insertion. At each station, pressure recording is obtained for 1–2 min until the catheter exits the zone. The resting duodenal pressure is recorded at that time. The basal SO pressure is averaged from all three recording tips measured between phasic waves and this value is subtracted from the duodenal pressure. Phasic wave amplitudes are measured from the basal pressure "plateau" to the peak height of the contraction.

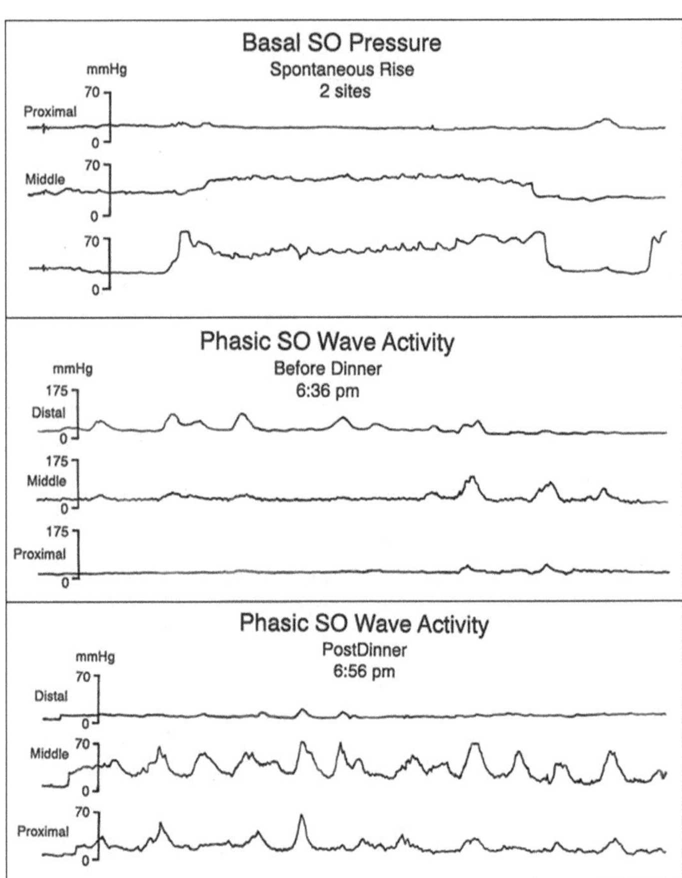

FIG. 16.9 Mealtime changes in SO pressures. Notable is the increase in phasic contractile activity post-dinner to enhance delivery of bile and pancreatic secretion into the duodenum. TOP: Basal SO pressure elevation noted in two recording tips during a 6 h recording period. MIDDLE: SO phasic activity prior to dinner. BOTTOM: SO phasic wave activity increased following a meal

Caveat: To adequately perform SO manometry it is necessary to have knowledge and past experience with basic manometry techniques and their subsequent application to pancreaticobiliary pressure recording. An effective communication and interaction between the SO dysfunction (SOD) manometrist and endoscopist is critical. A patient endoscopist is essential to acquire an accurate trace recording.

- Investigations.
  - If the patient's gallbladder has been removed and the patient meets the Rome III symptom criteria for suspected SOD, these patients can be stratified according to the Milwaukee classification (Table 16.3). At the time of ERCP, the basal pressure, amplitude, duration, frequency, and propagation pattern of phasic sphincter of Oddi contraction waves is obtained. Basal sphincter pressure higher than 40 mmHg is used to diagnose sphincter of Oddi dysfunction. CCK can also be administered to determine if there is an atypical contraction compared to normal relaxation. The reproducibility of SO motor function recording was verified in 47 healthy patients who had a repeat manometric study after a 1 year interval. There was a significant correlation in basal SO pressure obtained over that period of time in this group of patients [9].
  - SO manometry results have been validated in helping detect both Type I and Type II (according to the Milwaukee criteria) SOD [10, 11]. The latter group of patients has been more thoroughly studied and reported [12]. Unfortunately, SO manometric pressure abnormalities have not been successfully correlated with positive sphincterotomy results in Type III functional patients.
  - The landmark 1989 Geenen-Hogan randomized controlled trial showed sphincterotomy during ERCP provided long term benefit in Type I and II patients with basal pressures >40 mmHg [11]. However, EPISOD, a 2014 multicenter, sham-controlled, randomized trial, did not show that manometry predicted which Type III patients would benefit with sphincterotomy in patients with abdominal pain after cholecystectomy [4]. EPISOD also did not show symptomatic benefit after sphincterotomy. However, this study did not make use

of a triple catheter manometry technique and suffered from lack of standardized techniques in the multicenter study. At this time there remains no sufficient diagnostic alternative for Type III patients. Craig et al. compared scintigraphy to manometry in patients with suspected SOD, and found scintigraphy correlated poorly with manometry [3]. Pereira et al. showed secretin-stimulated magnetic resonance cholangiopancreatography was insensitive in predicting abnormal manometry but useful in selecting patients who would benefit from sphincterotomy [13]. This MRI technique is not yet standardized or widely accepted however.

- SO manometric studies have demonstrated unique features in patients with suspected Type III symptoms. Rapid phasic wave activity (tachyodia) (Fig. 16.10) and a paradoxical response (contraction) to CCK injection (Fig. 16.11) have been recorded in patients with this suspected problem. However, the clinical significance of this has not been established.

Fatty Meal Ultrasound Study

A fatty meal stimulated assessment of the biliary system utilizes transabdominal US to assess the

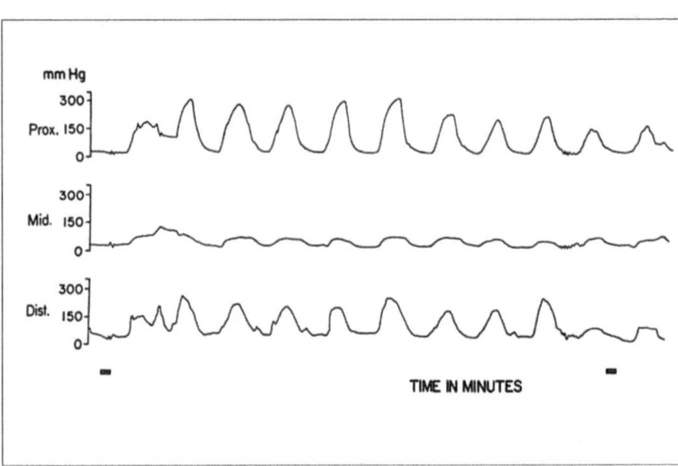

FIG. 16.10 Rapid SO phasic wave activity (tachyodia)

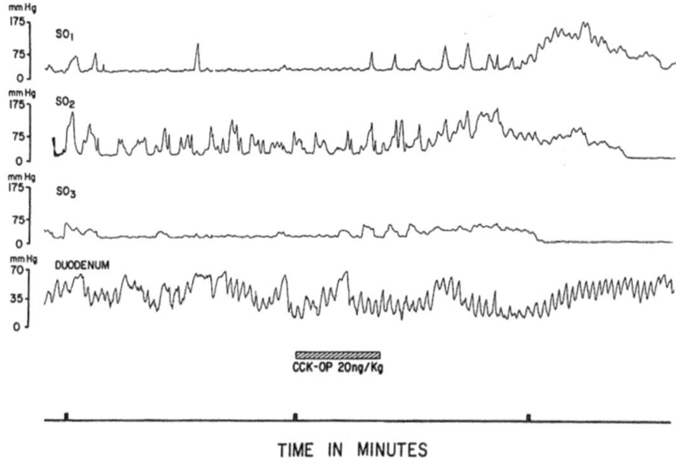

Fig. 16.11 SO paradoxical contraction following CCK infusion

GBEF in response to a fatty meal in patients who have *had their gallbladder removed*. Evaluation of the CBD diameter takes place before and 45 min after a fatty meal (Fig. 16.12) [14], to determine if dilation has occurred.

Darweesh et al. compared quantitative hepatobiliary scintigraphy (QHS) and fatty-meal sonography (FMS), for evaluating patients' status post cholecystectomy with suspected partial common duct obstruction [15]. Each patient with suspected partial common duct obstruction underwent a negative endoscopic retrograde pancreaticobiliary test. Each test had a 67 % sensitivity that improved to 80 % when the findings from both test results were combined. This finding was confirmed by Rosenblatt et al. [16], who examined 304 patients after cholecystectomy who had been evaluated by manometry, US, and HIDA. Using manometry as the gold standard, sensitivity for US was 21 % and for HIDA 49 %. Specificity for US was 97 % and for HIDA 78 %. When used together, the sensitivities of these tests increased.

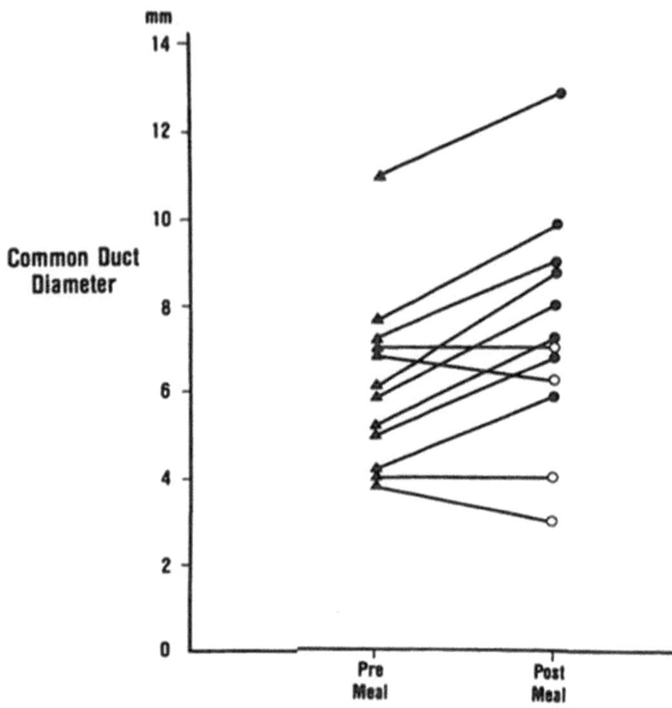

FIG. 16.12 Common bile duct diameter in patients with suspected partial common duct obstruction on the basis of ERCP and/or manometric findings, before fatty meal and 45 or 60 min after fatty meal. Of 12 patients, 8 (solid circles) were judged to be true-positives with a CBD diameter increase of ≥2 mm

Accuracy decreased across the spectrum from type I to type III, according to Milwaukee criteria (Table 16.3).

- Management.
    - The management differs depending on the SOD classification (Table 16.2). Type I and Type II patients should undergo sphincterotomy. Treatment for Type III patients remains unclear. SO manometry has shown past benefit in biliary type II patients, as indicated in the Geenen-Hogan trial (as above).

In patients with suspected biliary type III, invasive procedures should be avoided unless a proper clinical assessment has concluded that potential benefits exceed the risk of complications. Noninvasive measures (see below) should be attempted before performing ERCP and manometry.

- Medical therapy has been investigated in limited studies and is currently not considered standard of care. Vitton et al. examined 59 patients treated with trimebutine and nitrates over 1 year [17]. Medical treatment was effective in 50 % of patients initially, and 62.7 % a 1 year. Only 14 patients then underwent sphincterotomy, with an immediate efficacy of 86 %. Khuroo et al. examined 28 patients with elevated SOD pressures who received nifedipine for 12 weeks and placebo for 12 weeks [18]. The cumulative pain score during nifedipine therapy was significantly less than during the placebo period. No further validation of these treatments has occurred however.

- Differential Diagnosis.
  - The location of abdominal pain does not confirm a biliary disorder. The Rome III criteria are useful in determining which patients can be classified as having functional gallbladder or SO pain. If a patient does not meet Rome III criteria for biliary dysfunction, the chances that this is the etiology of his/her pain are slim to nonexistent.

References

1. Gani JS. Can sincalide cholescintigraphy fulfill the role of gallbladder stress test for patients with gallbladder stones? Aust Nz J Surg. 1988;68:514–9.
2. Yap L, Wycherley AG, Morphett AD, Toouli J. Acalculous biliary pain: cholecystectomy alleviates symptoms in patients with abnormal cholescintigraphy. Gastroenterology. 1991;101(3):786–93.
3. Craig AG, Peter D, Saccone GTP, Ziesing P, Wycherley A, Toouli J. Scintigraphy versus manometry in patients with suspected biliary sphincter of Oddi dysfunction. Gut. 2003;52(3):352–7.

4. Cotton PB, Durkalski V, Romagnuolo J, Pauls Q, Fogel E, Tarnasky P, et al. Effect of endoscopic sphincterotomy for suspected sphincter of Oddi dysfunction on pain-related disability following cholecystectomy: the EPISOD randomized clinical trial. JAMA. 2014;311(20):2101–9.

5. Dave RV, Pathak S, Cockbain AJ, Lodge JP, Smith AM. Chowdhury, Toogood GJ. Management of gallbladder dyskinesia: patient outcomes following positive 99mtechnetium (Tc)-labeled hepatic iminodiacetic acid (HIDA) scintigraphy with cholecystokinin (CCK) provocation and laparoscopic cholecystectomy. Clin Radiol. 2015;70(4):400–7.

6. Yost F, Morgen Thaler J, Presti M, Burton F, Murayama K. Cholecystectomy is effective treatment for biliary dyskinesia. Am J Surg. 1999;178:462–5.

7. Skipper K, Slyh S, Disun E, Schwartz A. Laparoscopic cholecystectomy for an abnormal hepato-iminodiacetic acid scan: a worthwhile procedure. Am J Surg. 2000;66:30–2.

8. Kingham JG, Dawson AM. Origin of chronic right upper quadrant pain. Gut. 1985;26(8):783–8.

9. Guelrud M, Mendoza S, Rossiter G, Villegas MI. Sphincter of Oddi manometry in healthy volunteers. Dig Dis Sci. 1990;35(1):38–46.

10. Rolny P, Geenen JE, Hogan WJ, Venu RP. Clinical features, manometric findings and endoscopic therapy results in group I patients with sphincter of Oddi dysfunction. Gastrointest Endosc. 1991;37:252–3.

11. Geenen JE, Hogan WJ, Dodds WJ, Toouli J, Venu RP. The efficacy of endoscopic sphincterotomy after cholecystectomy in patients with sphincter-of-Oddi dysfunction. N Engl J Med. 1989;320(2):82–7.

12. Kaikaus RM, Jacob L, Geenen JE, Catalano MF, Schmalz MJ, Johnson GK, et al. Long-term outcome of endoscopic sphincterotomy in patients with group II sphincter of Oddi dysfunction. Gastroenterology. 1995;108:A419.

13. Pereira SP, Gillams A, Sgouros SN, Webster GJM, Hatfield ARW. Prospective comparison of secretin-stimulated magnetic resonance cholangiopancreatography with manometry in the diagnosis of sphincter of Oddi dysfunction types II and III. Gut. 2007;56(6):809–13.

14. Darweesh RM, Dodds WJ, Hogan WJ, Geenen JE, Lawson TL, Stewart ET, et al. Roscoe Miller award. Fatty-meal sonography

for evaluating patients with suspected partial common duct obstruction. Am J Roentgenol. 1988;151(1):63–8.

15. Darweesh RM, Dodds WJ, Hogan WJ, Geenen JE, Collier BD, Shaker R, et al. Efficacy of quantitative hepatobiliary scintigraphy and fatty-meal sonography for evaluating patients with suspected partial common duct obstruction. Gastroenterology. 1988;94(3):779–86.

16. Rosenblatt ML, Catalano MF, Alcocer E, Geenen JE. Comparison of sphincter of Oddi manometry, fatty meal sonography, and hepatobiliary scintigraphy in the diagnosis of sphincter of Oddi dysfunction. Gastrointest Endosc. 2001;54(6):697–704.

17. Vitton V, Ezzedine S, Gonzalez J, Gasmi M, Grimaud JC, Barthet M. Medical treatment for sphincter of Oddi dysfunction: can it replace endoscopic sphincterotomy? World J Gastroenterol. 2012;18(14):1610–5.

18. Khuroo MS, Zargar SA, Yattoo GN. Efficacy of nifedipine therapy in patients with sphincter of Oddi dysfunction: a prospective, double-blind, randomized, placebo-controlled, cross over trial. Br J Clin Pharmacol. 1992;33(5):477–85.

Index

© Springer International Publishing Switzerland 2016

K. Dua, R. Shaker (eds.), *Pancreas and Biliary Disease*,
DOI 10.1007/978-3-319-28089-9